Applications of Deep Learning and Big IoT on Personalized Healthcare Services

Ritika Wason
Bharati Vidyapeeth's Institute of Computer Applications and Management (BVICAM), India

Dinesh Goyal
Poornima Institute of Engineering and Technology, India

Vishal Jain
Bharati Vidyapeeth's Institute of Computer Applications and Management (BVICAM), India

S. Balamurugan
QUANTS IS and Consultancy Services, India

Anupam Baliyan
Bharati Vidyapeeth's Institute of Computer Applications and Management (BVICAM), India

A volume in the Advances in Medical Technologies and Clinical Practice (AMTCP) Book Series

IGI Global
DISSEMINATOR OF KNOWLEDGE

Published in the United States of America by
IGI Global
Medical Information Science Reference (an imprint of IGI Global)
701 E. Chocolate Avenue
Hershey PA, USA 17033
Tel: 717-533-8845
Fax: 717-533-8661
E-mail: cust@igi-global.com
Web site: http://www.igi-global.com

Library of Congress Cataloging-in-Publication Data

Names: Wason, Ritika, 1982- editor. | Goyal, Dinesh, 1976- editor. | Jain, Vishal, 1983- editor. | Balamurugan, S. (Shanmugam), 1985- editor. | Baliyan, Anupam, 1976- editor.
Title: Applications of deep learning and big IoT on personalized healthcare services / Ritika Wason, Dinesh Goyal, Vishal Jain, S Balamurugan, Anupam Baliyan, editors.
Description: Hershey : Medical Information Science Reference, [2020] | Includes bibliographical references and index. | Summary: "This book explores the different applications of deep learning algorithms in implementing big data and IoT enabled smart solutions for personalized healthcare services"-- Provided by publisher.
Identifiers: LCCN 2019036402 (print) | LCCN 2019036403 (ebook) | ISBN 9781799821014 (hardcover) | ISBN 9781799821021 (ebook)
Subjects: MESH: Deep Learning | Personal Health Services | Internet | Big Data
Classification: LCC R858 (print) | LCC R858 (ebook) | NLM W 84.1 | DDC 362.10285--dc23
LC record available at https://lccn.loc.gov/2019036402
LC ebook record available at https://lccn.loc.gov/2019036403

This book is published in the IGI Global book series Advances in Medical Technologies and Clinical Practice (AMTCP) (ISSN: 2327-9354; eISSN: 2327-9370)

British Cataloguing in Publication Data
A Cataloguing in Publication record for this book is available from the British Library.

Advances in Medical Technologies and Clinical Practice (AMTCP) Book Series

Srikanta Patnaik
SOA University, India
Priti Das
S.C.B. Medical College, India

ISSN:2327-9354
EISSN:2327-9370

Mission

Medical technological innovation continues to provide avenues of research for faster and safer diagnosis and treatments for patients. Practitioners must stay up to date with these latest advancements to provide the best care for nursing and clinical practices.

The **Advances in Medical Technologies and Clinical Practice (AMTCP) Book Series** brings together the most recent research on the latest technology used in areas of nursing informatics, clinical technology, biomedicine, diagnostic technologies, and more. Researchers, students, and practitioners in this field will benefit from this fundamental coverage on the use of technology in clinical practices.

Coverage

- Nursing Informatics
- Biomedical Applications
- Neural Engineering
- Biometrics
- Patient-Centered Care
- Diagnostic Technologies
- E-Health
- Clinical Nutrition
- Medical Imaging
- Medical Informatics

IGI Global is currently accepting manuscripts for publication within this series. To submit a proposal for a volume in this series, please contact our Acquisition Editors at Acquisitions@igi-global.com or visit: http://www.igi-global.com/publish/.

The Advances in Medical Technologies and Clinical Practice (AMTCP) Book Series (ISSN 2327-9354) is published by IGI Global, 701 E. Chocolate Avenue, Hershey, PA 17033-1240, USA, www.igi-global.com. This series is composed of titles available for purchase individually; each title is edited to be contextually exclusive from any other title within the series. For pricing and ordering information please visit http://www.igi-global.com/book-series/advances-medical-technologies-clinical-practice/73682. Postmaster: Send all address changes to above address.

Titles in this Series

For a list of additional titles in this series, please visit: www.igi-global.com/book-series
http://www.igi-global.com/book-series/advances-medical-technologies-clinical-practice/73682

Communicating Rare Diseases and Disorders in the Digital Age
Liliana Vale Costa (University of Aveiro, Portugal) and Sónia Oliveira (University of Aveiro, Portugal)
Medical Information Science Reference • © 2020 • 412pp • H/C (ISBN: 9781799820888) • US $295.00

Exploring the Role of ICTs in Healthy Aging
David Mendes (Universidade de Évora, Portugal) César Fonseca (Universidade de Évora, Portugal) Manuel José Lopes (Universidade de Évora, Portugal) José García-Alonso (University of Coimbra, Spain) and Juan Manuel Murillo (University of Coimbra, Spain)
Medical Information Science Reference • © 2020 • 300pp • H/C (ISBN: 9781799819370) • US $285.00

Artificial Intelligence Paradigms in Smart Health Informatics Systems
Abdel-Badeeh M. Salem (Ain Shams University, Egypt) and Senthil Kumar A V (Hindusthan College of Arts and Science, India)
Medical Information Science Reference • © 2020 • 300pp • H/C (ISBN: 9781799811015) • US $265.00

Incorporating the Internet of Things in Healthcare Applications and Wearable Devices
P. B. Pankajavalli (Bharathiar University, India) and G. S. Karthick (Bharathiar University, India)
Medical Information Science Reference • © 2020 • 288pp • H/C (ISBN: 9781799810902) • US $285.00

Impacts of Information Technology on Patient Care and Empowerment
Roger W. McHaney (Kansas State University, USA) Iris Reychev (Ariel University, Israel) Joseph Azuri (Maccabi Healthcare Services, Israel) Mark E. McHaney (U.S. Air Force, USA) and Rami Moshonov (Assuta Medical Centers, Israel)
Medical Information Science Reference • © 2020 • 452pp • H/C (ISBN: 9781799800477) • US $295.00

Handbook of Research on Clinical Applications of Computerized Occlusal Analysis in Dental Medicine
Robert B. Kerstein, DMD (Tufts University School of Dental Medicine, USA & Private Dental Practice Limited to Prosthodontics and Computerized Occlusal Analysis, USA)
Medical Information Science Reference • © 2020 • 1356pp • H/C (ISBN: 9781522592549) • US $765.00

Early Detection of Neurological Disorders Using Machine Learning Systems
Sudip Paul (North-Eastern Hill University Shillong, India) Pallab Bhattacharya (National Institute of Pharmaceutical Education and Research (NIPER) Ahmedabad, India) and Arindam Bit (National Institute of Technology Raipur, India)
Medical Information Science Reference • © 2019 • 376pp • H/C (ISBN: 9781522585671) • US $265.00

IGI Global
DISSEMINATOR OF KNOWLEDGE

701 East Chocolate Avenue, Hershey, PA 17033, USA
Tel: 717-533-8845 x100 • Fax: 717-533-8661
E-Mail: cust@igi-global.com • www.igi-global.com

Table of Contents

Preface xii

Chapter 1
Automation in Healthcare Services 1
Vijay Prakash Gupta, Institute of Technology and Science, Ghaziabad, India
Amit Kumar Arora, KIET Group of Institutions, Ghaziabad, India

Chapter 2
Deep Data Analytics: Future of Telehealth 20
Madhulika Bhatia, Amity University, Noida, India
Madhurima Hooda, Amity University, Noida, India
Priya Gupta, All India Institute of Medical Sciences, New Delhi, India

Chapter 3
Emergence of IoT and Big Data: A Study in the Healthcare Industry 42
Gurinder Singh, Amity University, Noida, India
Vikas Garg, Amity University, Greater Noida, India
Pooja Tiwari, ABES Engineering College, India
Richa Goel, Amity University, Noida, India

Chapter 4
Automation in Healthcare: A Forecast and Outcome – Medical IoT and Big Data in Healthcare 55
Alankrita Aggarwal, IKG Punjab Technical University, India
Kanwalvir Singh Dhindsa, Baba Banda Singh Bahadur Engineering College, India
P. K. Suri, Kurukshetra University, India

Chapter 5
An Effective Diagnostic Model for Personalized Healthcare Using Deep Learning Techniques......... 70
Parul Agarwal, Jamia Hamdard, India
Syed Imtiyaz Hassan, Maulana Azad National Urdu University, India
Syed Khalid Mustafa, University of Tabuk, Saudi Arabia
Jawed Ahmad, Jamia Hamdard, India

Chapter 6
Real-Time Mental Health Monitoring: The Indian Scenario 89
Ritika Wason, Bharati Vidyapeeth's Institute of Computer Applications and Management (BVICAM), India
Prashant Singh Rana, Thapar Institute of Engineering and Technology, India
Vishal Jain, Bharati Vidyapeeth's Institute of Computer Applications and Management (BVICAM), India

Chapter 7
Disease Diagnosis and Treatment Using Deep Learning Algorithms for the Healthcare System........ 99
Nirbhay Kumar Chaubey, Ganpat University, India
Prisilla Jayanthi, K. G. Reddy College of Engineering and Technology, India

Chapter 8
Elderly Behavior Prediction Using a Deep Learning Model in Smart Homes 115
Sridevi U. K., PSG College of Technology, India
Sophia Sudhir, Sri Krishna College of Engineering and Technology, India
Shanthi Palaniappan, Sri Krishna College of Engineering and Technology, India

Chapter 9
A Surrogate Data-Based Approach for Validating Deep Learning Model Used in Healthcare 132
Meenakshi Srivastava, Amity University Uttar Pradesh, Lucknow, India

Chapter 10
Managing the Scarcity of Monitoring Data Through Machine Learning for Human Behavior in Mental Health Care 147
Nitesh Kumar Dixit, Bhartiya Institute of Engineering and Technology, Sikar, India
Dileep Kumar Agarwal, Bhartiya Institute of Engineering and Technology, Sikar, India
Mahendra Kumar, Bhartiya Institute of Engineering and Technology, Sikar, India

Chapter 11
Machine Learning Is the Future for Lung Cancer Prognosis and Prediction...................................... 176
Ayshwarya Balakumar, Kristu Jayanti College, India
Senthil S., REVA University, India

Chapter 12
Effective and Accurate Diagnosis Using Brain Image Fusion 197
Sivakumar Rajagopal, Vellore Institute of Technology, India
Babu Gopal, Velammal Institute of Technology, India

Compilation of References 218

About the Contributors 241

Index 247

Detailed Table of Contents

Preface xii

Chapter 1
Automation in Healthcare Services 1
Vijay Prakash Gupta, Institute of Technology and Science, Ghaziabad, India
Amit Kumar Arora, KIET Group of Institutions, Ghaziabad, India

The health care service industry (also known as a medical industry) is an industry that is comprised of the services related to the safeguarding or enhancement of patient health or provides services to treat patients with medicinal, protective, rehabilitative, and analgesic care. For the last two decades, it has been seen that there are drastic changes in healthcare services through automation, digitalization, technological innovation, and communication. Automation has made a revolutionary change in the healthcare industry and allowed for it to be more cost-effective for the industry to run day-to-day operations. Automation-driven health care activities are free from human fatigue and error, so they can help out to provide consistency, accuracy, and potentially lead to a reduction in patient complications, infections, and deaths. Besides, automation can help hospitals, professionals, and doctors for cost-reduction measures and increased efficiency as part of their monetary benefits.

Chapter 2
Deep Data Analytics: Future of Telehealth 20
Madhulika Bhatia, Amity University, Noida, India
Madhurima Hooda, Amity University, Noida, India
Priya Gupta, All India Institute of Medical Sciences, New Delhi, India

In the past, doctors and specialists were not connected to patients through telemedicine for providing virtual health and medicine. In rural areas, where experts in medical fields were not able to reach or be present at, telemedicine proved a great benefit. As the years passed, the explosive use of the internet brought profound changes to telemedicine practices. The escalation of smart devices with the capability of delivering high quality video and audio raised the possibilities of delivering remote healthcare. Telehealth care helps patients at home or at assisted living facilities as a revolutionary alternative to personal visits for both basic as well as expert care. Applying deep data analytics to telemedicine will create new horizons in telehealth by analyzing large data sets of patients using live video streaming to predict the health challenges of patients.

Chapter 3
Emergence of IoT and Big Data: A Study in the Healthcare Industry 42
Gurinder Singh, Amity University, Noida, India
Vikas Garg, Amity University, Greater Noida, India
Pooja Tiwari, ABES Engineering College, India
Richa Goel, Amity University, Noida, India

The main focus of this research paper is to understand the use of IoT in healthcare to achieve sustainable development. This paper has used the descriptive method to collect the data for study. The research methodology is FAHP, which is a cross-sectional research survey in nature. After data collection, the agreed paired comparison matrices, which are then further allocated to the weighted criteria and then accordingly a priority for the IoT usage is judged. According to the findings of the research, it has been identified that "profit maximization" and "quality of life" were on the top for priority for IoT in the healthcare sector for sustainable development, although, three major areas were identified. Additionally, if we consider according to usage then it is mostly used by the health care sector as UV radiation, dental care, and fall detection.

Chapter 4
Automation in Healthcare: A Forecast and Outcome – Medical IoT and Big Data in Healthcare 55
Alankrita Aggarwal, IKG Punjab Technical University, India
Kanwalvir Singh Dhindsa, Baba Banda Singh Bahadur Engineering College, India
P. K. Suri, Kurukshetra University, India

Major challenges to the society are the people have aging populace and occurrence of continual diseases and eruption of transferable diseases. to embark upon these unmet healthcare desires for the quick guess and therapeutic of all the important diseases a new area called health informatics is emerging as an interdisciplinary research which is dealing with the getting hold of, spread, dispensation, to store as well retrieve. Particularly when the industry is acquired the health information by using the unassuming sense and wearable technology is well thought-out as groundwork stone in healthiness industry. According to a reports, sensors can be worn and hooked on clothes which can acquire the health information uninterrupted.

Chapter 5
An Effective Diagnostic Model for Personalized Healthcare Using Deep Learning Techniques 70
Parul Agarwal, Jamia Hamdard, India
Syed Imtiyaz Hassan, Maulana Azad National Urdu University, India
Syed Khalid Mustafa, University of Tabuk, Saudi Arabia
Jawed Ahmad, Jamia Hamdard, India

This chapter discusses a deep learning and IoE (Internet of Everything) based analytical model for disease detection, prediction and correct treatment for the patient would be proposed. In the proposed model, all the stakeholders, namely doctors, patients, medical staff within a clinic, hospital or a medical institute, would be embedded with micro-sensors. The sensors would in turn sense and capture the information gathered from these sources and the surrounding environment and then send it to a single repository, a base or a server, where it would be stored for further processing. These sensors produce massive amounts of data, which needs to be encrypted as well. Then, in order to improve the effectiveness and accuracy of prediction from the data received from these sensors, deep learning methods are used. Further, the advantages of the proposed model would be explored. To conclude, the limitations, opportunities and future applications of deep learning techniques would be discussed in this chapter.

Chapter 6
Real-Time Mental Health Monitoring: The Indian Scenario 89
Ritika Wason, Bharati Vidyapeeth's Institute of Computer Applications and Management (BVICAM), India
Prashant Singh Rana, Thapar Institute of Engineering and Technology, India
Vishal Jain, Bharati Vidyapeeth's Institute of Computer Applications and Management (BVICAM), India

Mental disorders have been identified as one among the leading causes of the global disease burden. Despite being one of the first nations in the world to identify mental health as an important indicator of personal well-being and having adequate plans and policies for ensuring the same, one in every seven Indians is affected by mental disorders of varying severity. Through this manuscript we try to analyze how real-time mental health monitoring has helped improve productivity among the global workforce as well as prevented deterioration of individual mental health across the globe. Our main plan of this study is to identify the significant efforts in mental health monitoring across the globe and then chalk out a real-time mental health monitoring framework for India. We also propose a real-time mental health monitoring smartphone-based framework for India we name as SmartMHealth. We describe the basic components of this framework in this study itself.

Chapter 7
Disease Diagnosis and Treatment Using Deep Learning Algorithms for the Healthcare System........ 99
Nirbhay Kumar Chaubey, Ganpat University, India
Prisilla Jayanthi, K. G. Reddy College of Engineering and Technology, India

This chapter explicates deep learning algorithms for healthcare opportunities. Deep Learning is a group of neural network algorithms and learns from various levels of representation and abstraction to aid in the data interpretation. Since the datasets get bigger, computers become more powerful, and the training of the datasets (images or numeric) gets much easier and the results achieved using deep learning are better. In contrast to machine-learning algorithms that rely on large amounts of labelled data, human cognition can find structure in unlabeled data, a technique known as unsupervised learning. It was noted that using deep learning algorithms on the dataset will reduce the number of unnecessary biopsies in future. In this chapter, the authors study deep learning algorithms to diagnose diabetic retinopathy retinal images and training a convolution neural network (CNN) algorithm to identify object tumors from a large set of brain tumor images.

Chapter 8
Elderly Behavior Prediction Using a Deep Learning Model in Smart Homes 115
Sridevi U. K., PSG College of Technology, India
Sophia Sudhir, Sri Krishna College of Engineering and Technology, India
Shanthi Palaniappan, Sri Krishna College of Engineering and Technology, India

The goal of a smart home is to keep track of the behaviors of the older adults with disabilities within the home, and then anticipate their activity to help with other actions. Elderly and disabled people have problems with their daily lives, while most other people are unaware of their difficulties. Helping the elderly to live independently allows them to lead their daily lives in a better manner. The implementation of analytics and machine learning algorithms leads to a predictive approach to health care services. In this chapter, a learning model in a smart home concept focuses on making it possible for the elderly to remain safe and comfortable at home. The transformative home security device learning architecture of the smart home platform is a valuable solution to studying mobility patterns at home, with the ability to identify behavioral changes related to issues of wellbeing. A predictive learning system can effectively recognize and identify the behavior of the elderly. A learning model, a recurrent neural network (RNN) is proposed to evaluate the people's activity. The focus of the present study is to forecast the deterioration in mental function and give warnings for the benefit of seniors.

Chapter 9
A Surrogate Data-Based Approach for Validating Deep Learning Model Used in Healthcare 132
Meenakshi Srivastava, Amity University Uttar Pradesh, Lucknow, India

IoT-based communication between medical devices has encouraged the healthcare industry to use automated systems which provide effective insight from the massive amount of gathered data. AI and machine learning have played a major role in the design of such systems. Accuracy and validation are considered, since copious training data is required in a neural network (NN)-based deep learning model. This is hardly feasible in medical research, because the size of data sets is constrained by complexity and high cost experiments. The availability of limited sample data validation of NN remains a concern. The prediction of outcomes on a NN trained on a smaller data set cannot guarantee performance and exhibits unstable behaviors. Surrogate data-based validation of NN can be viewed as a solution. In the current chapter, the classification of breast tissue data by a NN model has been detailed. In the absence of a huge data set, a surrogate data-based validation approach has been applied. The discussed study can be applied for predictive modelling for applications described by small data sets.

Chapter 10
Managing the Scarcity of Monitoring Data Through Machine Learning for Human Behavior in Mental Health Care 147
Nitesh Kumar Dixit, Bhartiya Institute of Engineering and Technology, Sikar, India
Dileep Kumar Agarwal, Bhartiya Institute of Engineering and Technology, Sikar, India
Mahendra Kumar, Bhartiya Institute of Engineering and Technology, Sikar, India

Nowadays, in many fields, including medicine and public health, developments in information and communication technology have introduced a revolution. Due to the absence of effective machinery algorithms and many possibilities to enhance patient understanding of chronic diseases, information gathered from the distinct sources were ignored. Therefore, researchers are investigating information shortages of computer training methods. This work recommends a fresh strategy to produce stronger predictive models specifically intended for the problems. In order to address the scarcity of data, works propose to make use of a semi-managed learning environment while using all unlabeled data sets. The techniques suggested were implemented in the mental health care field of bipolar disorder. The methods suggested enhancing the efficiency of ranking to the accuracy of $\approx 73\%$ to $\approx 90\%$. The results have been achieved by overcoming previous methods that use traditional monitored methods of learning.

Chapter 11
Machine Learning Is the Future for Lung Cancer Prognosis and Prediction 176
Ayshwarya Balakumar, Kristu Jayanti College, India
Senthil S., REVA University, India

Lung cancer is one of the major reasons for the death if it is not diagnosed in the early stages of cancer. It is the one among the most dreadful disease which affects in the lungs function. It can be identified only after the disease spread into the deeper parts of the lungs and then only it will make a life threading problem. Lung cancer prognosis which was done based on the various parameters such as age, sex, condition of smoking, duration of smoking and count of smoking per day. The proceedings were done using the algorithm for the time to first cigarette after awakening which is represented as TTFC. The expert doctor says that the back-propagation network is a great deal in the recognition of the lung cancer without any involvement by them. This research is based on the classification of lung cancer and its stages using the establishment of the BPN and predicts the recurrence. Similarly, with this BPN, an algorithm that is inspired from its habitat known as ant lion optimization algorithm is also used in the optimization of weights and parameters of the BPN. The use of the ALO algorithm provides an improved convergence mechanism by improving the proposed technique's accuracy. The use of this proposed method with the BPN optimizes the network and the ALO optimizer provides an accurate prediction of the lung cancer by the earlier stage and even predicts the changes for reoccurrence after diagnosis. The prognosis analysis was made by the various comparative study between the characteristic features of HIV and the unaffected person using the algorithm such as the Wilcoxon rank-sum test. This algorithm will continuously classify the viral load and CD4 count which is based on factors such as age, sex, and smoking activities. It will be useful for early diagnosis and future prediction. Lung cancer rates can be analyzed based on the incident rates of affected and unaffected persons to HIV infections.

Chapter 12
Effective and Accurate Diagnosis Using Brain Image Fusion 197
Sivakumar Rajagopal, Vellore Institute of Technology, India
Babu Gopal, Velammal Institute of Technology, India

Medical imaging techniques are routinely employed to create images of the human system for clinical purposes. Multi-modality medical imaging is a widely used technology for diagnosis, detection, and prediction of various tissue abnormalities. This chapter is focused on the development of an improved brain image processing technique for the removal of noise from a magnetic resonance image (MRI) for accurate image restoration. Feature selection and extraction of MRI brain images are processed using image fusion. The medical images suffer from motion blur and noise for which image denoising is developed through non-local means (NLM) filtering for smoothing and shrinkage rule for sharpening. The peak signal to noise ratio (PSNR) of improved curvelet based self-similarity NLM method is better than discrete wavelet transform with an NLM filter.

Compilation of References 218

About the Contributors 241

Index 247

Preface

It gives us immense pleasure to put forth the book *Applications of Deep Learning and Big IoT on Personalized Healthcare Services*. Healthcare is an industry that has seen great advancements in personalized services through big data analytics. With the application of smart devices to the medical field, massive volume of data is being generated. The humongous data has further added to the challenge of correctly diagnosing patients as early as possible. This has resulted in the implementation of precise, machine learning based algorithms that can process large amounts of information and successfully apply smart living and diagnosis to medical environment. Professionals worldwide are involved in relevant research for successfully empaneling these smart technologies within their own personalized healthcare processes. The book *Applications of Deep Learning and Big IoT on Personalized Healthcare Services* is a pivotal reference source that provides a collection of innovative research on the analytical methods and applications of deep learning based smart algorithms for the personalized treatment of patients. While highlighting topics including cognitive computing, big data analytics, and IoT, this book is ideally designed for network designers, analysts, technology specialists, medical professionals, developers, researchers, academicians, and post-graduate students seeking relevant information on smart developments within individualized healthcare. It is a collection of innovative research chapters that explores global concerns in the applications of information technology to businesses and the explosive growth that resulted. Highlighting a wide range of topics such as Clinical Data, Cognitive Computing, Effective Algorithms, Healthcare Claim Management, Natural Language Processing, Network Security, Pharmaceutical Application, Predictive Analytics, Supply Chain Optimization, Timely Diagnoses, this book is ideally designed for engineers, manufacturers, technology managers, technology developers, IT specialists, productivity consultants, executives, lawyers, programmers, managers, policymakers, academicians, researchers, and students. Topics presented in each chapter of this book are unique to this book and are based on unpublished work of contributing authors. In editing this book, we encouraged researchers and practitioners from both academia and industry to present their latest state-of-art research results and methodologies addressing top concerns in areas of applications of Deep Learning and Big IoT on Personalized Healthcare Services and to establish worldwide cooperative research and development. We believe the book is ready to serve as a reference for larger audience such as system architects, practitioners, developers, and researchers.

Chapter 1

This chapter highlights the importance of real-time mental monitoring for attaining sustainable development of a nation. It further proposes a real-time mental health monitoring smartphone-based framework for India coined as Smart mHealth.

Chapter 2

This chapter discusses the benefit of Applying Deep data analytics in telemedicine by analyzing large data set of patients using live video streaming to predict the health challenges of patients.

Chapter 3

In the current chapter classification of breast tissue data by NN model has been detailed. In absence of huge data set, Surrogate data-based validation approach has been applied. The discussed study can be applied for predictive modeling for applications described by small data sets.

Chapter 4

This chapter explicates the emergence and application of Big Data and IoT in the field of healthcare applications. In this chapter, authors analyze how Big Data and IoT are altering the semantics of the healthcare industry.

Chapter 5

This chapter emulates the smart home environment to enable the elderly people spend their lives at their homes through what we term as assisted living.

Chapter 6

Automation-driven health care activities are free from human fatigue and error, so they can help out to provide consistency, accuracy and potentially lead to a reduction in patient complications, infections, and deaths. Besides, automation can help hospitals, professionals, and doctors for cost-reduction measures and increased efficiency as part of their monetary benefits.

Chapter 7

This chapter examines a Deep learning and IoE (Internet of Everything) enabled analytical model for disease detection, prediction and correct treatment of the patients. In the proposed model, all the stakeholders, namely doctors, patients, medical staff within a clinic, hospital or a medical institute, would be embedded with micro-sensors using some fixed devices.

Chapter 8

This chapter presents a comprehensive overview, market shares and growth opportunities of Robotic Process Automation in Healthcare market by product type, application, key companies and key regions. Automaton technology is an area of evolving escalation, remarkably as they congregate miscellaneous functionalities together.

Chapter 9

This chapter proposes a BPN based mechanism to optimize the underlying network. The ALO optimizer provides an accurate prediction of the lung cancer at earlier stage and even predicts the chances for re-occurrence of the same after proper treatment.

Chapter 10

This work recommends a fresh strategy to produce stronger predictive models specifically intended for the healthcare problems. In order to address the scarcity of data, the work proposes to make use of a semi-managed learning environment while using all unlabeled data sets.

Chapter 11

This chapter elaborates deep learning algorithms for healthcare opportunities. In this chapter, authors also study deep learning algorithms to diagnose diabetic retinopathy retinal images and training a CNN algorithm to identify the object tumor from a large set of brain tumor images.

Chapter 12

This Chapter is focused on the development of an improved brain image processing technique for the removal of noise from Magnetic Resonance Image (MRI) for accurate image restoration. Feature selection and extraction in MRI brain images are processed using image fusion.

We further also express our sincere thanks to Mrs. Jan Travers, IGI-Global, for giving us an opportunity to convene the book in his esteemed publishing house and Ms. Courtney Tychinski, IGI-Global, for her kind cooperation in completion of this book. We thank our esteemed authors for having shown confidence in the book and considering it as a platform to showcase and share their original research work. We would also wish to thank the authors whose papers were not published in this book, probably because of their minor shortcomings.

Editors:

Ritika Wason
Bharati Vidyapeeth's Institute of Computer Applications and Management (BVICAM), India

Dinesh Goyal
Poornima Institute of Engineering and Technology, India

Vishal Jain
Bharati Vidyapeeth's Institute of Computer Applications and Management (BVICAM), India

S. Balamurugan
QUANTS IS and Consultancy Services, Coimbatore, India

Anupam Baliyan
Bharati Vidyapeeth's Institute of Computer Applications and Management (BVICAM), India

Chapter 1
Automation in Healthcare Services

Vijay Prakash Gupta
Institute of Technology and Science, Ghaziabad, India

Amit Kumar Arora
https://orcid.org/0000-0001-9311-0740
KIET Group of Institutions, Ghaziabad, India

ABSTRACT

The health care service industry (also known as a medical industry) is an industry that is comprised of the services related to the safeguarding or enhancement of patient health or provides services to treat patients with medicinal, protective, rehabilitative, and analgesic care. For the last two decades, it has been seen that there are drastic changes in healthcare services through automation, digitalization, technological innovation, and communication. Automation has made a revolutionary change in the healthcare industry and allowed for it to be more cost-effective for the industry to run day-to-day operations. Automation-driven health care activities are free from human fatigue and error, so they can help out to provide consistency, accuracy, and potentially lead to a reduction in patient complications, infections, and deaths. Besides, automation can help hospitals, professionals, and doctors for cost-reduction measures and increased efficiency as part of their monetary benefits.

INTRODUCTION

The health care service industry (also known as a medical industry) is an industry that comprises the service related to the safeguarding or enhancement of the health of the patient or that provides the services for health care of patient with medicinal, protective, rehabilitation, and analgesic care.

The delivery of modern health services is based on an intensifying group of trained and dedicated professionals, doctors and specialists coming together as an interdisciplinary team.

For the last two decades, it has been seen that there are drastic changes in healthcare services through automation, digitalization, technological innovation, and communication.

DOI: 10.4018/978-1-7998-2101-4.ch001

Automation is considered as revolutionary changes to trace out the present and past data which are stored as a history of medical diagnosis of patients.

Automation in health care service make easier to share any data or information among healthcare professionals and enhanced the proficiencies of patient results. Automation has made the revolutionary change in the healthcare industry and finished it more cost-effective for the industry to run day-to-day operations.

The present business models of the health care industry are more in jeopardy of competition, increasing the pressure of cost-cutting and meet patient's demands on time without any gap.

Automation in the health care industry is now recognized as the tools of instantaneous access to information and treatment with the help of digital and automatic machinery, robots, etc. Automation helps to get rid of searching the data from the pile of files and old records stored and kept in physical form in hospitals as well as the traditional method of surgery and treatment of the patient.

Even the Government of all nations is also focusing on digitalization and computerization particularly in healthcare facilities with a dream to convert the industry into a computerization system because it will help in the wisdom of punctuality and cost-effective health care facilities for manufacturing, patients as well as civilization.

To deal with these confront, businesses are now implementing the dynamic business scenario in health care industry by digital alteration and automation that connect the industry with every unit of data and information across channels, operation, and patient outreach.

Because of the above context and background, primarily this chapter will give complete information about the market of health care industry in India, benefits of automation as cost-effective health care services for industry as well as its patients.

Secondly, it discusses how automation has improved the patients' health and their life style as and promptness in medical services facilities.

GROWTH STORY OF HEALTH CARE INDUSTRY IN INDIA

In the various service industries, the healthcare sector plays a very important role and contributing a good percentage in the GDP of the economy.

As per the data of various service industries, healthcare has to turn into one of the major sectors both in terms of Return on Investment as well as generation of employment.

The health care sector consists of Hospitals, telemedicine, clinical practices, and automated medical apparatus and tools, etc

Now a day's increasing population and Growing incidence of lifestyle diseases is increasing the need for affordable health care services due to an increase in medical expenses. Technological advancements, an automaton in diagnosis and cure of the disease as well as the use of technology, Artificial Intelligence, and robot surgery, telemedicine, health insurance penetration and the initiative was taken by the government driving the healthcare market in India.

This service industry consists of several components like trained doctors, nurses, intern people, some special medical automated machine operators, etc. Each one has their specified roles and responsibilities to perform. The definition of healthcare can differ across countries based on their utility, but the outcomes and the working are remaining the same.

MARKET SIZE OF INDIAN HEALTH CARE INDUSTRIES

Health Care Industries in India is projected to be a US$9 billion opportunity by 2020. Currently, Health Care Industry is pegged at US$3 billion. Considering the entire globe, the medical tourism market is estimated at around US$40-60 billion. As per the data of the Confederation of Indian Industries (CII), the main agenda that attracts medical tourism to visit India is the most cost-efficient, and treatment is very low as compared to other developed nations.

As per the present global Tourism Index, currently India's ranks is 5th and in Asia its ranks 2nd as per International Healthcare and Research Centre statistics. This rank shows a good choice for India in becoming a future leader in medical tourism and Health care Industry given the fact that it focuses on building infrastructure, technology & services, and seamless experience for patients.

It has been observed that the healthcare service market can increase threefold by 2022. As per the scenario of the medical tourism market of India, it has been expecting that across 22-25 percent of the growth in the medical care industry is expected by 2020. There are most of the chances to boost health care service by spending the budget and its GDP share in health care. It has been found that the expenditure on the health sector by the Indian government has increased in the budget to approx 1.4 percent in Financial Year 2018 from 1.2 percent in Financial Year 2014. The GOI is decided to add more money and spending for public health i.e. 2.5 percent of the country's GDP by 2025.

MILESTONES OF HEALTHCARE INDUSTRY IN INDIA.

As per the data published on INVEST INDIA, there is some growth story of India's Health Care Industry which are mentioned below:

- The healthcare industry in India, it has been projected that the market may see a tripartite bounce in value terms to reach $ 372 bn by 2022.
- In the year 2017, India has become the fourth largest industry in terms of employment generation, as the sector employed a total of the number of 319,780 people.
- By the end of 2020, India is anticipated to make its position amongst the top list in healthcare service provider in terms of market share growth.
- By the end of 2020, the healthcare market is anticipated to grow by 150 percent compared to the current ratio.
- By 2022, the diagnostics market share of in Indian health industry is anticipated to grow at a Compounded annual growth rate of more than 20.0% to reach the level of 32 billion dollars from 5 billion dollars in 2012.
- Comparing the period from 2015 to 2020, the in-patient market share is expected to increase with a compound annual growth rate of 13%.

EXISTING HEALTHCARE ENVIRONMENTS

In recent years there has been a concerted move towards the adoption of automation in health care in systems in hospitals but still, the healthcare industry is lacking in some areas which are given below:

Manual Record of patient Information: It seems that now a day's in the health care industry most of the hospitals are recording medical information and patient records manually.

Dependency on Nurses Only: The current health care industry in India has been observed that most of the hospitals are having a huge dependency on nursing staff those who are responsible for the take care of patients.

Lack of ICU: There is very little use of Intensive care units in hospitals now days especially in rural areas, as well as it is not run by an automated machinery system.

Inefficient Medical Staff: Medical staffs are unable to diagnose the abnormality, disease and past health records of patients.

Lack of Automated Health Care Services: In present health care services in rural and semi-urban areas as well as in government hospitals also there are no automated systems to diagnose and care for the patient. In most hospitals, the patient is not getting immediate health care services also because of the non-availability of proper resources and technology.

Extra effort put by Doctors: Because of the lack of automated tools and techniques in hospitals especially in rural areas the physician has to do extra effort and repeatedly visit the patient to diagnose and asses the current recovery and sickness conditions of patient to know the various basic parameters such as body temperature, blood pressure, drip level, etc.

Lack of Resources during emergency care: In case of emergencies, the nursing staff is not too competent to take care of the patient they frequently approach doctors to give information about the patient current conditions and recovery status with the help of telephonic communication or by direct meetings.

Lack of Continuous Monitoring System: In most of the hospitals the continuous patient monitoring system is used only in the Intensive Care Unit (ICU) not for all wards.

Chances of Human Error: From the problems identified, the existing health care systems are manual inspections, labor-based work, chances to human errors, judgments based on experiences without analysis and observations from clinicians and nurses finally ineffective. It introduces a huge amount of pressure on clinicians and nurses as stated by Mengling Feng et al (2011). Hence, here promptly we need an effective mechanism to address affordable and quickly available healthcare for all.

HEALTH CARE INDUSTRY IN INDIA

It seems since the last decades, the healthcare industry is escalating day by day. In these decades the health care industry is growing at a fast speed which is happed only due to the increase in investment and expenditure from the government as well as private players also.

It has been observed that in the year 2018, there was an increase in investment in healthcare by the private sector. So many famous international business firms are investing in the healthcare industry through FDI, which acts as a catalyst in the success and growth of the health care industry.

In the current scenario, the increases in diseases due to changes in the lifestyle of people, the demand for affordable healthcare services are increasing. The new technologies like telemedicine and expenditure through the budget done by the government in the healthcare service industry are also acting as the major driving forces for the growth of the healthcare industry in India.

As the country is becoming more digitalized due to which Telemedicine technique has also come into existence in the healthcare service industry. Now a day due to changes in the business environment and consumer preference the government of India has more focused on the growth and development of telemedicine and initiated investment in various health care services to provide better health care medical facilities in rural India as well. From the below graphs we can see that the per capital healthcare expenditure is increasing and in India 40% share is of government hospitals followed by Mid-tier, top tier, and nursing home.

EMERGING TRENDS IN INDIAN HEALTHCARE IN INDIA

Automation in health care has made revolutionary changes in the health service industry and it has a diverse advantage in the way where healthcare services provided in India. In the current economic scenario of the Indian healthcare segment, the private players will be the major adaptor of technology and automation in his services. Automation in health care will become an inseparable part of the health care services which is provided by the hospitals or patient care units. Automation in health care will help to minimize the costs and manage the operations effectively due to this benefits the health care industry is expected to attain a big transformation, profitable and grow in the forthcoming coming days.

Figure 1. Share in healthcare spending in India, 2015

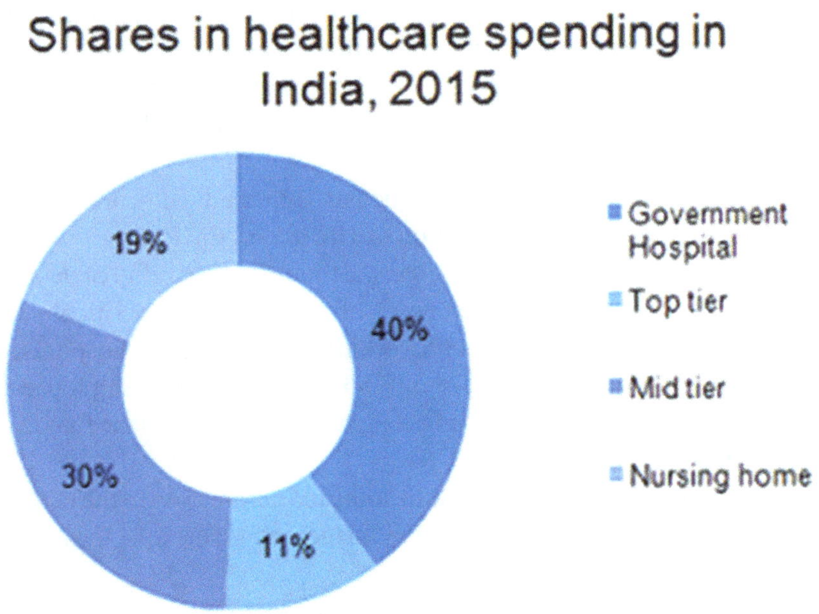

Figure 2. Per-capita healthcare expenditure

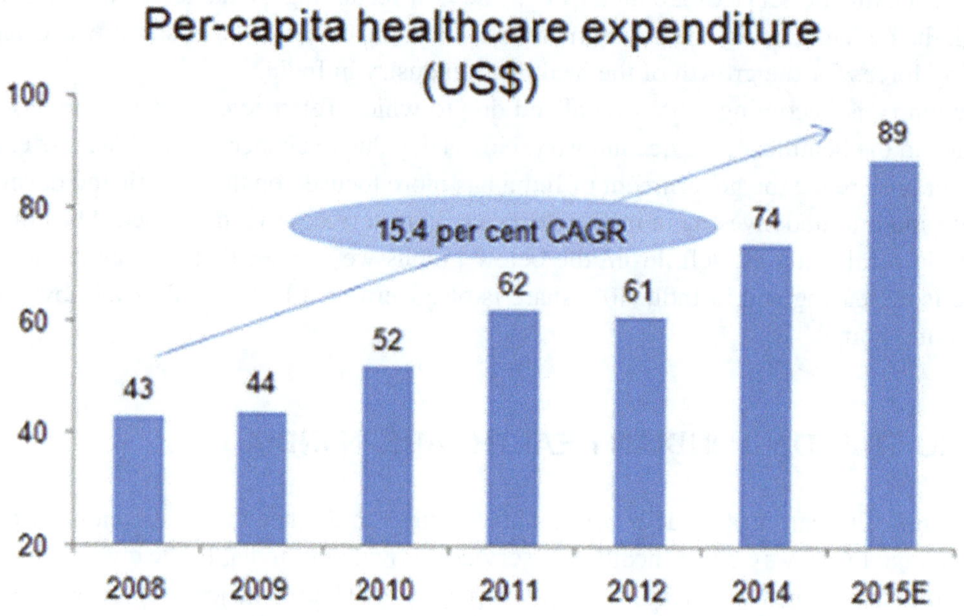

The business environment is so dynamic and demand in the health care sector is increasing very tremendously these days. With the increasing demand in health services, it has also expected by the patient that they would be treated more efficiently with modern, automatic, digital and innovative methods. For getting the above systems for diagnosis and treatment, the patient is putting pressure on hospitals to implement automation and technology to modernize traditional service patterns.

So due to the patient demand and pressure nowadays the healthcare industry are now equipped with innovative tools and techniques with added information technology system such as automation and digitalization in health care services, which are playing a major role in the growth of medical services in India as well as in other developing countries in the globe.

The healthcare industry in India is expected to greater deployment of various innovative medical tools such as telemedicine, hospital management information system (HMIS), online or electronic medical records (EMR), etc.

Now a day's cloud computing-based techniques used in the healthcare industry are one of the best tools to be applied progressively in the adoption of HMIS and EMRs.

The advantages of these are easy and error-free and timely accessibility of data without any geographical and location barriers with fast response in case of emergencies for critical patients.

To adopt the more improved and efficient working system in their hospitals, most of the hospitals are using full automation system for seeking full information of their employees and staffs, as well as a settlement of bills, keeping and maintaining the patient records, finance and in operation as well as treatment of the patient.

Along with the growing popularity of digitalization and automation in the health care industry, market penetration of robotic surgery will increase in the forthcoming years.

INNOVATIONS IN HEALTH CARE INDUSTRY

Automated health Monitoring System: Automated health tracking and monitoring system are being used to overcome the various problems of the patient like convenient to use, size of utensils are handy, lightweight and mobile. The automated monitor is also used as a tool to keep watch on the patient's pulse rate and indicators related to diseases.

The high degree of professional competence: Nowadays in the modern era and the era of digitalization and automation all health professionals are very expert and using the technology to deliver patient-centered care as well as more focused on quality improvement approaches, and informatics.

Healthcare facilities through telemedicine: In the current scenario of automation in the healthcare industry, Telemedicine has emerged as one of the innovative health care tools Telemedicine helps to solve the clinical problems from da distance especially for the people of rural areas. Telemedicine is helping the patient to consult his doctor at their home as per his convenience and comfort without visiting a doctor's clinic.

Automated Paperless admit and discharge of patient: With the introduction of automation, internet and technology now a day's hospitals are adopting the paperless system of admitting and discharge of patients as well as to reduce time spent by patients in doing paper-based formalities. In addition to that, health the insurance claim process was also very lengthy and uses of too many paper formalities for a claim but due to the automation system in the healthcare industry, the claim of medical insurance has also become very easy and quick.

Automated and digitized Medical records management: Automated and digitalized Medical records management help to collect, sort and take data from patient records by scanning the bar code which is pasted at the time of admission of the patient on the prescription. It is easy for hospital officials to eliminate the time taking exercise by manual feeding of data, data classification, and data indexing of patient records which causes delays in getting critical patient information on time especially in case of emergency cases.

Some other benefits of Automated and digitized Medical records management are given below:

- Minimize the time consumption of manual work of documentation
- Reduce the costs of labor for manual data entry
- Quick response to the patient about their query and history of health.
- Improve patient care with prompts services with the help of the quick sorting of their health records.
- Required less space for the storage of Physical documents and records of a patient as well as reduce the cost also associated with the storage of documents and records.

Applications of AI in Healthcare and Research: The main focus of Artificial Intelligence in health care is to analyze relationships between prevention or treatment techniques and patient outcomes. In today's health care services AI is now become one of the important parts of Industry and is used to improve the patient experience.

Super Specialty hospitals with digital and automated technology: Super Specialty hospitals in India have emerged an institution of healthcare services provider under one roof where a patient can get all services and facilities Medical Stores, Primary Health Care & various diagnostic centers like pathology, X-Ray, Ultrasound etc. The main focus of Super Specialty hospitals with digital and automated technology is to achieve excellence in medical services with affordable, costs effective methods of diagnosis and treatment of a patient.

Advancement of research and development in scientific medicine: Due to the addition of automation in healthcare industry Healthcare changes radically because of technological developments in every area related to health care systems like new drugs and treatments, new devices, new AI and digital support for healthcare, etc. Nowadays due to innovative research technological advancement is increasing day by day which is benefited to hospitals, doctors the staff as well as the patient.

DEFINITION OF *AUTOMATION*

Automation can be defined as the use of automatic equipment, its application and uses technologies in machines and tools for self-performing to reduce the effort and errors of human beings and to provide effective services.

ABOUT AUTOMATION IN HEALTH CARE

The words Automation was a term used earlier in other manufacturing industries. But due to advancements in healthcare technology in the past decade, healthcare automation is quickly becoming the norm.

By implementing automation successfully, the patient is now more efficiently being treated by the healthcare service industry can be getting much satisfaction because of efficient and modernize processes of treatment, including a simplified and faster process of health care as well as cost savings benefits also.

Nowadays in Indian as well as a foreign business, it has been pragmatic that more than 75% of hospitals and health centers focused on overall cost discounts and advanced medical services with efficiency is the main focus area. Healthcare industries are continually looking to reduce costs by reducing the wastage of time and money both. Whereas automation of physical work can also be an important part of a strategy for better services and improved performance.

With the help of automation diagnosis of diseases and its route cause is now become easier and convenient. Diagnosis by an automated system made more accurate and efficient in both monetary terms and in reduced time which gives accurate information about the medical condition.

TYPES OF AUTOMATED MACHINES USES IN HEALTH CARE

Diagnosis in Medical Imaging

Medical imaging refers to a type of unique technology that is used to scan the human body to analyze, screen, or treat medical conditions. Medical imaging gives diverse evidence about the area of the body and disease being studied or treated, related to possible disease.

Robotic Surgery

Robotic or Robot-assisted surgery is just like an assistant with advanced computer technology and Artificial Intelligence with the experts of professional surgeons. These technologies assist the surgeon with a 10x overstated, high-definition, 3D-image of the body's difficult anatomy.

Uses of Robotics in the healthcare industry as introduced with great potential for increasing the productivity of health care and patient welfare service. Robot-assisted surgery helps surgeons to ease to do critical and complex operations through tiny incisions using robotic technology.

Surgical robots are much intelligent due to enabled AI system is controlled by computer commands and devices that can be programmed to aid in the positioning and manipulation of surgical instruments. Robot-assisted surgery assists surgeons with to do their work in more refined ways within the stipulated time without error to gain better accuracy and results.

COMPUTER-AIDED DIAGNOSIS

Computer-aided diagnosis (CAD) has emerged as one of the innovative tools in the medical imaging and diagnostic radiology field. CAD is a concept recognized by taking into account equally the roles of both doctors and computers. Now a day's CAD is being used to ensure proper surgery and prediction of how organs will perform as well as it has been also used for the detection of cancer and other diseases in any part of the human body with accuracy. So, the above tools and technologies in medical diagnostics and operation is a way for possible cost reduction and improving accuracy by using technology instead of human doctors.

ADVANTAGES OF AUTOMATION TO HEALTHCARE

- **Labor Savings**

Uses of automation in healthcare with the help of computers, robots and the use of Artificial Intelligence (AI) replaced the labor considered as a substitute with automated machines for the benefits considering cost and time saver.

- **Faster data to enrich**

Medical Professionals are working now a day on automation techniques to produce and data mining within time and a new method to find out the existing data. Such efforts could reduce unnecessary physician and mental frustration and enhance patient care as practitioners get the evidence they need at just the right time in just the right setting.

- **Improvement in Quality of Standard of living and death rate.**

Automation tools reduced human error or fatigue up to the zero levels, and also help to provide a basis of care activities. In most of the cases in the medical industry, it has been found that Quality improvement and Consistencies in the health industry will result in a reduction of death rate and Improvement in Quality of Standard of living.

- **Reduce wastage paper, manpower and time**

The use of expensive stationery and other materials like booklet, form, file, etc needed for documentation of records of patient history and summary can lead to a lot of wastage of paper, manpower and time both. But with the help of automation, we can save the wastage of stationery and manpower, which is some of the biggest costs that we have seen heavily weigh on healthcare providers.

- **Positive Outcomes**

When any patients follow a uniform care path reinforced by the automation system, it is more likely they will get positive outcomes. It gives better results with accuracy, increased operational efficiency, productivity, and cost-savviness. Today's there is demand for automated techniques of treatment and diagnostic procedures by the patient as well as it has also been demanded by the healthcare service industry to upgrade their medical facilities to facilitate their patients for getting the positive results and satisfaction to their customers to this end.

- **Automation streamlines medical billing.**

Using the automation system in health care services will help the health care organization to make proper calculations of bills of their patients. In the modern digitalized era and automation in health care services, now it is very much convenient for hospital officials to make the bill of admitted patients instantly while the discharge of patients after his treatment. With the help of uses of automation in health care services, there are minimum uses of paperwork in the accounting and billing system of hospitals as well as chances of error and any disputes are also negligible.

- **Automation allows for accurate information capture**

Data, records and disease or treatment history of the patient in the healthcare industry is very vital for further analysis and it helps to take exact decisions to doctor for the wellness of the patient. So the data, records and treatment history of all patients must be safe and easily traceable with the help of automation.

Any slight errors or wrong information about the records and treatment history of the patient can cause serious problems for patients and may grounds for the source of legal repercussions also. Such conditions will need to be the focus and solve which is expected by effective hospital management software and automation system which provides opportunities for easier and with fewer errors.

Other advantages are:

- Guarantee a patient's wellbeing and keeps living healthy.
- Reduced risk of any casualty during the critical care of the patient.
- Minimize workload and boost the efficiency of hospital personnel.
- Improve the comfort level of the patients and enhance mobility.
- Minimize the cost and provide health care services with higher efficiency.
- Continuous monitoring of patients and updating in data of health recovery.

ADVANCING THE HEALTHCARE SERVICE INDUSTRY WITH ROBOTIC PROCESS AUTOMATION (RPA)

India is adopting technological advancement especially health care services and the growing adopting technological advancement has a lot to do with it. In Indian current health care industry scenario is now more efficient, effective and affordable by patients as well as adopting and innovative technologies in health care analysis and dialysis. Advancing in the Healthcare Service Industry with Robotic Process Automation helps in the transfer of various information from multiple Electronic Health Records, other various concern departments and specialty units. Now, the healthcare industry has shifted towards digitalization and has started to adopt RPA (Robotic Process Automation) with an escalating rate. With robotic process automation in health care increases efficiency, productivity and outcome, as well as improved customer experience, will be the top priorities for the healthcare service industry. In the current dynamic environment, healthcare service providers are exploring the different opportunities and ways to provide the best patient treatment, care, and diagnosis with objectives to reduce costs, improve productivity, and intensify operational efficiencies. Along with these advances in the healthcare service industry they are facing lots of challenges, specifically the management of information and data as well as their distribution in various Intra and Inter platforms. Healthcare Service Industry is also exploring the different opportunities to advancing the healthcare service industry with robotic process automation (RPA) in other various areas including clinical applications, lab information systems, third-party portals, insurance portals, radiology information systems, scheduling applications, etc. These systems' integration is typically intricate, and most care providers still rely on humans to act manual labor-intensive tasks to process information. It has seemed that with the help of RPA, healthcare institutions can improve their efficiency and deliver better medical care to their patients.

THE FUTURE APPLICATIONS OF AUTOMATION

In the future, the medical automation system has great potential to revolutionize clinical practices in a sense of safety, consistency, and improved quality health care services with refined productivity and cost-effectiveness of patient care. With the use of automation along with AI & Digitalization in health care, the patient will get prompt services in their treatment which will save his life, time and money. Automation in the health care system will be easy to access the history or records of patients related to his disease and treatment done. In this way in the future by exploiting technology and automation system in the health care industry will go beyond human limitations in treating patients and will be easy to diagnose disease and cure it timely.

RENOVATION IN PATIENT MONITORING BY AUTOMATION SYSTEM

The advancement and automation in creative medicinal services frameworks for diagnosis of disease and critical cases necessitate automatic monitoring of the patient, automatic health record indicators, automatic record of data and its communication across different concern departments such as hospitals, Intensive critical care units, and outpatient clinics. Nowadays with advanced technologies and automation in health care services, the number of patient monitoring systems is developed and utilized effectively. Some of them are listed here.

Remote patient monitoring: is a type of innovative monitoring system of patient admitted in various wards and care units with the help of remote technology. It is also beneficial for those patients who are outside the hospital clinic especially in remote and rural areas where people are not in reach with hospitals. It may increase accessibility of patient and which increase the care and reduce the cost of moving from one place to other places.

Home-based patient monitoring: In this monitoring system the aging population and those who have chronic diseases prefer to receive care in their homes instead of in a hospital.

Mobile-based patient monitoring: is a type of monitoring system in which patient can be monitored anywhere any time with the help of GPS enabled small compact unit like a cell phone or a wrist watch which will also convenient for patients to carry this device with them wherever they are moving and specialist can also able to gain the proper information about their current health status.

Internet-based patient monitoring: In today's business scenario, the uses of IoT with different types of sensors are increasing significantly including the health care services industry also. IoT with different types of sensors run through the internet helps people to provide medical healthcare services anywhere, any time. Now a day's IoT technology has introduced many types of medical facilities for both doctors and patients. Now with help and uses of IoT, patient can be monitored and tracked by the physicians on internet. IoT has becomes the middle chain between physician and patient to transfer the data related to their illness and cure.

Uses of Cloud Computing

Cloud computing is becoming a very vital part for each and every service industry including the healthcare service industry also. The uses of cloud computing make easy for hospital officials to manage and optimize information that can be stored in the cloud database as well as it can be easily accessible whenever needed at anytime, anywhere. Cloud computing offers the instant access and availability of various data of past history and treatment of a patient which is stored in a cloud system for the best care to their patients in an economical way. It helps doctors and specialists to access and compare patient data to give better diagnosis and treatment to their patients. Apart from the storage function, the cloud can also be used for the knowledge-sharing platform by which specialists or doctors can get information all around the world at any time, which results in getting the information about the illness, cure, and treatment for the well being of a patient.

Uses of Big Data in Healthcare: Nowadays due to an increase in client base in the service industry the volume of data and its size is increasing day by day in big amounts which are usually generated from diverse sources. In the case of the health care industry also the database is an important tool to provide better services to the patient such as patient past records, case history, hospital admission notes, discharge summaries, insurance reports, etc. So, the management and handling of such big data is a very complex and difficult task. As a result of the excess pile-up of records and data of the patient in the healthcare service industry, there is the problem of backup and storage of data in paper or document form. However, the handling of day to day and a large amount of data makes it difficult to processed and analyzed by traditional techniques. Consequently, technologies such as cloud computing are now gradually is being used by various service industry along with the health care industry which makes easy for the processing of massive data effectively and securely within instant time. Hence, the healthcare service industry is now gradually becoming a big data industry. So, the uses of big data in the healthcare industry are introduced and it benefits the hospital's officials to manage the data with the help of the Data Base Management system, big data and cloud computing techniques to get information anywhere, any time. So, efficient management of big data can change the scenario of modern service providers with new opportunities for modern healthcare service providers also. The uses of big data can be considered as steps to convert this potential into better services and financial advantages.

IoT Based ICU Patient Monitoring System: Intensive Care Unit or ICU is a unit of hospitals where critical cases and patients are admitted for their treatment. So due to the critical conditions of a patient the doctors need to have very active and vigilance in all-time as well as always tries to remain updated with changes in the health status of patients including records like sugar level, blood pressure, pulse rate, and temperature, etc.

So, this physically with manual methods of updated records of multiple patients admitted in ICU is too much time taking and hectic task. So, in this type of situation, the IoT based system can make the task easy and convenient for the hospital's administration and doctors to update all-time records over the internet. IoT based ICU Patient Monitoring System collects various information on patient health status with the help of a few sensors, wi-fi, and internet. There are various updated records of blood pressure and heartbeat of an admitted patient which can be monitored with an electronically connected module to provide information to concerns person. On the press of a button, the sensor senses of the blood pressure in diastolic along with the heartbeat and sends it to the central controller. Thus, the doctor can get access to these vital parameters pertaining to the patients' health over the IoT from anywhere over the world. In this way, IoT based ICU Patient Monitoring System is an enhanced system that helps in monitoring ICU patients without any manual intervention.

Contactless heart rate and respiration rate monitoring system: It is a unique innovation came into existence in the health care industry, which can be made to measure the accuracy of the rate of heartbeats and respiration of patient etc without coming into the contact of the patient. This can be used in case of a sensitive patient where one can not touch the patient, especially in burn or injury.

Elderly patient monitoring: This type of monitoring system is specially designed for physical disabilities and also physically challenged people who are not in a condition of visiting the doctor's clinic or hospitals. It is an internet-based house automation system in health care is designed to assist the people to support and also monitor and control the values of the device using smart phones.

Agent-based patient monitoring: In current health care industry Agent-based patient monitoring system is acting like a third party agent who is experts of various health care professionals collects data with the help of innovative and digital tools from various patients and gives prescriptions to patients as per their diseases and recommends measures to hospital's staff.

Figure 3. Remote pain monitoring in hospital for inpatients and ICU patients.
Source: *Published in IEEE Journal of Biomedical and Health Informatics 2018.*

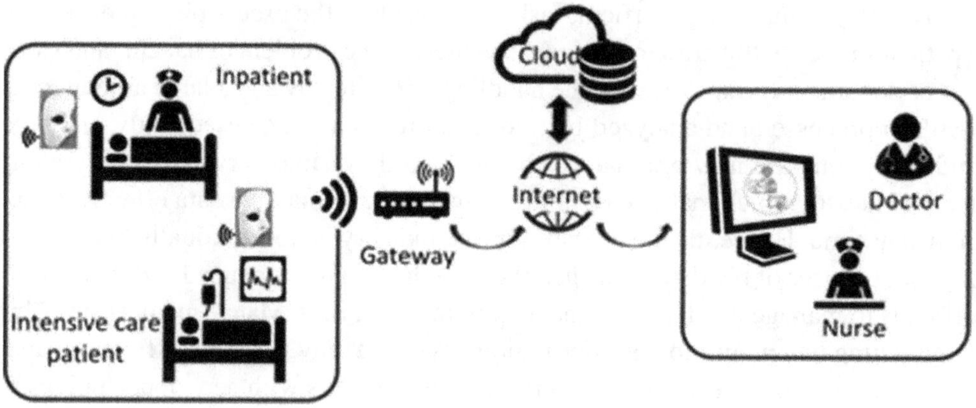

TRENDS AND PROSPECTS OF TELEMEDICINE

Due to a lack of resources in the current health care industry, a new system is introduced i.e is called as 'Telemedicine' which has been defined as the uses of telecommunication to diagnose the disease of a patient across the globe without any limitations and barriers. It is considered as the delivery service in the healthcare industry reachable to all at any place without any barrier of distance even in remote areas also. By seeing the advantages of these prospects in telemedicine, nowadays so many healthcare professionals are started the use of information and communication technologies for the exchange of valid information and diagnosis of a patient who is not in their reach.

In the current health care business scenario, Telemedicine is considered as an innovative system of giving the best healthcare services across the globe. The use of this technique is considered as Cost-adaptive, in terms of money and time. So, the use of this technique is mostly acceptable in developing countries, especially in rural areas.

Remote sensors wearying by patients pass on imperative signs to an individual server, which is activated on PDA gadgets, for example, tablets, advanced cells or workstations. In the arrangement, the information is transfer to the room server (clinic server) of the social insurance framework from an individual server, for example, a restorative database or crisis server over in Network. From the server, the patient's information is examined by healthcare networks (like Doctors, Experts or Nurse).

WIRELESS SYSTEMS IN HEALTH CARE

The monitoring of the patient in the health care service industry is one of the major concerns and it can be provided at the best level by health care service provider with the help of new innovative tools and technology in which wireless system is also considered as a new tool because of its innovative technology. So, by seeing the advantages of this wireless health care system, the current health care industry is now adopting this system in their hospitals.

An automatic wireless monitoring system is one of the important needs to organize a complete wireless sensor network in the healthcare system.

Figure 4. sensor network application in medical
Source: *https://www.cse.wustl.edu/~jain/cse574-08/ftp/medical/figure2.jpg*

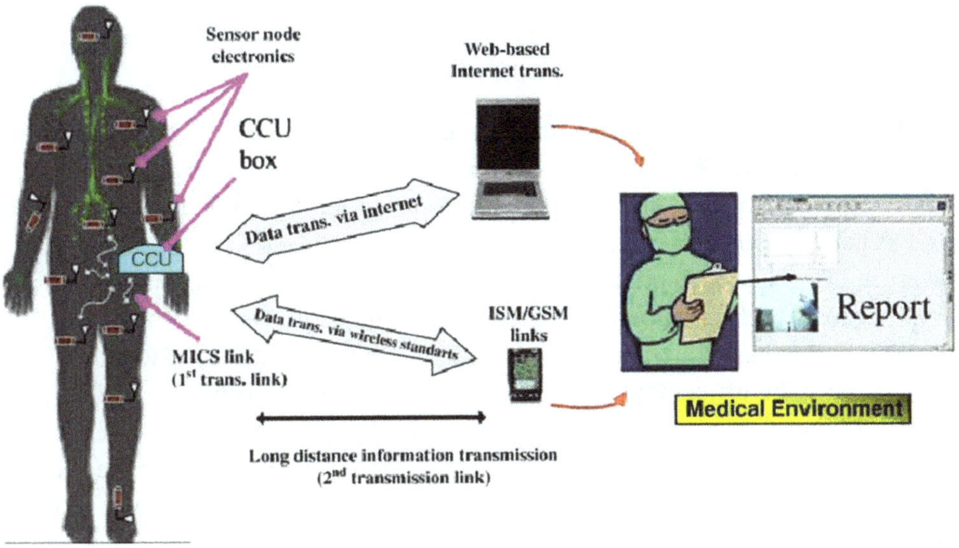

Health care is using the sensor to measure the patient's body temperature and pulse rate with the help of wireless devices in hospitals. These sensors are also used to monitor the condition of the multiple patient at time without labour and effort as well as need not to visit frequently to the patient in every ward of hospitals because all wards are equipped with wireless systems and connected with internet by which the health care professionals and specialist are able to get information of their patient online and prepare a report of their recovery or health conditions on regular interval of time.

Moreover, all of these concealed wireless systems in health care for medicinal applications are now not only listening carefully by healthcare peoples and the government but also by researchers and businesses.

PROSPECTS AND CHALLENGES OF WIRELESS HEALTH CARE SERVICES.

With the set up new tools and technologies in the current health care industry, along with the service providers patient also much benefited in terms of cost-saving, time-saving and instant error-free services with more comfort. Hospitals or health care industries are using wireless technology and devices to reduce human errors, increase the quality of patient care, improve efficiency, as well as to provide more comfort to the patient. Although, apart from the various benefits of this technology, it has been also observed that it is not effective in some fields especially in critical cases where the patient requires much vigilance and facing various challenges while implementing and operating this system.

AUTOMATED HEALTH CARE SERVICES 2019 (TRENDS, OPPORTUNITIES, AND OUTLOOK)

Trends

Automated and Digital health services promise to change the appearance of the healthcare service industry. The growing demand for Automated and Digital health services has been noted as an emerging development in the medical field. Automation has introduced a range of benefits to both the service provider as well as patient both.

The healthcare industry has been progressively adopting automation in various several areas such as robotic surgery, diagnosis of disease, patient record, and telemedicine, etc.

The healthcare industry has witnessed so many changes that occur due to automation i.e. the newer approaches characterized by efficiency. Automation in health care also helps medical professionals, doctors, and nurses to focus on better and improved patient care services.

Increasing demand for automation with internet technology in health care services is considered as opportunities and important trends nowadays. Moreover, it helps to hospital industry to provide improved health care facilities as compared to traditional technologies. Additionally, these technologies are found very successful in remote monitoring and clinical care also.

Opportunities

Now a day's changes in population demographics, such as aging populations with an increasing prevalence of chronic diseases, is become a better opportunity in the market of automated health care services.

Automation and digitalization in health care services have brought in a range of benefits. The healthcare industry has been progressively adoption automation in several areas such as during operations, monitoring of patient's blood pressure, heartbeats and temperature as well as it is been also demanded by patient to save time and money both during the services of health care So, due to these benefits for both service providers as well as patient it is considered as an opportunities for this industry.

The areas in which automated health care services have emerged as opportunities are:

- Automated medical diagnosis.
- Automated medication delivery systems.
- Automated laboratory testing and analysis.
- Automated home monitoring and telemetry.
- Automated medical imaging and image analysis.
- Automation in monitoring patient conditions.
- Automated operating rooms and related equipment.
- Automated healthcare logistics, resources, and patient tracking.

OUTLOOK

Automation and digitalization in the health care industry are helping to "connect the dots" between service providers and patients. To gauge the economic benefit of digital transformation in health care services health care service industry plays a major role in the delivering of sustainable health care. Automated technology such as telemedicine could expand services while also helping hospitals bend the cost curve. If we talk about the business outcome approach is focused on solution acceleration, including continuous improvement in each and every aspect of health care services. So, in a dynamic business scenario, every outcome-based solution requires a detailed understanding of customers or patient needs.

CONCLUSION

India is having a population of approx 1.30 billion people with a predominantly rural population. As we know that in more than 65% of the population of India are residing in rural areas who often have limited access to automated healthcare services.

Due to these challenges, the healthcare industry has adopted mobile services which are primarily managed by the government and complemented by various private healthcare service providers. Delivering automated medical services to rural areas is extremely painstaking and often not viable for government and as well as private healthcare providers alone. So, there is an imminent need for innovation and digitalization in the health care industry especially in rural areas to maximize outreach and provide healthcare services to a wider population. So, this problem can be solved only by proper implementations of policy, strategy, management, and innovation of technologies like automation, digitalization, IoT, and Big data in the health care industry in India.

In view of the above issues, The Indian government and other various private players of the health care industry has done the so many efforts and adopted the automation and digitalization techniques to health care to deliver the cost-effective healthcare services in India. Telemedicine is considered as one such project, which may be able to facilitate healthcare services to a patient who is an outreach to hospitals even to the remote areas of India. It has been observed that over the last ten years, the Indian government, along with private healthcare providers, has invested a huge amount in health care services and exploring the possibility of providing medical services and healthcare by using other innovative tools and techniques apart from automation and digitalization. Automation and digitalization in the hospital allow the exploration of current assets and the exploration of new ways of using them, with the end result of tangible improvements in both quality enhancement and cost rationalization.

Automation-driven health care activities are free from human fatigue and error, so it is much useful to provide instant and cost-effective methods to go ahead in the reduction of complications in health care services.

Somewhere it has been also observed that as the results of the digitalization processes accomplished within the hospital especially in rural areas are tremendously variable and hospital managers experience pitfalls and shortcomings in their implementation.

In conclusion, from an empirical point of view, the chapter directs healthcare practitioners and service provider with clear guidelines to leverage on automation and digitalization in health care services not only use asset automation and digitalization as a driver of cost reduction, but also as a tool to control the financial situation of their hospitals in order to increase the quality of healthcare services offered in their hospitals.

REFERENCES

Analytic Insight. (n.d.). Advancing healthcare industry robotic process automation. Retrieved from https://www.analyticsinsight.net/advancing-healthcare-industry-robotic-process-automation/

Badawi, O., Brennan, T., Celi, L. A., Feng, M., Ghassemi, M., Ippolito, A., & Moses, C. (2014). Making big data useful for health care: A summary of the inaugural mit critical data conference. *JMIR Medical Informatics*, *2*(2), e22. doi:10.2196/medinform.3447 PMID:25600172

Ben-Ari, J., Zimlichman, E., Adi, N., & Sorkine, P. (2010). Contactless respiratory and heart rate monitoring: Validation of an innovative tool. *Journal of Medical Engineering & Technology*, *34*(7-8), 393–398. doi:10.3109/03091902.2010.503308 PMID:20698739

Chan, V., Ray, P., & Parameswaran, N. (2008). Mobile e-Health monitoring: An agent-based approach. *IET Communications*, *2*(2), 223–230. doi:10.1049/iet-com:20060646

Divakaran, S., Manukonda, L., Sravya, N., Morais, M. M., & Janani, P. (2017, September). IOT clinic-Internet based patient monitoring and diagnosis system. In *Proceedings of the 2017 IEEE International Conference on Power, Control, Signals and Instrumentation Engineering (ICPCSI)* (pp. 2858-2862). IEEE. 10.1109/ICPCSI.2017.8392243

Elprocus. (n.d.). Automatic wireless health monitoring system circuit. Retrieved from https://www.elprocus.com/automatic-wireless-health-monitoring-system-circuit/

Gastaldi, L., & Corso, M. (2012). Smart healthcare digitalization: Using ICT to effectively balance exploration and exploitation within hospitals. *International Journal of Engineering Business Management*, *4*, 4–9.

IBEF. (n.d.). Healthcare India. Retrieved from https://www.ibef.org/industry/healthcare-india.aspx

Idtechex. (n.d.). Digital health 2019 trends opportunities and outlook. Retrieved from https://www.idtechex.com/en/research-report/digital-health-2019-trends-opportunities-and-outlook/660

Ilahi, L., & Ghannouchi, S. A. (2013). Improving telemedicine processes via BPM. *Procedia Technology*, *9*, 1209–1216. doi:10.1016/j.protcy.2013.12.135

India Times. (n.d.). Indian healthcare in 2018 and forecast for 2019. Retrieved from https://health.economictimes.indiatimes.com/news/industry/indian-healthcare-industry-in-2018-and-forecast-for-2019/6726959

IndiaPKI. (n.d.). Patient Admission & Discharge. Retrieved from www.indiapki.org

National Health Portal, India. (n.d.). Retrieved from https://www.nhp.gov.in/

Nevon Projects. (n.d.). Iot based ICU patient monitoring system. Retrieved from https://nevonprojects.com/iot-based-icu-patient-monitoring-system/

Nuffield Bioethics. (n.d.). Artificial intelligence in healthcare and research. Retrieved from https://nuffieldbioethics.org/wp-content/uploads/Artificial-Intelligence-AI-in-healthcare-and-research.pdf

Pinto, S., Cabral, J., & Gomes, T. (2017, March). We-care: An IoT-based health care system for elderly people. In *Proceedings of the 2017 IEEE International Conference on Industrial Technology (ICIT)* (pp. 1378-1383). IEEE. 10.1109/ICIT.2017.7915565

Rao, P. B., & Uma, S. K. (2015). Raspberry Pi home automation with wireless sensors using smart phone. *International Journal of Computer Science and Mobile Computing*, *4*(5), 797–803.

Travel trends Today. (n.d.). Medical tourism emerging as a next growth driver. Retrieved from https://www.traveltrendstoday.in/news/india-tourism/item/5792-medical-tourism-emerging-as-a-next-growth-driver

Yang, G., Jiang, M., Ouyang, W., Ji, G., Xie, H., Rahmani, A. M., ... Tenhunen, H. (2018). IoT-Based Remote Pain Monitoring System: From Device to Cloud Platform. *IEEE Journal of Biomedical and Health Informatics*, *22*(6), 1711–1719. doi:10.1109/JBHI.2017.2776351 PMID:29990259

Zhang, W., & Li, Y. (2014). A Study on Consumer Behavior of Commercial Health and Fitness Club--A Case of Consumers in Liverpool. *American journal of industrial and business management, 4*(1), 58.

Chapter 2
Deep Data Analytics:
Future of Telehealth

Madhulika Bhatia
https://orcid.org/0000-0001-6833-5657
Amity University, Noida, India

Madhurima Hooda
Amity University, Noida, India

Priya Gupta
All India Institute of Medical Sciences, New Delhi, India

ABSTRACT

In the past, doctors and specialists were not connected to patients through telemedicine for providing virtual health and medicine. In rural areas, where experts in medical fields were not able to reach or be present at, telemedicine proved a great benefit. As the years passed, the explosive use of the internet brought profound changes to telemedicine practices. The escalation of smart devices with the capability of delivering high quality video and audio raised the possibilities of delivering remote healthcare. Telehealth care helps patients at home or at assisted living facilities as a revolutionary alternative to personal visits for both basic as well as expert care. Applying deep data analytics to telemedicine will create new horizons in telehealth by analyzing large data sets of patients using live video streaming to predict the health challenges of patients.

INTRODUCTION

The merging of technological applications with health called Telehealth. The face of health care is totally changing as it was in earlier days. The need for merging technology with health is rising day by day. The popularity of Telehealth is increasing rapidly and accepted in large part. In cluster of health care Telemedicine and Telehealth used interchangeably (Priyanka & Kulennavar, 2014).

DOI: 10.4018/978-1-7998-2101-4.ch002

Figure 1. Disciplines accepted Telehealth

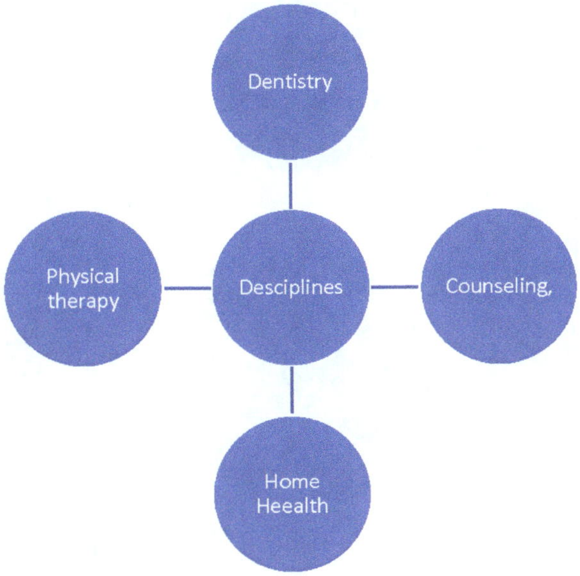

Telemedicine is defined as an application of tools, techniques and technology in medicine so that people can take advantage from it from any part of the world and round the clock, where as Telehealth is having a wider scope related to many techniques and approaches to deliver clinical services, enhancing knowledge and know how about health and medicine.

Telehealth is adopted worldwide and to be used by all disciplines related to health. Below are many health disciplines where Telehealth has been widely accepted shown in Figure 1.

- Dentistry
- Counseling
- Physical therapy
- Home health, etc.

To educate medical professionals and stack holders, Telehealth changes the era from transforming the scene from activities related to diagnostic used in traditional era regarding monitoring health of patient.

The delivering mode which helps in delivering health care services and public health with the use of information and communication technologies to pursue below services as shown in Fig 2.

- Treatment
- Consultancy
- Suggestion and advices
- Individual Care
- On time treatment without delays

Figure 2. Services provided by Telehealth

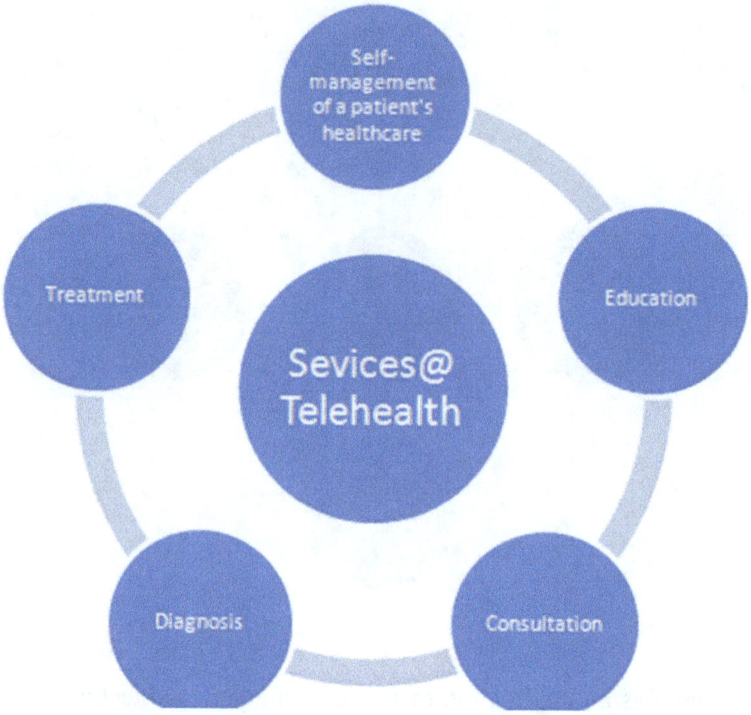

In this scenario the patient is at their own location and the health service provider is at other remote location.

The National Business Group on Health is providing Telehealth services are provided to their employees. But by 2019 the number will increase by ninety seven percent.

In India the population with old age are increasing day by day, population is increasing, less doctor to patient ratio. There is hard need of medical experts to cure chronic diseases. The cost to health diagnosis is also increasing day by day. The innovation in technology is constantly improving and patient care systems is improving day by day to assist the system from isolated locations.

The facts shows that Telemedicine hits will capture in billions by 2021.The visualization of these figures are shown in Figure 3.

Goals Telehealth

The goals of Telehealth, also called e-health or m-health (mobile health) which includes the following:

- Accessibility of health solutions to patients living in remote areas.
- The people having less mobility to travel and less options for transportation, Telehealth is a boon for them.
- A very convenient access medical specialists.

Figure 3. Market potential of Telehealth by 2021

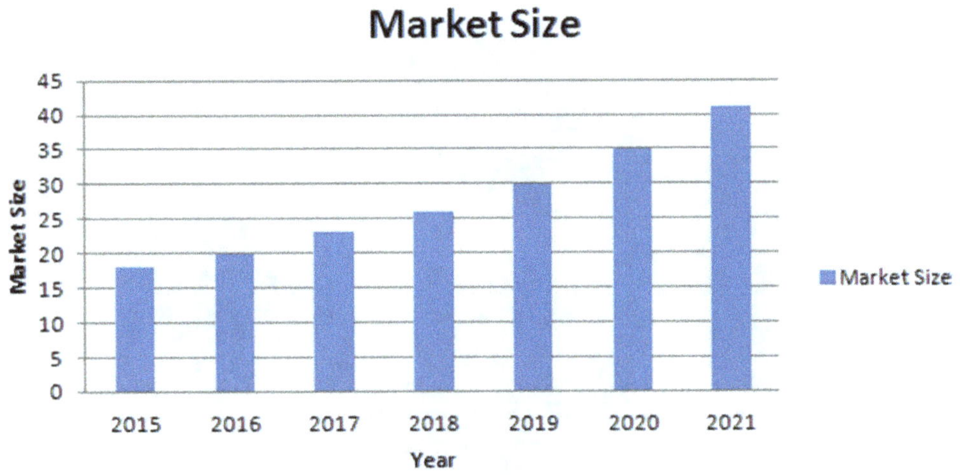

With the help of Telehealth services there is improvement in communication and coordination between team of healthcare providers and health care seekers. Telehealth support self health management.

Telehealth Services

Telehealth provide various services shown in Figure 4.

Patient Portal

A patient Portal is a kind of online portal. This portal is a good choice over e-mail service for secure sharing of information about various medical information. It's a more secure online tool that provides services

In a big system patient can make a lot of communication and can choose expert for particular disease.

Virtual Appointments

Online video conferencing can be opted for making appointments virtually, the patient can see medical practitioners, experts via video conferencing. Some time physical visit is not compulsory, in that case Virtual appointments can be opted.

These visits include appointments which are web based. These can be opted for some minor illness. Some big companies offer doctors virtual services to employee. Medical care is given in the form of home medicines or prescriptions.

Health Remotely

There are variety of technologies exist which a doctor can choose and give care to the patient to keep check on the health of patients. These technologies include:

Figure 4. Telehealth services

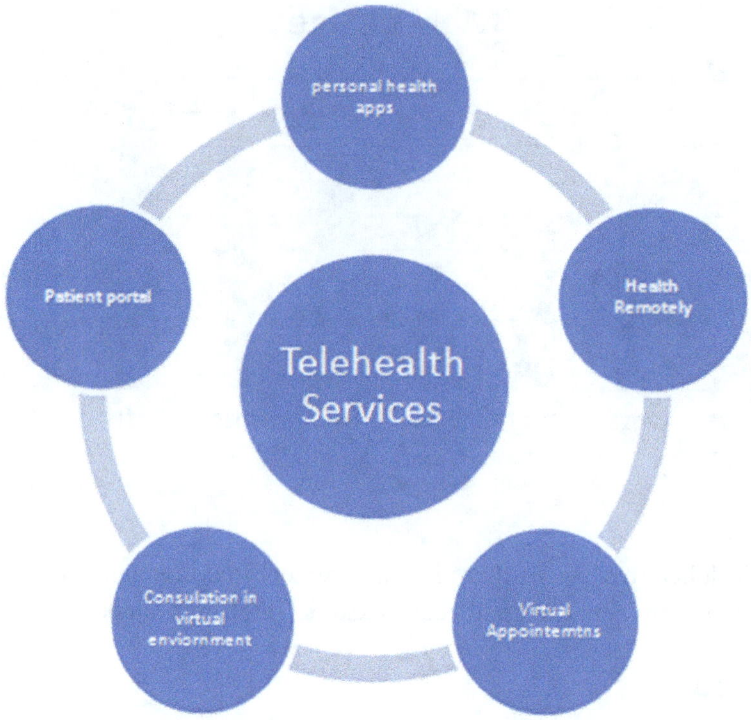

- Portals which are based on web sites.
- Applications which are based on mobile to upload the data related to medical condition of patient like information, such as levels of glucose in blood so that the team of doctors and care taker can check and take decision promptly and advise proper treatment.
- There are many devices which are wireless in nature and available supporting telehealth and helping experts to quantify pressure in blood, how the lung is functioning as well as transfer information related to these levels remotely to be shared among various experts.
- There are devices which can be wore by patient and it spontaneously documenting and transfer information, such as heart beat, glucose level in blood, gait, controlling of posture, shaking, body activity and patterns of sleep.
- There are monitoring devices which can be installed for old age people or people with chronic mantle disorders. These devises can detect abnormalities in normal activities of these people.

Consultation in Virtual Environment

Technology is proved to be very useful in providing better care to health seekers. Consultation can be done in virtual environment and team of doctors can discuss to settle on one decision about treatment.

The images like MRI, CT-SCAN can be shared among experts for special reviews. The expert can take virtual consultation on video conferencing to discuss in detail.

These prevent patients to avoid queues and waiting times to avoid useless travels.

Personal Health Records

There are health record system which collect information about health of a patient. This system is accessible to a patient by any smart device. An electronic personal health record system often called a PHR system — is a collection of all data and information related to our health that can control and help in maintaining information. An application based PHR system can be accessible to anytime from anywhere via a mobile web-enabled device, such as your computer, laptop, tablet or smart phone(Gagnon et al., 2005).

In critical situations this record can give all detailed description about patient.

Personal Health Apps

There are number of applications which are developed to keep the health record of patients securely.

- Keep record of medical status of individuals.
- Keep record of important symptoms.
- Keep track of calories.
- Manage reminders and important reminders.
- Keep record of physical activities.

Background

The traditional healthcare system needs a transformation towards a new face totally that give direction towards opting of new communication technologies as a tool for this. Various E-health programs showing a major change in medicine field and truly use of analytics is surely proved a innovative change in the framework.

There are many Medical consultation forum providing assistance through audio and video to the patient. Below are few facts about popularity of Telehealth.

The users of Telehealth are increasing day by day.

Millions of members are there and applications are downloaded and expecting to more in coming year for the use of virtual consultation on audio and video platforms. The landscape of Telehealth is changing in future.

Doctors are reporting that they have more Telehealth patients transacting then patients coming for physically for checkups and consultancy.

For example if some patient have Diabetes, then how technology can help the patient to provide Telehealth services merged with analytics.

The mobile phone and applications are being used to monitor logs of food intake, medicine intakes and blood pressure levels and sugar levels to be reviewed by nurses who responds in a virtual environment to the patient sitting at remote location. Following are the services that Telehealth provides. Popular Mobile applications are shown in Fig 5 below.

- Mobile application can be used to get estimation of diet and level of physical activity is required and how frequent insulin can be taken.

- Various web based portal exist to check the tests perform on patients, appointment tracking and automatic reminders to doctors and patients.
- E-Medicine services.

Telemedicine and Telehealth Inception

True meaning of Tele health and medicine is healing from a distance adopted majorly through the military and space industries.

"Services related to healthcare deliver majority of services where factor like distance by most of the medical professionals using Information technology techniques for the exchange of correct facts for curing and preventing disease and impairment.

Proposed Work: Fortification and Atrophy of Telemedicine

The shape and face of Health care sector is moving to broad surface. The era of charge based care is changing to outcome based care. The use of advanced Tele methods for health care that can be facilitated to the customers is done only because of involvement of various telecommunication technologies like e-mail, smart phones and wireless tools(Gale et al.,2013).

Figure 5. Popular Mobile Apps

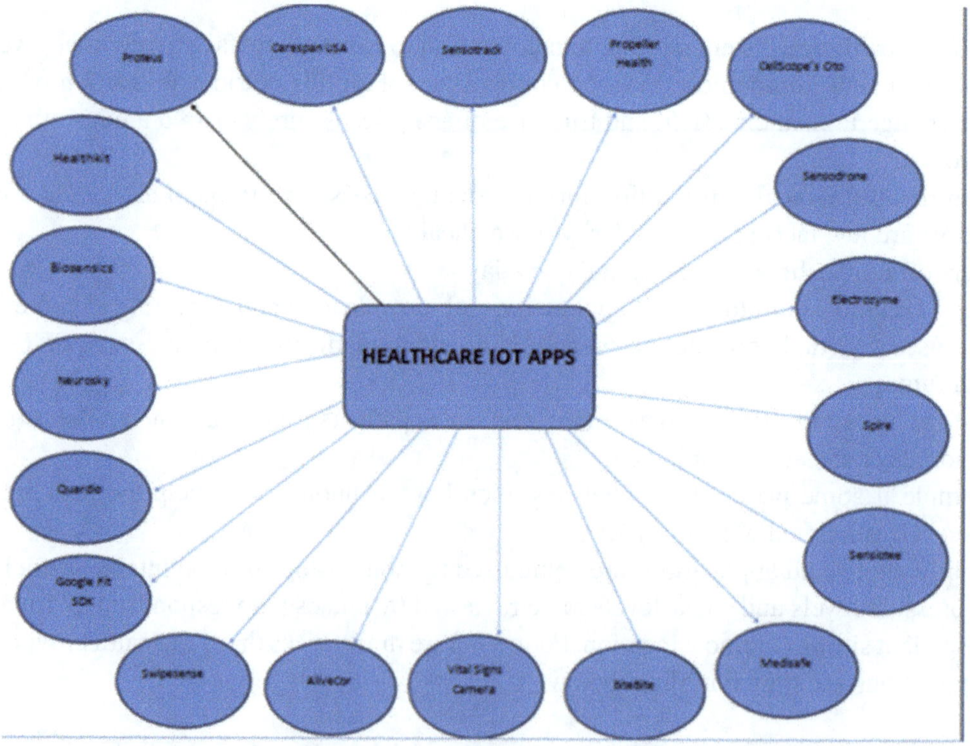

Telehealth is implemented totally by using ICT in medical fields as well as for prescribing medicine as shown in Figure 6.

- Patient consultations
- Video conferencing
- Transmission of still images,
- E-health including patient portals,
- Remote monitoring of vital signs,
- Continuing medical education,
- Consumer-focused wireless applications
- Nursing call centers

Brackets of Telehealth

Telehealth is categorized into four different categories, according that are detailed below as shown in Figure 7.

- mHealth,
- Keeping an eye on Patient from doctors location,
- Saving status and taking decision,
- Video in real time mode.

Figure 6. Implementation of ICT in Healthcare

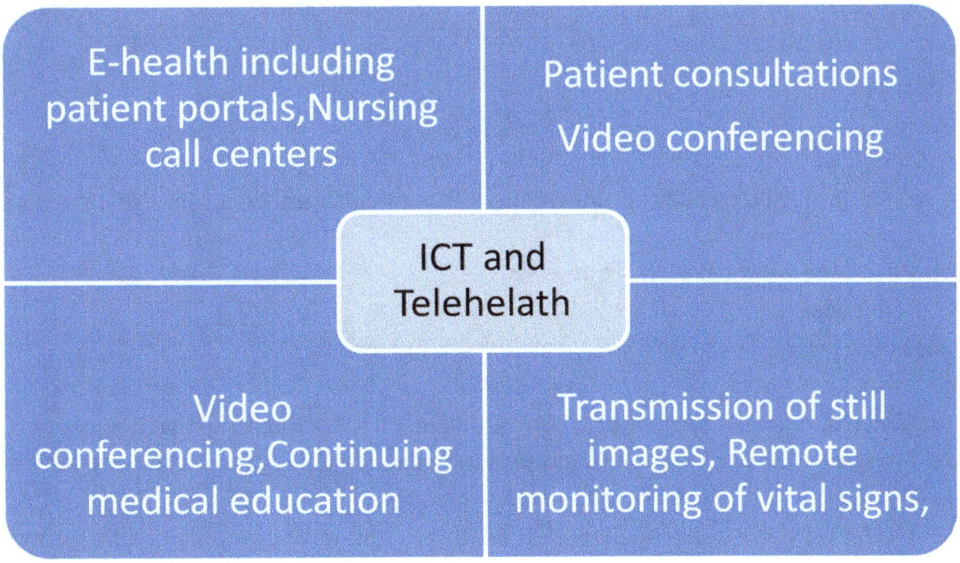

Figure 7. Categories of Telehealth

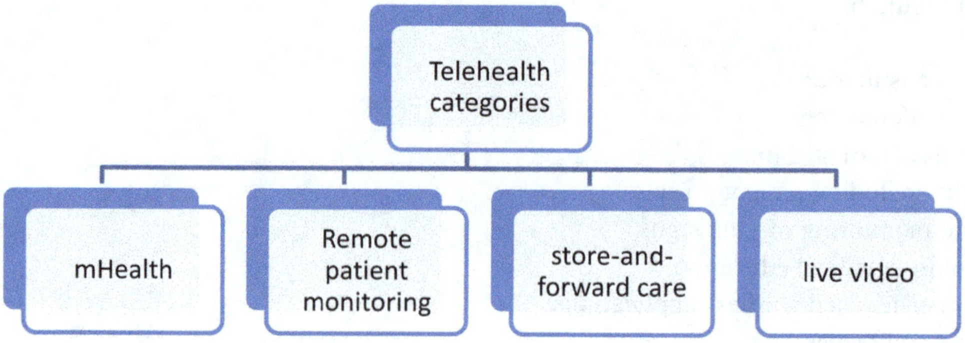

The Distinction

A conversation and discussion— whether in physical presence, via use of various technologies or on the telephone — between a health service user and a doctor can be benefitted. The important bullet is the providing a prescription for medication to a unknown person who the doctor has never examined and patient health record is not accessible to doctor. When there is a telemedicine visit, the curer is observed by the healthcare people. The person accompany patient follow instruction of provider from a far away remote location and place a stethoscope or exam camera on the body of health seeker (McLean et al.,2011).

Deep Data Analytics: The Need in Telehealth

A remote patient monitoring collect huge amount of data related to health from various devices and sources. In India one fourth of the Indian living alone and fifteen million elderly people living alone India. The assistance to them through their daily health has proven the need of Deep data analytics to Telehealth

The Telehealth system make use of smart devices like as shown in Figure 8.

- Smartphones,
- Fitbits,
- Bluetooth
- Sensors

All these devices are used to acquire information about health information. Pressure on Blood

- Activities that take physical work from body
- Levels of Glucose
- Body Mass of patient

This accumulated data related to health is then published on a dashboard so that doctors of patient, their near ones and providers can track on them and provide advance care, even from very far location(Gale et al., 2013).

This proved to be very advantageous solution for those who have complex health records.

Figure 8. Telehealth Devices

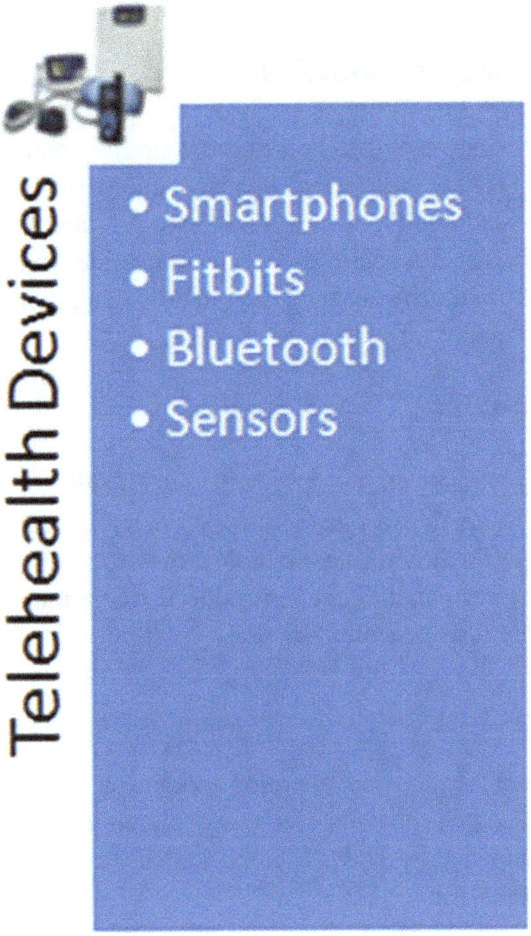

Presence of Big Data in Tele Health

The company has tie ups with services like Big Data Analytics. It will provide more useful details from such massive data coming from different sources(Dubey, 2015).

With the help of Deep Data analytics and Big data techniques the health data can be deeply analyze to ensure customized notification and health recommendations for patient and their dear ones.

The famous Big Data systems are show below:

- IBM Watson,
- Cloudvara
- Hortonworks

The Prediction about medicine is collected to provide clinical decisions about Health data.

The use of deep data analytics proves in practicing the patient care and health care operations. It leads to identification of disease fast and introducing advance drugs to cure the problem.

Some companies monitor rate of heart beat of a patients from a remote distance and analyze the data on an analytical platform to provide smart

The Power of Telehealth Merger with Analytics

Technology merged with Health care sector has given more strength and pillars to Health care industry with round the time accessibility. New innovations Research about Telehealth is still relatively new and merging it with Analytics provided Intelligence to Healthcare data and Information.

In 2016, Some studies shows that Telehealth and monitoring system has drastically reduced the death due to heart attacks because of monitoring system, tracking the dangerous signs of heart attack on time which have surely changed the quality of living.

Current Scenario - Telehealth

Most of developed nations have already started 'test beds' which helped many people to provide health care solutions in real time environment. National Health Service proposed seven projects to test Mobile Health and Telehealth technology for monitoring remotely providing many people to take access resources monitoring health. A self health care era has been introduced where many smart devices developed by big health care companies . The data generated by these health devices are analyzed using deep Data analytics (Koch, 2006).

The projects are stated below:

- In some country some mental illness is planning to connect through an a platform invented by Accenture immediately dispatch specialists in critical situations.
- An intelligence centre launched by IBM, GE and will use remote monitoring platform to help mental health problem of patients.
- A remote monitoring program by HP will monitor the people suffering from diabetes.
- In a project by remote monitoring help dementia patients at home.
- In a project Telehealth is merged with predictive analytics to target serious health issues in residents with chronic conditions like **COPD** and heart failure. The analytics will take sue of medical document to take factors like weather and socio-economic data to predict in advance that which patient is at risk and at what time.
- A project helped elderly residents to live independently by use of mobile phones.

What are the Technical Infrastructure Requirements of Telehealth

Rural health provider finding Telehealth a very important tool for patient assistance. Infrastructure requirements for implementing Telehealth depending upon the category of services are being provided by Telehealth. There is a need of Internet for transmitting data in the form of audio and video. Peripherals that are digitally sound is also required and to be part of infrastructure. The availability of Technical support staff is also required twenty four by seven (Bowonder,2005).

Below are the details of infrastructure required for Telehealth.

Broadband internet. Need of broad band internet is must as a part of Telehealth Infrastructure. Need of sufficient bandwidth to transmit audio and video data. But there is a challenge for a rural health care organization. It create a lot of problems and issues while connecting it to broadband service.

Imaging devices These devices are very important part of telehealth. Many rural health organizations want to assist patients when they are living far. Now a days medical devises like Digital stethoscopes can transmit organ sounds like heart beat etc to remote health providers.

Technical support staff. Technical staff members who support and help answer questions twenty four by seven about programs related to Telehealth. To help with efficiency, technical support staff may be shared across collaborating organizations.

Staff Learning and Training to implement telehealth we need to give proper training to staff about how to use telehealth technology which is very important and take time. The staff involved in training should be fully trained to assist, practice with the use of telehealth.

Telehealth Services

There are lot of clinical Telehealth services that can be offered.

- **Live, interactive video consultation**: With the use of videoconferencing technology which facilitate service seeker to visit physician in a virtual environment.
- **Storage and forwarding consultation**: Store and forward is a telecommunication technique which captures information of patient then it is analyzed and evaluated by a service provider at another site.
- **Hybrid consultation**: There are many consultant which use of interactive videos, consultation and storing - forwarding consultancy to Patient as well as making a hybrid team of consultancy.
- **Telehealth vs Telemedicine**?

The long distance health assistance using various electronic means and information to assist long-distance clinical health care, patient and professional health-related education in addition to using technologies like video conferencing, the internet and storing-and-forwarding imaging then streaming of patient data and health records.

Telehealth is a broader scope of *healthcare services* that are provides remotely. Telemedicine refers specifically to various clinic that are remote and provide services to patient (Hebert, 2006).

Telemedicine Programs: Success

The IT infrastructure of health is majorly effected by the grown popularity of telemedicine along with clinicians and patients that are ready to take full use of novel tools that are used in Telemedicine.

In a common practice the patient and care takers are implementing telemedicine programs get a cut on the costs related to patients who are visiting telehealth providers physically. There are telehealth programs who are helping care seekers like patients residing in remote areas to have access to seek care without traveling to clinic.

Network remote connect allow various organizations to consider and facilitate various clinicians, health center and patients to connect securely with the network(Gagnon et al.,2005).

According to reports telemedicine market is rising to touch almost $64 million by 2022 because of adoption of more and more industries, hospitals adopting Telehealth.

The rise of telemedicine also because of population increase as well as rise in chronic disease and willingness of people to consult various specialist. There is trend of common platform which allow various health specialist to adopt telemedicine as well as talk on common platform.

Video conferencing is one of the most data intensive obstacles facing telehealth. When visiting a remote patient, clinicians need a secure connection on which to share PHI. Clinicians also need a reliable connection so the video is clear.

Telemedicine Equipment

Mostly all people have access to use basic telecommunications technologies like telephones, internet, and computers. But most of the solutions related to telemedicine need more technology equipment than those require for traditional care. Below are the few telemedicine equipment a provider providing health care need to purchase to get initiate telemedicine(Chen et al., 2016).

Mobile frame

- Storage system
- Telemedicine cart,
- Mobile frame storage system to carry cameras,
- Computers monitors,
- Keyboards,
- Computers,
- Mobile medical devices,
- Computer monitors.
- Telemedicine Kiosks
- Digital Camera
- Webcam,
- High-resolution digital cameras for crystal-clear video capture.

There are many other equipments that are required for implementing telemedicine

Telemedicine Kit

These Telemedicine kits containing big medical kit inside it having a small computer with an inbuilt camera screen with mounted camera, along with basic mobile medical devices.

Telemedicine Software

As more and more people are adopting Telemedicine. The rate of data explosion is also there. The challenge of handling and storing this data in a most optimize way pushing adoption of cloud. Due to increase of data by telemedicine solutions, data should be moved to the cloud. There are requirement of installing software system on telemedicine providers system along with software may require additional equipment like data storage, servers, hardware devices. The software solution should be compatible with system software's installed on health provider system. There are variety of telemedicine software serving different purpose like live chat, storing forwarding health record, visualizing analyzing medical data of patient who need assistance from a remote area. So it's advisable to look for an integrated software solution for providing Telemedicine services (Gianvecchio et al., 2008).

Moreover Health care providers often adopt Mobile medical devices which are used to capture health seeker data and sharing it with other medical expert at remote area to get advice. Patient who is having heat problems can be monitored for heart beats using these devices. The activity of heart can be monitored using ECG device.

Some personalized and customized telemedicine solutions are also there to assist and question patient regarding their health in the form of questions. Then there can be a record of responses and approach like deep data analytics can be applied to the responses collected so far to know the pattern and trend of health state of patient. This data is sent to medical expert to check continuous monitoring on health of patient living in a remote areas. There can also be a vital signal monitor equipped with ECG device (Mohr et al., 2013).

Store and Forward kind of solution related to telemedicine where doctors and care experts consulting, sharing solutions related to healthcare and looking in to patient conditions at some place and try to share the data, medical record of patient visually with another doctor at some other place. The devices related to telemedicine are more complex. Various devices that are used in telemedicine provide a much wider category of medical scopes which include combination of visual and audio recording devices. Some devices have feature of capturing images of the patient examination and there is a facility of sharing these visual data to other location on cloud or via storage peripherals like USB port. Digital stethoscopes let physicians record and share a patient's heart and lung sounds.

Possible Course of Action: The Right Telemedicine Solution

As the field is rising day by day and medical experts as well care seekers are adopting it in many ways to get the health solutions at their very step. So there are lot of new, precise, Telemedicine equipment out there but we don't require most of this telemedicine equipment to get started. There will be more and more queries to adopt telemedicine solution as well as equipment. what will be the quantity of telemedicine equipment that is required to purchase? How the Telemedicine being implemented in hospital and organization and how it will practiced on what scale and level. Who will be the experts to use telemedicine? As well as what will be the application areas to apply and utilize telemedicine? What's the minimum amount of equipment someone need to buy to first initially implementing telemedicine (Islam et al., 2015)

There should be a proper selection of vendor while buying these equipment and as the equipment are costly there is a need of proper training to the staff is required. The implementing environment can go under special demo if software and equipment before and after buying the telemedicine infrastructure.

Telehealth now and Towards Eternity: Deep Data Analytics

The effectiveness of health care depending upon anytime accessibility of data and saving of data on daily basis and representing it to the medical experts: The Deep Data is the solution. Smart devices generating and storing massive amount of data. Using Deep Data it categorize this data into meaning full sections and discarding redundant data.

The Variance: Big and Deep Data

Big and deep data both take huge amount of data collected every single moment from various sources from various location. Industry combine this with analytics and use it to predict the trends or differences to take intelligent decisions.

Deep Data analyzed specific information.

The Deep data analytics can be applied to healthcare industry. The trail on health care and medicine can be more accurate and up to date(Bhatia & Mittal, 2017).

The Choice

There are two options opting Big data or Deep data depending on the requirement as well as property of data. As suggestions and predictions about patient health to make out more specific trends then Deep data is best option(Gale et al., 2013).

Results and Discussion: Deep Data Analytics (Computing + Machine learning + Analytics): Need in Telehealth

The use of smart devices to keep track of important patient measurements such as blood pressure and heart rate. These smart devices allow doctors and patients to collaborate one to one and keeping real time eye on health of patient. The data collected in a real time mode assist the doctors to keep eye on exact quantity of medicine hence providing virtual health care. The researcher announced that by 2020, half of the IoT devices will have healthcare applications. The data generated by health care smart devices is in Exabyte only deep data analytics is the right choice for finding intelligent solution (Dimitrov, 2016).

Reasons: Opting Deep Data Analytics Uncommon property of Health Data

The application of linear analytics on data collected by health care system is very tough because the data is not structured. There is a need of different and complex methods to handle data. The properties of health care data are described in Fig 9 below:

Smart devices generating data from many sources and saved at many locations in different format example text, images, scan formats so there is a strict need to apply Technology applications like deep data analytics to health care industry for making lives of health seeker more comfortable (Munten, 2013).

The medical findings after retrieving data and capturing health data demands consistency in data. The collection and storing of data is done without keeping fact that how the data is aggregated and analyzed later by opting intelligence. Opting a standard method of digging deep into unstructured data make it better data for analytics (Ong et al., 2012).

CONCLUSION: EVIDENCE: IMPACT OF ANALYTICS ON TELEHEALTH

In a country there was an initiative taken up to reduce the c-sections. The practice of storing indication about c-Section is indication by fetal or maternal indication. The analytics were applied on the data stored in textual form. The wisdom was added in the data and health providers and doctors gain insight

Figure 9. Multiple sources of data

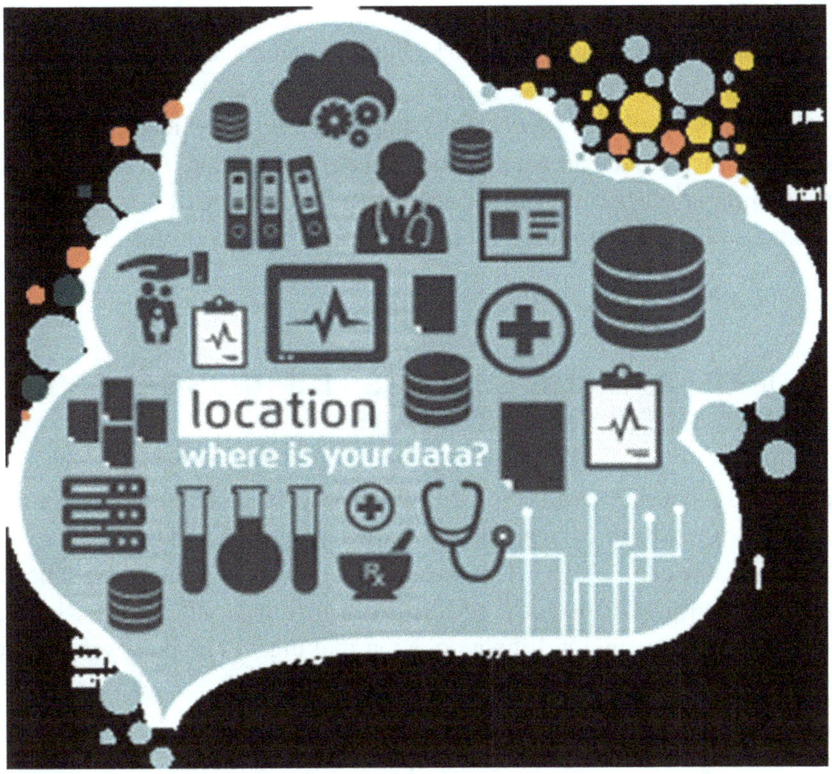

inside data and established opportunities to standardize the decision making and reduces unnecessary C-sections(Belle et al., 2015).

"Testimony: Research in Telehealth- Deep Analytics"

The data related to health is abstract and having some erratic definitions. The decision about a person is diabetic or not can be collaborated by two experts through Tele methods. Right Prediction about measurement of values can be done using analytics (Greenhalgh et al., 2012)

"Applying Deep Data Analytics: Adding Functionality to Telehealth: Success Stories"

The data generated from multiple sources is converted into Big Data in the same way health data is also going very big in terms of size and volume because of using smart devices and adoption of Telehealth and Telemedicine. This data is to be used for intelligent decision making but it create challenge for analyst to take decision on it. To solve the problem Deep learning Techniques can be applied to support this data. The data can be labeled or unlabeled inside big data. So it is very difficult to process this data. So Deep Learning proving and playing an important role in getting solutions for Big Data analytics (Priyanka & Kulennavar, 2014).

Below are some success stories shown in Table 1-3 and is visualized in Fig 9-11.

- **Telehealth Users**

Number of Telehealth users 0.3 millions in 2013 but it is increased to 7 millions in 2018. Telehealth adoption among users

Total eleven Telehealth Companies successfully implementing Telehealth.

An average wait time for a doctor in Major cities is twenty minutes. As the diseases and unhealthy life style is being adopted in Metropolitan cities, there will be shortage of doctors by 2025. In this cases the Telehealth and smart solutions provided by analytics is proved boon for health seekers (Bowonder et al., 2005).

CONCLUSION: DEEP LEARNING SUCCESS - IMPRESSIVENESS OF DEEP LEARNING IN TELEHEALTH CARE

Health care industry needs accuracy and Deep Learning network are accurate and gain accuracy at each level. To monitor health of a person in routine or at critical stages in real time, data is updated through cloud and other devices (Gale et al., 2013). This meet expectations of patients with health care industry. The most latest advancement in Deep Learning has given insight to situations where experts out performs and removed the delays in any intelligent decision making. Some points that support perfectness of applying Deep learning to Telehealth (Roine et al., 2001).

- Labeled data from Big data is extracted as deep learning techniques require Labeled Data. hence leads to intelligent solutions in quick mode and less with errors (Belle et al., 2015).

Table 1. Adoption of Health Plans

Health Systems	Need of Video Visit (%)
Consumers would switch to a PCP	20
Seek care	20
Regular check-ins	60
Completing post-surgical follow-up or hospital discharge visits	52

Table 2. Adoption of telemedicine in urgent cases

Health Plans	Need of Video Visit (%)
Seeing their PCP	65
Routine needs	78
Getting birth control	33
Manage a chronic condition	60

Table 3. Adoption of telemedicine in urgent cases

Employers	Need of Video Visit (%)
Urgent care needs such as a fever	39
Prescription renewals	78
Getting birth control	33
Night care	20
Caring for an ill/aging relative	79

Figure 10. Success Stories in adoption of Telehealth

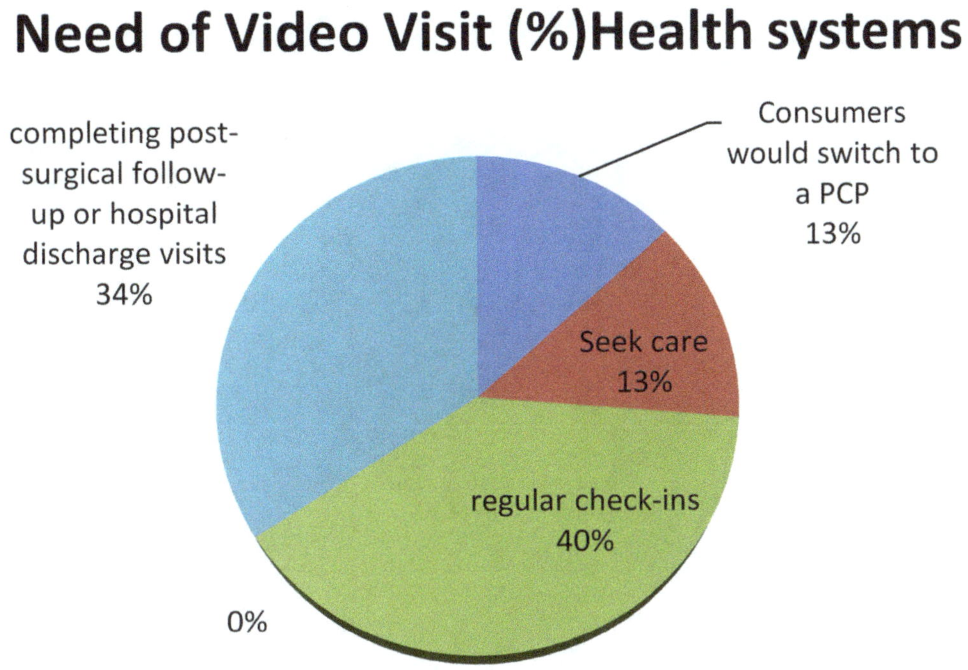

Figure 11. Need of video visit by Plans

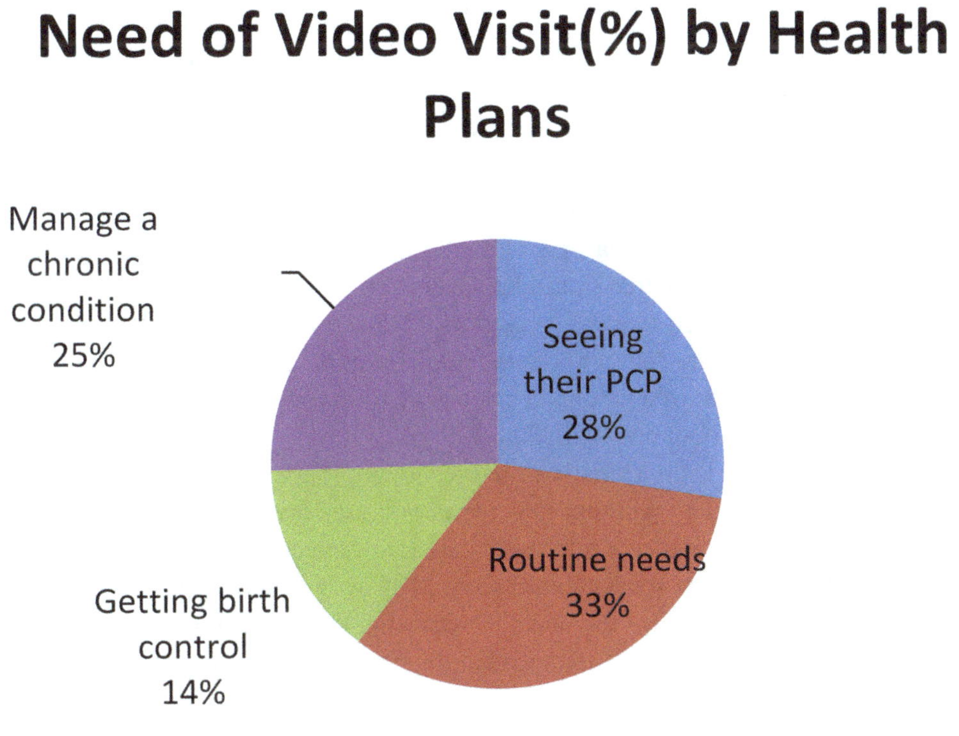

Figure 12. Need of video visit by employers

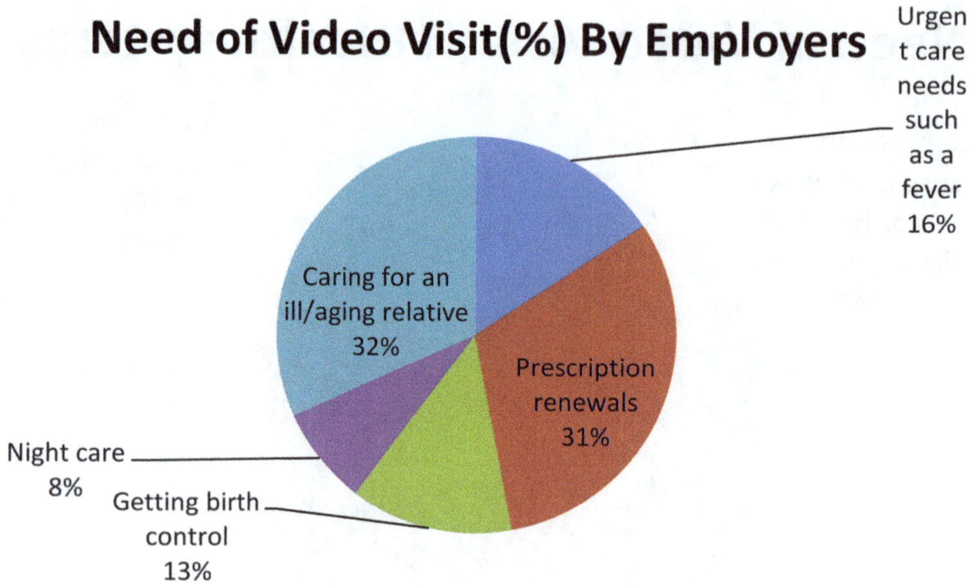

- Telehealth devices generating massive amount of data. To train and generate patterns and significance, there is a need of high computational power. Parallel computing have and parallel architecture and is required for deep learning. To train the network for such a huge amount of data require weeks but with clusters and power of cloud it reduces to hours (Hendy et al., 2012).

The research in Medical field proved that a deep learning has a capability to identify cancer cells and training is done on high dimensional data set.

Industrial Automation: Deep learning is helping to improve worker safety around heavy machinery by automatically detecting when people or objects are within an unsafe distance of machines (Mofatt et al., 2010).

The accuracy and deepness of Deep learning networks applied to Telehealth complex data is that the network is trained with around a hundred of hidden layers (Munten, 2013).

Deep learning models are trained by using large sets of labeled data and neural network architectures that learn features directly from the data without the need for manual feature.

Deep neural networks are organized in several layers which contains set of linked nodes. This network consist of several hidden layers (Copper et al., 2008).

Convolution neural network is an example of deep network that can be applied to Telehealth data. The feature learning with data that was input to network and uses two dimensional convolution layers, making this framework perfect to process telehealth data (Dinesen et al., 2016).

This network can also be used to extract feature from MRI images, scans etc. to automatic extract the features from medical images to reduce the need of extracting feature manually. One powerful feature of this network is it can be applied directly to medical images (Wootton, 2001).

Internet of Humans: A support to Deep Learning for Telehealth

There are number of things that are available free on internet. The way data is collected and being used commercially leads to era of Internet of Humans.

The data capturing is done very easily through mobile applications. Mobile applications take permission from users to access the information stored in users mobile phone (Sanders et al., 2012).

Use of bots, many human wearable devices and personal digital assistants collect data, derive data according to patterns. Many types of watches are in the market which collect data related to health of patient (Sanders et al., 2012).

With the help of massive amount of data related to user profiles are captured with the help of temporary files, applications, social media, web sites and the data collected is for some useful findings. The reason for this is world wide web organizes information as a structure of data and not the meaning of the data. So, while the data is captured, the semantic link is missing for realizing "Internet of humans (Gianvecchio et al., 2008).

The web of connecting users according to data structuring not the semantics of that data. That is why it is called Internet of Humans.

It has been observed by researchers that each step of every user on internet create a data point and multidimensional views of data. So the Telehealth relating to Internet of Humans generating data and Deep Data analytics giving more support to Telehealth (Dagon et al., 2007).

REFERENCES

Belle, A., Thiagarajan, R., Soroushmehr, S. M., Navidi, F., Beard, D. A., & Najarian, K. (2015). Big data analytics in healthcare. *BioMed Research International*. PMID:26229957

Bhatia, D.M. & Mittal, D.M. (2017). Big Data & Deep Data: Minding the Challenges. *Deep Learning for Image Processing Applications*, *31*, 177.

Bowonder, B., Bansal, M., & Sharnitha Giridhar, A. (2005). A telemedicine platform: A case study of Apollo hospitals telemedicine project. *International Journal of Services Technology and Management*, *6*(3-5), 449–466. doi:10.1504/IJSTM.2005.007420

Chen, M., Ma, Y., Song, J., Lai, C. F., & Hu, B. (2016). Smart clothing: Connecting human with clouds and big data for sustainable health monitoring. *Mobile Networks and Applications*, *21*(5), 825–845. doi:10.100711036-016-0745-1

Cooper, D. L., Smith, G. E., Regan, M., Large, S., & Groenewegen, P. P. (2008). Tracking the spatial diffusion of influenza and norovirus using telehealth data: A spatiotemporal analysis of syndromic data. *BMC Medicine*, *6*(1), 16. doi:10.1186/1741-7015-6-16 PMID:18582364

Dagon, D., Gu, G., Lee, C. P., & Lee, W. (2007, December). A taxonomy of botnet structures. In *Proceedings of the Twenty-Third Annual Computer Security Applications Conference (ACSAC 2007)* (pp. 325-339). IEEE. 10.1109/ACSAC.2007.44

Dimitrov, D. V. (2016). Medical internet of things and big data in healthcare. *Healthcare Informatics Research*, *22*(3), 156–163. doi:10.4258/hir.2016.22.3.156 PMID:27525156

Dinesen, B., Nonnecke, B., Lindeman, D., Toft, E., Kidholm, K., Jethwani, K., ... Gutierrez, M. (2016). Personalized telehealth in the future: A global research agenda. *Journal of Medical Internet Research, 18*(3), e53. doi:10.2196/jmir.5257 PMID:26932229

Dubey, H., Yang, J., Constant, N., Amiri, A. M., Yang, Q., & Makodiya, K. (2015, October). Fog data: Enhancing telehealth big data through fog computing. In *Proceedings of the ASE Big Data & Social Informatics 2015* (p. 14). ACM.

Gagnon, M. P., Lamothe, L., Fortin, J. P., Cloutier, A., Godin, G., Gagné, C., & Reinharz, D. (2005). Telehealth adoption in hospitals: An organisational perspective. *Journal of Health Organization and Management, 19*(1), 32–56. doi:10.1108/14777260510592121 PMID:15938601

Gale, N. K., Heath, G., Cameron, E., Rashid, S., & Redwood, S. (2013). Using the framework method for the analysis of qualitative data in multi-disciplinary health research. *BMC Medical Research Methodology, 13*(1), 117. doi:10.1186/1471-2288-13-117 PMID:24047204

Gianvecchio, S., Xie, M., Wu, Z., & Wang, H. (2008, July). Measurement and Classification of Humans and Bots in Internet Chat. In Proceedings of the USENIX security symposium (pp. 155-170). Academic Press.

Greenhalgh, T., Procter, R., Wherton, J., Sugarhood, P., & Shaw, S. (2012). The organising vision for telehealth and telecare: Discourse analysis. *BMJ Open, 2*(4), e001574. doi:10.1136/bmjopen-2012-001574 PMID:22815469

Hebert, M. A., Korabek, B., & Scott, R. E. (2006). Moving research into practice: A decision framework for integrating home telehealth into chronic illness care. *International Journal of Medical Informatics, 75*(12), 786–794. doi:10.1016/j.ijmedinf.2006.05.041 PMID:16872892

Hendy, J., Chrysanthaki, T., Barlow, J., Knapp, M., Rogers, A., Sanders, C., ... Newman, S. (2012). An organisational analysis of the implementation of telecare and telehealth: The whole systems demonstrator. *BMC Health Services Research, 12*(1), 403. doi:10.1186/1472-6963-12-403 PMID:23153014

Islam, S. R., Kwak, D., Kabir, M. H., Hossain, M., & Kwak, K. S. (2015). The internet of things for health care: A comprehensive survey. *IEEE Access: Practical Innovations, Open Solutions, 3*, 678–708. doi:10.1109/ACCESS.2015.2437951

Koch, S. (2006). Home telehealth—Current state and future trends. *International Journal of Medical Informatics, 75*(8), 565–576. doi:10.1016/j.ijmedinf.2005.09.002 PMID:16298545

McLean, S., Protti, D., & Sheikh, A. (2011). Telehealthcare for long term conditions. *BMJ (Clinical Research Ed.), 342*(5), 449–457. PMID:21292710

Moffatt, J. J., & Eley, D. S. (2010). The reported benefits of telehealth for rural Australians. *Australian Health Review, 34*(3), 276–281. doi:10.1071/AH09794 PMID:20797357

Mohr, D. C., Burns, M. N., Schueller, S. M., Clarke, G., & Klinkman, M. (2013). Behavioral intervention technologies: Evidence review and recommendations for future research in mental health. *General Hospital Psychiatry, 35*(4), 332–338. doi:10.1016/j.genhosppsych.2013.03.008 PMID:23664503

Munten, G. (2013). An organisational analysis of the implementation of telecare and telehealth: The whole systems demonstrator1. *Nederlands Tijdschrift voor Evidence Based Practice*, *4*(11), 9–10. doi:10.100712468-013-0032-0

Ong, M. E. H., Ng, C. H. L., Goh, K., Liu, N., Koh, Z. X., Shahidah, N., ... Lin, Z. (2012). Prediction of cardiac arrest in critically ill patients presenting to the emergency department using a machine learning score incorporating heart rate variability compared with the modified early warning score. *Critical Care (London, England)*, *16*(3), R108. doi:10.1186/cc11396 PMID:22715923

Priyanka, K., & Kulennavar, N. (2014). A survey on big data analytics in health care. *International Journal of Computer Science and Information Technologies*, *5*(4), 5865–5868.

Roine, R., Ohinmaa, A., & Hailey, D. (2001). Assessing telemedicine: A systematic review of the literature. *Canadian Medical Association Journal*, *165*(6), 765–771. PMID:11584564

Sanders, C., Rogers, A., Bowen, R., Bower, P., Hirani, S., Cartwright, M., ... Chrysanthaki, T. (2012). Exploring barriers to participation and adoption of telehealth and telecare within the Whole System Demonstrator trial: A qualitative study. *BMC Health Services Research*, *12*(1), 220. doi:10.1186/1472-6963-12-220 PMID:22834978

Wootton, R. (2001). Telemedicine. *BMJ (Clinical Research Ed.)*, *323*(7312), 557–560. doi:10.1136/bmj.323.7312.557 PMID:11546704

Chapter 3
Emergence of IoT and Big Data:
A Study in the Healthcare Industry

Gurinder Singh
Amity University, Noida, India

Vikas Garg
https://orcid.org/0000-0002-1421-5980
Amity University, Noida, India

Pooja Tiwari
ABES Engineering College, India

Richa Goel
Amity University, Noida, India

ABSTRACT

The main focus of this research paper is to understand the use of IoT in healthcare to achieve sustainable development. This paper has used the descriptive method to collect the data for study. The research methodology is FAHP, which is a cross-sectional research survey in nature. After data collection, the agreed paired comparison matrices, which are then further allocated to the weighted criteria and then accordingly a priority for the IoT usage is judged. According to the findings of the research, it has been identified that "profit maximization" and "quality of life" were on the top for priority for IoT in the healthcare sector for sustainable development, although, three major areas were identified. Additionally, if we consider according to usage then it is mostly used by the health care sector as UV radiation, dental care, and fall detection.

INTRODUCTION

In the healthcare industry which includes the personal healthcare and different applications related to healthcare has increased in the tremendous amount in the respect to the usage of Internet of Things and big data particularly. Despite of so many challenges, even during present times how other services in

DOI: 10.4018/978-1-7998-2101-4.ch003

the healthcare sector is accelerating and they are connecting. It can be observed that the application of Internet of Things will surely increase as it is one of the crucial components in the industry of health care with reference to digital transformation and in these other stakeholders are also supporting and coming together.

Additionally, consumers are very much engaged and involved in the activities which are related to the their health, rather requirement regarding rural and home facilities are quite increasing, different players in the field of healthcare ecosystem are coming up with the innovative approaches and partnerships, and the main goal of the healthcare sector is to keep the expenditure in control, keeping in consideration the quality care. It is becoming essential that more integrated approach is required in IoT enabled e-health.

For the past so many decades, in the sector of health care technology has become integral part in many processes. Although, the circumstances have changed a lot in so many years. There are immense novel opportunities have evolved due to paradigm shift in the area of Internet of Things (IoT). In addition to advances in the area of IoT and big data with special reference to the data handling, multiscale, multimodal, data sets which are heterogeneous in nature have actually created the opportunity for eHealth and mHealth which are comparatively better tailored and accurate than previously. But based on the growth observed in the IoT a paradigm shift can be observed in the health care sector which in turn ensure the accessibility and availability, and during delivery it improves the rules as well. Additionally, existing health care requirements can be satisfied due to broadened horizon in the IoT health, there are many crucial challenges for providing the appropriate, risk free, consistent, supple and power-efficient solutions exist to provide solution to many medical demands. The only solution to this particular problem and challenges is the integration and coordination between the software and hardware sector, which can motivate the movement of technology forward. Remarkable advancement is required in the different areas such as bioelectronics, communication devices, networks and different software, pattern recognition, data analytics which is sophisticated in nature, cloud computing, big data, cloud computing, information technologies and development, before the emergence of truly IoT health care world. Research in the field of health care sector bring together different disciplines on one platform such as researchers in the area of engineering, medicines, engineering in the biomedical sector, computer science, and big data analytics can be easily located working on the associated projects.

Improvement in health has become a prime issue; there are many physicians and microbiologist who are working together on lab studies. For the creation of the new therapeutic approaches and novel diagnostic new tools are used by the different biomedical engineers. The behaviour of the different diseases are analysed by the different computer scientists, and according to the various symptoms infections can be predicted based on the algorithm by the help of artificial intelligence and different computer systems. On the other hand, research in the pharmaceuticals are conducted to cure the different diseases like cancer and Ebola, by the help of collaboration with the different hospital and clinics for the collection of the data with reference to health care, geolocation and different other connected fields. If we integrate the expertise together and consider them, a gap is quite clearly observed between them, and these gaps clearly indicates the challenges in the field of technology challenges for developing the unified, and highly adaptive framework for health care. This kind of framework will be able to maintain the correlation towards the molecular physiology, behaviour and also considering the specific diseases are emerging. According to our thoughts, the solo unwavering method to cultivate this framework is that interactive cyber physical solution can be constructed in the form of cloud based health care service, so as to provide the breakthrough in the different areas which are mentioned above which enables to construct the cyber physical solution which is interactive in nature through the cloud based services in the sector of health, which helps to enable the health care which is more intelligent in nature by using the different technologies like smart molecular sensing, therapeutics control, and computational bioinformatics.

The linkage of different devices which are physically present and other objects, which are incorporated with different software, electronics, network connectivity and sensors which help these items to gather and exchange the data is known as IoT, i.e., Internet of Things. IoT will have a very crucial and private effect on the medicines. By 2020, most of the Internet of Things, i.e., IoT technology will be associated to the healthcare sector as compared to any other sector which will be approximately 40% and will end up in making a billionaire market of $117. The combination of IT, i.e., information technologies with medicine, like medical informatics, will bring out a change in the prevailing healthcare sector as well as will give out positive impact such as reduction in the cost, decrement in the incompetency, and savings lives. Fig.1 demonstrates the actual picture of the future hospitals using IoT technology and the change in the medicine by using IoT technology. With the help of this technology every diabetic patient will get an ID card which when will be scanned will provide an access to the patient's medical history, prescription provided to them, laboratory results and other medical details which will get stored on a cloud with complete security so as to maintain patient's health records electronically. This will provide an easy accessibility of the health records to the concerned nurses and physicians on different devices. It seems to be simple but involvement of EHR, i.e., Electronic Health records will bring a huge change. Digitalisation will take over the place of normal pen and paper in a very less span of time, which are used now days for maintaining records. There are many pros linked with this technology. There are many cons related with usual way of maintaining records such as they mostly written as in a questionable form, require huge spaces to keep, unreachable to the concerned person that are the health care providers and the researchers. Other than providing easy accessibility to the records and ease in sharing it, EHR's will remove various incompetencies. Rather now a day's various devices contain sensors in themselves and communicate in their own coded language but in the implementation of this technology communication will still act as a barrier. Different manufacturers own their registered protocols due to which sensors manufactured by different makers doesn't inevitably communicate with each other. This all different software combined with the privacy apprehensions and the official capacity to handle all the information collected, usually abandons important information on small databases, which discourages the use of the IoT. The term which will be popularised in future is precision medicine. The cycle starts with genomics which is further followed by the omics platforms, giving different type of data for analysis purposes and for interpretation. In the year 2015, there was a joint project launched by the Oregon Health and Science University and Intel named as the Collaborative Cancer Cloud which was a highly performing analytical platform which not only collects as well as provide storage to the private medical data with full security which is quite useful to conduct the research for patients who are suffering from cancer. Although the project was launched with cancer as the main concern, but Intel plans to expose the merged cloud network for other institutions which includes the institutions which are occupied with work of the cure of the diseases such as Parkinson. With the usage of Internet of Things, i.e., IoT technology, solutions via engineering imitations are producing the medicines to be P4 medicines, which are personalized, preventive, participatory and predictive.

IoT Application in Healthcare Sector

The boundaries of the healthcare and healthcare communication have extended and moved ahead as compared to the traditional view in terms of the digital technologies (Palfrey and Gasser, 2011; Schiavo,

2013). Healthcare industry is totally transformed due to Internet of Things (IoT) (Bhatt et al., 2017). There are numerous devices of IoT which are linked to each other and other data which is physiological in nature which includes monitoring temperature, glucose level of blood and other important data which are gathered by the help of big data (Dey et al., 2018). The prime objective and concern is to deliver the innovative service in the healthcare sector for the patients; who include regular monitoring and detecting the lethal disease at the initial level (Mandler et al., 2015). Extensive growth can be observed and analysed in the sector of healthcare with regard to digital data and information and IoT (Ustundag and Cevikcan, 2017).

Healthcare industry can get the advantage by the use of IoT in different ways, which includes the managing different diseases, preventative care, using the technology of automation for the patients in clinical, and giving assistance in living and clinical monitoring remotely (Dey et al., 2018) and help in giving the valuable insights in healthcare, minimizing the cost and also leading to the advent of the systems of well-care (Holler et al., 2014). Also conducting the in-depth assessment of innovative market which also includes the analysis of vendor, which promotes the growth, quantitative assessment of the company and also value chain (Dey et al., 2018). An inclusive grouping of different areas which are relevant in the areas of IoT in the smart health in the healthcare sector has been presented by IoT European Research Cluster (IERC). There can be several usages some can be in the form of services and some can be in the form of products. Additionally, some of the areas which are related to the health sector are:

- Fall Detection: It is basically useful for the people who are physically challenged and for the elderly people so as to make their life easy and independent.
- Medical Fridges: Some conditions are controlled (temperature) and organic elements are kept in the container (Internal temperature protective control). This task can be well assumed by the help of IoT and can cause objects interaction.
- Sportsmen Care: This application is really useful for the measurement of sleep, weight, blood pressure and other parameters which are required for professional athletes.
- Patient Surveillance: This technology is quite beneficial in monitoring the in-hospital from remote places and particularly for the aged individuals for their home care.
- Chronic Disease management: This is used when there is no requirement of the physical attendance and the patient is suffering from the chronic disease. As the less people will be present in the hospital which will result in reducing the cost.
- Ultraviolet Radiation: This technology helps to measure and give notifications to the people regarding their entry in some area which have revelation to the rays of UV at a certain time.
- Hygienic Hand Control: RFID is used for emission measurement and this device can be linked which will help to identify the pollution in the environment.
- Sleep Control: If this is linked to the different individuals it can help us to identify the signs of pulse rates, while sleeping assessing the blood pressure and this data can be further be collected and analysed
- Dental Health: The brushing information of the individual can be recorded by the help of Bluetooth enabled toothbrush. It also helps to study the brushing habit of the individual and statistics can be shared with the dentist.
- IoT application in different cases in healthcare sector
- If analysed from the perspective of spending in IoT it is manly applicable for monitoring the health (remote) and

- Very soon it can be analysed that IoT will not be unique rather it will become a pervasive issue in case of healthcare and activities and processes related to it at different levels.

Additionally, it can be observed that application of IoT, which previously used to fit in the context of the consumer, is now getting the different and special place between the patients or consumers and provider of healthcare services. The role of engagement of patient and awareness of consumers plays a crucial role and it includes the premiums and incentive s related to healthcare sector.

If we discuss beyond the scope of the IoT there is a possibility of tremendous growth in different area of healthcare such as hospitals and IoT application can be leveraged by combining it with artificial intelligence, robotics and big data type of technologies.

IoT: The Future of Pharma?

In the year 1999 for the very first time IoT was used to describe the entire world. This world includes many things such as individuals, plants, animals and even non-living items such as vehicles, which allow them to have identity in digital way and which can be organized and managed. In the present era of digitalization all the individuals are connected to each other through internet but IoT is able to make the connection between all the objects, and it can be easily accessed by the people by managing and controlling the different applications in the electronic gadgets and smart devices [10]. In the modern era of digitillization the concept of IoT is considered as new technology and a mode of communication which gives the benefit of sending data related to anything (living and non-living object) through the network connection such as internet or intranet [11].

Development of Electronic business (E-business) is coming up in many cases as more and more business are relying upon the IoT and it is also making easy to maintain relationship with customers [13]. Indeed, the interoperability between different objects, objects with humans, and humans with object and with this kind of approach there is a possibility that new services will come into practice [14]. Additionally, one of the main aims of the IoT is to escalate the level of intelligence in every sphere such as life, business and economy [15].

Long way back the existing pharma understood that there will be no growth as well as will not even have a sense of competitiveness just by trading in the basic medicines. The basic modification which is known as moving “beyond the pill”, basically came out of two recognitions: (1) usually usage of only medicines are not enough to get the desired results for patients, and (2) “beyond the pill” concept can add new ways of revenues as the traditional pharmaceuticals become an old fashioned concept. Due to this new technology pharma Internet of Things, i.e., Pharma IoT is being created as it has increased the attention in the techniques of using the new technologies for developing the business processes and patient care. The concept of Pharma Internet of Things (Pharma IoT) includes products of medical and its associated processes of care being digitalised via connecting various smart medical gadgets and IT gadgets which includes tools like cell phones, web, applications, etc. in the process of development of drugs, trials of clinical and caring the patients. The results of this technology, i.e., Pharma Internet of Things in the advancement and clinical trials can engage blends of new improvised services and technologies to generate entirely new types of illness treatment possibilities (for example, Treatment 2.0). With the usage of Pharma Internet of Things in patient care sector, health care professionals and the patients as well will get to utilise the medicines which will contain innovative sensor hardware and will be able to create customised care services and processes (Product 2.0). Some of the examples of

Pharma Internet of Things are the linked sensor wearables for Parkinson's illness and various sclerosis patients that give management of medicines, developing the patient results and their quality of life. In addition to this, prevailing equipment of medical products like the insulin sticks and the inhalers can be combined with the technology of sensor and connectivity so as to gather data for additional care analytics, and also for the customised therapy. With the use of this technology there will be a development in the process of private medication and processes of care, as the patient care gathered data will give new ways of competitiveness and inventions. With the pros of this technology, there are also some hurdles which are being faced, pharma organizations have to take upcoming EU, i.e., European Union, legislations regarding data privacy and protection into consideration, which will provide control to the patients regarding own care data. For instance, patients will be able to exchange their health and care information with various providers of service, which will lead to the development of completely new types of models of business and platforms of service, example, and brokers of data.

Healthcare- Mobile Application and Devices

We are moving into a generation of information, where the basics are the knowledge and the data. Now it is a generation where customer is the king and the wants of the products are determined by them more often as compared to the past. One illustration of this varying model of business is the My Tomorrows model, in which pharma and the customers are directly linked. In this upcoming generation, applications and tools will be utilised to make a "health selfie". For illustration: A device named the Myo, which was initially used to control the movements in the games, now is being utilised as an orthopaedic used for the patients who are required to perform exercises after any fracture. With the help of this device, the doctors can compute the movement angle and the patients can see their improvement. A device named The Zio Patch which is used for calculated the pulse rate and ECG, i.e., electrocardiogram and has been permitted by the US Food and Drug Administration. Now the question arises that where is pharma involved in this? Impressively, there are indications that pharma is moving ahead from its conventional approach centred on medicines.

In a recent time, Glaxo made an announcement that it is making an investment in two drugs, which are electroceuticals and bioelectrical which work by using nerves micro-stimulation. • Google and J&J has come together to evolve surgeries done by robots. That's not enough; they are also teaming up with Philips for their devices which can be wore like devices used to check the blood pressure. • Novartis is again collaborating with Google for sensor technologies, like wearable device used to compute levels of glucose in blood and the smart lens. A lot of information can be gained using sensors for the progression in the pharma, but it is most vital to hire the accurate patients for the exact clinical trials. There was once a device which was only used by the runners and the athletes, but now the situation is changed, now these devices have expanded their reach to the common market, and soon there will be a bundle of information availability with the pharma and the consumers not just limited to pulse rate, ECG, blood pressure and breathing rate, rather will have more progressed data like the sleeping patterns, and inflammation, etc. There are number of cell phone applications which have come together like MyDairo and SleepBot, which backup handling of devices. Recently, a program named RANKED Health is being launched by the Hacking Medicine Institute, which will help in evaluation and ranking the applications centred for health and the linked devices. It is being forecasted that in the upcoming time people will check their phones or smart watches more often to keep an eye on their health results as compared to prevailing situation in which they check their emails and WhatsApp. In a distinctive situation, which might include an old person, who is recuperating from any illness at home, connected to a group of various linked services cascading towards diverse parties, like physician, family members and tele- carer. In a recent time, there was announcement made regarding the collaboration of Medtronic with Canary Health, which is a digital health managing application, to be a distributor or reseller of the company's digital products like the programs managing the chronic diseases, which includes its CDC acknowledged Diabetes Prevention Program, which targeted at changing behaviours in people before diabetes. This partnership moved ahead of just reselling of the digital equipment of Canary Health. According to a news released by Canary health, both of the partnering companies strategize to form the solutions that, "leverage Medtronic's devices, services and infrastructure as well as Canary Health's suite of behaviour-change programs, design expertise, and deep user engagement experience," One of the reasons for Medtronic for finding attractiveness in Canary Health is that the organization's digital gadgets can be compensated. As these digital programs regarding health get established, investors are keeping an eye on different ways which are innovative in nature and are approved so as to decrease the burden of the cost incurred for long lasting illness such as diabetes. As suggested by the CDC, i.e., Centre for Disease Control and Prevention, programs created by the Canary Health and other platforms named as Omada Health and Noom Health, which provide an well-organized routine to the people which do not have diabetes, —"can cut their risk of developing type 2 diabetes by 58% (71% for people over 60 years old)." In addition to this CDC further said that, "this finding was the results of a program helping people lose 5% to 7% of their body weight through healthier eating and 150 minutes of physical activity a week". Diabetes is being expressed as one of the expensive and long-lasting illness, the doctors, hospitals, spenders and patients have equal curiosity to get this epidemic. In simple way, this program is supporting to change from just giving care to the ill to actual delivery of healthcare.

Big Data Analytics

The landscape of big data is quite big which consist of different layers which includes infrastructure, analytics, applications, open source, cross-infrastructure/analytics, data sources, and APIs. Map Reduce which is one of the technologies of Big Data is mainly used for extremely parallel analytics, data analytics of streaming data which is online, it also plays a crucial role in managing and analysing of large scale M2M or IoT data (Holler et al., 2014). Algorithms which are not supervised over the machine for example machine learning, cognitive and deep learning algorithm and networks which are neural and artificial in nature mainly works as a game changer in the analytics of healthcare. Big data is not similar to basic analytics. As the basic analytics is only confined to the analysis of number, data and strings unlikely big data analytics also analyses the documents, geospatial data, three-dimensional data, audio, photos and videos, and unstructured text, including log files and social media (Nicoletti, 2017). By the help of the different architectures, tools, algorithms and techniques the value of the big data analytics can be determined. Advanced analytics (including predictive and prescriptive analytics) can be defined as "a business -focused approach, comprising techniques that help build models and simulations to create scenarios, understand realities, and hypothesize future states" (Mullins, 2002).

To conduct the analysis of cloud analytics technology of cloud computing is used. On cloud systems for conducting the analysis of big data different models are used. The prime models which are used are Platform as a Service (PaaS) and Software as a Service (SaaS). For the analytics of Big Data the model of PaaS provides tools, programming suites, environments, and libraries which are already constructed and ride on cloud platform. The model of SaaS also provides end users the complete application so the work can be done on the substantial data through the function of scalability of system of clouds with regards to big data storage and processing (Zomaya and Sakr, 2017). Cloud has a main positive point that it basically provides the effective and cost-efficient way of pre operationalized analytics (Turkington et al., 2016).

Some modern methods of analytics are used by the big data. As (Natarajan et al., 2017) has given the description of learning by machine new case which are used by

- Some of the impact of limitation of humans can be enriched.
- By the help of learning and prediction new knowledge can be created and also the data can be reduced.
- It is learned that how and what way computational biomarkers can be generated.
- The data management task can be more effectively processed and with a higher degree of performance and consistency.
- It also serves as the foundation for the workflows in clinical manner and analytics in predicative and prescriptive analytics, intelligent search which are secondary in use.

Data, Data, Data

The main component of sensors which are wearable in nature is the gathered data, and several parties are putting their efforts to collect the data and get its control in their hands. Microsoft invented an electronic health safe named "Health Vault", which act as an EMR. Philips and salesforce collaborated with the Radbound University Medical Centre in Holland on the program "Here Is My Data", which is a record of the data where the data can be stored by the patients and thereafter access cab regulated. Salesforce plays an important role in this. This salesforce program influences Veeva, which is a CRM, i.e., customer relationship management system currently broadly utilized in pharma. This enables the salesforce to be capable of filling the space between pharma and the medical data of patient. "Big data" is a term which is being utilised extensively by the general public and the media since last few years. Although various interpretations have been anticipated, the most used terminologies includes the "3 V's", these V's are as follows: first is Volume which stands for huge quantity of data, second Variety stands for important diverseness in the kind of availability f the data in the set, and last V is Velocity which stands for the rate of speed at which any user or data scientist can get accessibility to the data for further analysing. This simply means that, one of the important upcoming users of the "big data" is the health care sector. For instance, Apple's Research Kit and Fitbit can give accessibility to the huge amount of data, which is available through biometric of the users, which further can be utilised so as to perform the hypothesis on fitness, disease development, nutrition, success rate of the treatment and many more. The highly complicated data sets with high dimension consist of imaging (which includes X-rays, slides, MRIs and photos), analysis of wave like ECG and EEG, transcripts related audio files, NLP outputs, i.e., Natural Language Processing, consisting free text notes, and plotting between structured concepts like the LOINC, i.e., Logical Observation Identifiers Names and Codes and the lab tests or the ICD9 and ICD10 codes. With the other things that the analysis data must give is the means to regularly updating the observations grounded on the knowledge acquired, at the same time maintaining the destination of the data at one place. The CMS, i.e., Centre for Medicare & Medicaid Services, has a huge amount of data of billing which can be extracted to advertise care, which is high in value, the same is applicable for insurers of private health. Also, hospitals made an effort to decrease the rate of re-hospitalising the patient by focusing on the patients through the forecasting AI, i.e., artificial intelligence programs which shows the patients who may have high risk involved according to the analysis done on the existing data gathered from the available records of the current patients. After all these and various other possible usages, there are a number of technologies, ethical and legal hurdles related to, with other things, differentiation, private issues, offence, intellectual property, and known consent, also clinical and research ethics.

Challenges for M-IoT

Top of the Internet sting, that is, through a procurement program IOT applications that provide basic information, but the powerful and the Internet of Things devices help designers instantly create analytical applications, display panels and the applications of the Internet-M. Skills that are of great importance to the main program, which are: (1) easily connectable, IO and service level of functional capability for association executives and machines, engines, and finding it lower cloud based services and applied research to gather and exchange achieve hierarchical recourse. (2) Simple management devices that can act as a study devices, have improved resource which enhances performance and expanded self-determination, as set out under the law limited blackouts maintenance costs. (3Incorporation of information: changes subtly and helps to store data. Separate and cloud APIs helps to connect the data, which facilitates the extraction of information required. Ingested different levels of information and data at that point, are the fundamental power which helps in extracting the information through a rich examination. (4) Information Analysis: Add knowledge of huge volumes of data IoT and allow more options to establish and upgrade activities. Apply a continuous current test conditions and to evaluate the consequences of our actions which he himself, however, in the same way. The conditions of the knowledge of the authority of reason, that may learn of the investigation the opinion of the fund is a good exchange of things and formless. Control panel that makes it easy to have an instinctive understanding. (5) Risk reduction, and to follow up and keep track anyway disconnect among government officers from the only online product support.

Road Ahead for Big Data in Healthcare Sector

The problems are divided into two key classes, money / design and development. In the conditions which are prevailing in the organization, the only way to get paid is that it requires a closed contact with the patients. In such circumstances it is very close encounters are taken mainly from the centre; centre benefits are not suitable for fertility and happiness after a fine to compensate the effect. Before things, as the best way to achieve this vision is information about the state of happiness. EHR systems, through his ambassador, were given to the happiness of the, so to speak, focused on the foundations of each of the storage facilities. Sometimes these storage facilities are enormous; storage facilities still remain the facilities of storage only. On the exchange, the individual records from the storage facilities, use of vocabulary dynamically systematized (codeset) structures provide (ADT, 100-CDA and Fhir objects), where it is provided as a current effort. In any case, it is the question of cutting data regular query response). The accumulated additional information is two central foci. (1) The problem of trade Communion with the Holy site. The databases systems do not need to build associated decode the information and data between two selective works are arranged; basically all interact with the 'plug' API standard media. Fittingly collected by processing them a rare Al.

New Generation of Digital Health Advisors

The complexity and growth of data in healthcare means that artificial intelligence (AI) will be increasingly implemented within the field. Many types of AI are already employed by payers and care providers and life sciences companies. Major categories of applications include diagnosis and treatment recommendations, patient engagement and adherence, and administrative activities. While there are many examples in which AI can perform health care tasks better than humans, the implementation factor will prevent automation of healthcare professional jobs on a large scale for the health period. What sets AI technology apart from ancient care technologies is the ability to obtain, process, and produce a well-defined end-user performance. AI will use machine learning algorithms to do this. These algorithms recognize behaviour patterns and kindle their own logic.

The primary purpose of applications for health-related AI is to examine the link between bar or treatment methods and patient outcomes. AI technologies were developed and applied to activities such as procedures for diagnosis, development of treatment protocols, development of medications, personalized medicines and monitoring and care of patients. Medical institutions such as the salad dressing clinic, the Sloan occupation Memorial have developed AI algorithms.

Large technology firms like IBM and Google and start-ups like Welltalk and Ayasdi have additionally developed AI treatment algorithms. In addition, unit area hospitals pursue AI technologies to support strategic programs that enhance cost efficiency, enhance patient satisfaction, and meet their staff and men want. Companies are working together to build prognostic analytics tools which allow care managers to enhance business operations through increased usage, reduced patient boarding, reduced length of stay and optimized staffing levels.

When technology evolves and is being applied in additional workplaces, there are several fears that robots or machines will replace their jobs. America's News Workers (2018) reports that doctor's victimization AI may not "win" over World Health Organization doctors in the near future. AI won't replace care staff, but it can give them more time to worry about the aspect of bed. AI burns care staff and causes overload of psychological features. Ultimately, as Kwan-Haase (2018) says, technology contributes to the achievement of social goals, together with higher levels of security, higher means of time-and household interaction, improved health care and increased autonomy.

With increased use of AI, there could also be a lot of care on the market in developing countries. AI continues to expand its capabilities and as it is ready to explain radiology, it will be able to diagnose a lot of folks with fewer doctors needed as many of those countries are deficient in area unit. AI aims at showing others in the world that can later lead to higher care and eventually global safety. Such victimization AI does not have the resources in developing countries of the World Health Organization would minimize the need for outsourcing and use AI to improve patient care.

One of the primary risks is that IoT provides security and privacy of data. IoT apps capture and communicate real-time data. Most IoT phones, however, lack protocols and levels of practice.

In addition, the implementation of multiple devices creates interruptions.

Artificial intelligence is not the production of a large part of the information, by means of a composite data set that shapes the mind, because the combination of all the data in that of the structure of the database at the point provides the opportunity that has developed a wide range of springs, HME data, performance data for the payer, and IOT information gadget, respond calmly, customer happiness information and information is that there is a united structure, an important data bits then AI can yield. The model became very considered and, taking a look in a particular case, information about an individual that the equivalent (not so uncertain) found in other places, such as the perception of the resolution subject to what happened with these different conditions of people. While individual clinicians need "clinical judgment". The recognition of an anxiety issue medical laboratories like every family resemblance to their parents standing models of association on the part of the therapist. Another period, "such as trainers, tele-carers digital health advisors can be set up for recommendations of support. Otherwise, the buyer may have a benefit of being able to interact with the people who were sitting next to Al's conventional machines at the same time. It may be that these types of buyers / patients and doctors commit to reduce discomfort. Physicians who are not listening? No individual will be able to accommodate it which is actually hindering the advisor as a digital security. This approach (we have to pay for human services) is necessary to participate in self-care and practices may be too strong movements to visits to authorized offices.

CONCLUSION

The M-IoT is fixing up restorative administrations' organizations, now people have initiated in utilising the Internet of Things so as to maintain their wealth needs. For instance, they (the people) can utilise Internet of Things contraptions to make themselves remember regarding courses of action, variations in heartbeat, calories devoured and fundamentally extra. There is a possibility that the foremost bit of the Internet of Things in the restorative administrations sector is the distant prosperity checking system, in which the patients can be watched and provoked from wherever. Progressing zone organizations are another genuine procedure IoT offers. By using the organization, experts can without quite a bit of a stretch track contraption regions, which direct lessens plenitude time spent. PDA use is growing very quickly, and the common person have already initiated in utilising compact applications for about everything. With respect to the human administrations sector, adaptable applications can improve trades among patients and experts over a checked affiliation. The basic commitment of DHA, that are the Digital Health Advisors and the doctors will be to progress agreeably when the connection is moving towards the system which is based on the Internet of Things. Authentic getting ready and information are necessary for better course of action. The standard system for record a patient's nuances, i.e., a bunch of paper tighten up on the bed of the patient, is not serious anymore, as this information can only be accessed by very few people, and sometimes these can be misplaced or blended. The support of this application in which active adaptable progression may act good, as they provide trouble free information the administrators on the application in the gadget. Prosperity data info will be available in just a click when the info is kept electronically, when safety and assurance hurdles are kept in mind.

REFERENCES

Auffray, C., Balling, R., Barroso, I., Bencze, L., Benson, M., Bergeron, J., ... Zanetti, G. (2016). Making sense of big data in health research: Towards an EU action plan. *Genome Medicine*, *8*(1), 71. doi:10.118613073-016-0323-y PMID:27338147

Filkins, B. L., Kim, J. Y., Roberts, B., Armstrong, W., Miller, M. A., Hultner, M. L., ... Steinhubl, S. R. (2016). Privacy and security in the era of digital health: what should translational researchers know and do about it? *American journal of translational research*, *8*(3), 1560. 1580. PMID:27186282

Bauer, H., Patel, M., & Veira, J. (2016). The Internet of Things: sizing up the opportunity. McKinsey & Company. Retrieved from http://www.mckinsey.com/industries/hightech/our-insights/the-internet-of-things-sizing-up-theopportunity

Canary Health. (n.d.). Retrieved from http://www.canaryhealth.com/

Centers for Disease Control and Prevention. (n.d.). Lifestyle change program details. Retrieved from http://www.cdc.gov/diabetes/prevention/lifestyle-program/experience/index. html

Cuba-Gyllensten, I., Gastelurrutia, P., Riistama, J., Aarts, R., Nunez, J., Lupon, J., & Bayes-Genis, A. (2014). A novel wearable vest for tracking pulmonary congestion in acutely decompensated heart failure. *International Journal of Cardiology*, *177*(1), 199–201. doi:10.1016/j.ijcard.2014.09.041 PMID:25499378

Dzubur, E., Li, M., Kawabata, K., Sun, Y., McConnell, R., Intille, S., & Dunton, G. F. (2015). Design of a smartphone application to monitor stress, asthma symptoms, and asthma inhaler use. *Annals of Allergy, Asthma & Immunology*, *114*(4), 341–2.e2. doi:10.1016/j.anai.2014.12.017 PMID:25661657

European Commission. (2014). Clinical trials - regulation EU No 536/2014. Brussels: European Commission. Retrieved from: http://ec.europa.eu/health/human-use/clinical-trials/regulation/index_en.htm

Famm, K., Litt, B., Tracey, K. J., Boyden, E. S., & Slaoui, M. (2013). Drug discovery: A jump-start for electroceuticals. *Nature*, *496*(7444), 159–161. doi:10.1038/496159a PMID:23579662

Flores, M., Glusman, G., Brogaard, K., Price, N. D., & Hood, L. (2013). P4 medicine: How systems medicine will transform the healthcare sector and society. *Personalized Medicine*, *10*(6), 565–576. doi:10.2217/pme.13.57 PMID:25342952

Foley, P., Steinberg, D., Levine, E., Askew, S., Batch, B. C., Puleo, E. M., ... Bennett, G. G. (2016). Track: A randomized controlled trial of a digital health obesity treatment intervention for medically vulnerable primary care patients. *Contemporary Clinical Trials*, *48*, 12–20. doi:10.1016/j.cct.2016.03.006 PMID:26995281

Giraldo-Rodriguez, L., Torres-Castro, S., Martinez-Ramirez, D., Gutierrez-Robledo, L. M., & Perez-Cuevas, R. (2013). Tele-care and tele-alarms for the elderly: Preliminary experiences in Mexico. *Revista de Saude Publica*, *47*(4), 711–717. doi:10.1590/S0034-8910.2013047004574 PMID:24346662

Hackl, W. O. (2016). Intelligent re-use of nursing routine data: Opportunities and challenges. *Studies in Health Technology and Informatics*, *225*, 727–728. PMID:27332320

HereIsMyData. (n.d.). Radboud University Medical Center. Retrieved from http://www.hereismydata.com/

INNT Foundation. (n.d.). Retrieved from https://www.innit.foundation

Kruse, C. S., Kothman, K., Anerobi, K., & Abanaka, L. (2016). Adoption factors of the electronic health record: A systematic review. *JMIR Medical Informatics*, *4*(2), e19. doi:10.2196/medinform.5525 PMID:27251559

MyDario.com. (n.d.). Retrieved from http:// mydario.com/

MyTomorrows. (n.d.). Retrieved from https://mytomorrows.com

Ranked Health. (n.d.). Retrieved from http:// www.rankedhealth.com/about/

Scheen, A. J. (2016). Precision medicine: The future in diabetes care? *Diabetes Research and Clinical Practice*, *117*, 12–21. doi:10.1016/j.diabres.2016.04.033 PMID:27329017

Senior, M. (2014). Novartis signs up for Google smart lens. *Nature Biotechnology*, *32*(9), 856. doi:10.1038/nbt0914-856 PMID:25203024

Sepah, S. C., Jiang, L., & Peters, A. L. (2015). Long-term outcomes of a Web-based diabetes prevention program: 2-year results of a single-arm longitudinal study. *Journal of Medical Internet Research*, *17*(4), e92. doi:10.2196/jmir.4052 PMID:25863515

SleepBot. (n.d.). Retrieved from https://mysleepbot. com/

Tung, C. E., Su, D., Turakhia, M. P., & Lansberg, M. G. (2015). Diagnostic yield of extended cardiac patch monitoring in patients with stroke or TIA. *Frontiers in Neurology*, *5*, 266. doi:10.3389/fneur.2014.00266 PMID:25628595

van Leeuwen, N., Swen, J. J., Guchelaar, H. J., & Hart, L. M. (2013). The role of pharmacogenetics in drug disposition and response of oral glucose-lowering drugs. *Clinical Pharmacokinetics*, *52*(10), 833–854. doi:10.100740262-013-0076-3 PMID:23719679

van Uem, J. M., Maier, K. S., Hucker, S., Scheck, O., Hobert, M. A., Santos, A. T., ... Maetzler, W. (2016, May 31). Twelve-week sensor assessment in Parkinson's disease: Impact on quality of life. *Movement Disorders*, *31*(9), 1337–1338. doi:10.1002/mds.26676 PMID:27241524

Zanella, A., Bui, N., Castellani, A., Vangelista, L., & Zorzi, M. (2014). Internet of things for smart cities. *IEEE Internet Things J*, *1*(1), 22–32. doi:10.1109/JIOT.2014.2306328

Chapter 4
Automation in Healthcare:
A Forecast and Outcome – Medical IoT and Big Data in Healthcare

Alankrita Aggarwal
https://orcid.org/0000-0002-0931-1118
IKG Punjab Technical University, India

Kanwalvir Singh Dhindsa
https://orcid.org/0000-0002-7911-9244
Baba Banda Singh Bahadur Engineering College, India

P. K. Suri
Kurukshetra University, India

ABSTRACT

Major challenges to the society are the people have aging populace and occurrence of continual diseases and eruption of transferable diseases. to embark upon these unmet healthcare desires for the quick guess and therapeutic of all the important diseases a new area called health informatics is emerging as an interdisciplinary research which is dealing with the getting hold of, spread, dispensation, to store as well retrieve. Particularly when the industry is acquired the health information by using the unassuming sense and wearable technology is well thought-out as groundwork stone in healthiness industry. According to a reports, sensors can be worn and hooked on clothes which can acquire the health information uninterrupted.

INTRODUCTION

The latest recent advancement in current know-how and the convenience of the internet is making it possible to bond an assortment of strategy to facilitate exchange a few words in the company of each other to contribute information. The Internet of Things (IoT) an innovative notion for the intention to allowing the user to join a variety of sensors and smart devices to bring together concurrent statistics on or after

DOI: 10.4018/978-1-7998-2101-4.ch004

the surroundings. On the other hand, it has been observed that all-inclusive raised area is motionless and misplaced in the electronic health and mobile health architectures to exercise. Here *e* and *M* are abbreviations of electronic and mobile respectively. Smartphone sensors are sensing and transmitting the data which is relevant to patient's health. In this chapter, our association is dual. Initially a critical analysis of existing literature that throws some light on the efficient methods to arrange IoT in the field of medicinal and smart clinical heed. Another is whether using IoT will be positive or negative outcome for the patient's health. Thus, by making healthcare the compulsory by the use of different sensors with the help of sensors, networking, internet services competently to offer a podium for accessing patients wellbeing data using smart phones.

There exist four key main beliefs of healthiness prediction

- The quantify of indecision and errors
- The most important objective
- The natural world of in sequence aggregation and the mode it affects accurateness and
- The scope of health forecasting.

The emergence of artificial intellect is remodeling industries in all circles of the world. The objective of the exploration suggested by (Winig, 2016; NIDEC, 2016; Bloom et al., 2011; Mayo Magazine, 1989) to take seize of increasing job of artificial intelligence in physical condition be concerned and organization alive and potential challenges to maximize reward associated to artificial intelligence and allied confluence technology

LITERATURE SURVEY

The use of computerization surrounded by the care do industry is usually controversial however this cannot be denied that this industry is to exist. Nearly every health trade professional asks the concerned to prepare things according to medical field but in automation tells concerning the advantages to prepare within the medical field. Automation within the care trade there are some positives and negatives of its impact are usually conflict-ridden. Although it is not clear how number of jobs can be created at the moment but the point that medical trade specialists will be helpful if automation will be bordered. Sensors can be embedded into clothing, frills, in the existing surroundings in order to gather health information flawlessly and pervasively in on a daily basis life. A study by (Winig, NIDEC, 2016) showed that designing of sensors can be done by means of electronic tattoos or it can be printed on human skin to facilitate long time vigor monitor. The chapter also aims at indication of up-and-coming inconspicuous wearable technology which is essential to the awareness of omnipresent healthiness data acquisition which also include:

- Unassuming sensing method
- Embedded fabric technology
- Bendable stretchable printable electronics
- Feeler synthesis to recognize a quantity of prospect guidelines of doing research.

OBJECTIVES OF THE CHAPTER

In order to revise and analyze the universal programmed progression Automation in health industry size increases to enter in solution region or countries, artefact kind in addition to relevance, times gone by figures from previous years and forecast to next coming years. In the direction of identifying the arrangement of robotic process mechanization in Healthcare marketplace by identifying its various secondary components. The focal point is on the input global Robotic Process Automation in Healthcare group of actors to characterize, explain, to discuss and solve the value, marketplace split, promote antagonism according to countryside, Strength weakness analysis and expansion plans in subsequently a small amount of years. Main aim is to analyze the programmed process computerization in health industry by means of admiration to human being intensification, upcoming prediction and the involvement in the complete market. Moreover, in the direction of contribute to comprehensive in rank effecting the enlargement of the market, different opportunity, drivers, manufacturing detailed confront to the threat. The expansion size of Robotic process Automation in healthcare submarkets along with the key regions with their respective key nation.

Analysis of aggressive progress such as expansion, agreement, innovative produce instigate and attainment within the marketplace. The deliberately outline of the major group of actors and scrupulously analyze their growth strategies. A lot of transformation is going in order to succeed in the extremely competitive environment. Most of the group needed to formulate major reserves in process and technology for cutting down the cost and to increase to lower down prices, increase admittance in delivery care products for improving medical.

According to (Celesti, 2019) most of the problems faced by the health care providers is that revenue generation ids major problem as they are shifting to new deliverance models and transforming to outpatient services to shrink managerial and other expenses.

Many of the forecaster firms and manufacturing expert such are emphasis on multinational company and medical industry forecast the subsequent medical technology trends are the prime boosters to resolve these challenges:

- Telehealth Devices
- Simulated Intelligence
- Humanoid
- Wearable devices and Internet of Things

Let us discuss these trends in brief:

Telehealth Devices

Growing requirement for telemedicine is escalating and is a immense approach to connection the break the space among medical practitioners and patients. The requirement to diminish health care expenses and increasing number of middle-aged customers are the major areas instilling the increase in Tele medicine services. According to a latest analysis from recommended panel that most of the clients are paying attention in getting healthcare virtually, and lesser number of clients has previously concluded in doing this. It is the clinical hesitation of a patient with a general practitioner, to maintain healthiness may be it is a prescription linked reminders, to track fitness indicator for e.g. blood pressure and blood sugars or getting every day hold up to administer continuing physical condition issues and patients have a first choice to avail it almost as telemedicine offers autonomy and convenience.

Simulated Intelligence

Internet of things (IoT) is shifting scenarios of e-health an m-health systems. This can be done by installing the permanent and portable health check devices in the clients body's to gather and propel the large amount of neighboring information to health care system for investigation. Presently work is going on fixing the moving medical instruments in patient's body so that a network can be created. This is done so that the nearby homely or clinical environment can be collected and similar type of health data can investigated. For this situation many machine learning with data extracting methods are becoming useful for solving real life problems. Nowadays many mobile applications called apps are designed for analysis and to process health data also for better medical interpretation and to find out the disordering of health patients. These techniques can be divided into two systems:

- Non-artificial intelligence systems
- Artificial intelligence systems.

The problem with the non-artificial intelligence systems have they give inaccurate results and also lack in convergence therefore such systems are substituted by Artificial Intelligence based systems over traditional systems. Artificial Intelligence based techniques are amalgam of different other algorithms like fuzzy, evolutionary algorithms, genetic algorithms, ANN (Artificial neural networks) and other soft computing techniques. Even though many of the artificial techniques are heard theoretically but if completely explored they can prove impending for practical purposes. It is stated by (Giovann et all, 2019) that the research is still going on in which mobility of patient is kept in mind based on machine learning and data learning to solve health problems.

The forthcoming years the situation of simulated intelligence (SI) is mounting and is likely to be one of the chief trends in healthcare manufacturing. Prime factors for command on accuracy tablets and price lessening are the key factors for SI in the healthcare business. SI know how to mould several areas of healthcare from hospice workflow tasks to make a diagnosis physical condition thereby provided on condition that progression should improve workflow efficiency with ever increasing indicative accurateness. Simulated in healthcare reveal that the SI physical condition market shows unpredictable intensification from billions to approximate trillions in approaching years of 2030. In latest survey volume of customers are enthusiastic to follow non-traditional techniques with the make use of artificial intelligence technologies. Because of service preference most of the patients are interested in using the following types of service:

- To keep an eye on the heart condition for example pulse, blood pressure, electrocardiograph and taking the reminder of the symptom and in receipt of counsel on heart stipulation cure.
- To administer an analysis with the intention of checking the heartbeat's beat and makes recommendation base on the results
- To give the customized advice may be provided for vigour and physical condition based on the individual preference and medical records.
- Taking the samples of the blood and provide the results.

Most of the startups companies to major players like Google, Microsoft, IBM or any other such corporations are almost in possession of SI healthcare project and have largely funded large money in these areas. In a little while, SI along with machine learning methods will survive in the industry of healthcare ecology which includes the undemanding customer health to multifarious illness administration and clinical judgment support. The purpose of artificial intelligence for to provide the health-related information on mobile information systems. So, there is a need to review the mobile information systems (MIS). A monitoring-based predictive model is used to explain and investigate a move toward to avert mobile heart failure patient's in valid moment.

One method suggested was based on mobile clinical data of more than 200 heart patients which was collected for about four years and the prediction model applied was a arrangement of alerts to monitor the data .A separate questionnaire was prepared with the help of Bayes classifier using Bernoulli distribution methods to reduce appreciably the false alerts.

Computer assisted analysis method for diabetic retinopathy based on fondues descriptions using a deep convolution neural network (DCNN) was proposed. Instead of long-established DCNN the usually used maxpooling layer amid unfinished max pooling have been replaced so that users can have identification rate is up to 90%. It is easy for a normal person to take fundus images by taking help of a handheld Hophthalmoscope and get the required results by the designed algorithm and name given to this app is Deep Retina.

One more mobile based device which is a mobile hardware-informational system in which a multifactorial neuroelectro stimulation is done. This is system is done with the help of two blocks. In first block a spatial distributed filed as low frequency pulses are put as multi element electrodes around the neck and second one is a control interface done with the help of a smartphone. Many online guiding platforms for elderly people have been developed using machine learning done using chats, videos, mails, blogging and different forums. The mentors are playing different roles by doctors, physiologist and other clinical staff providing formal and informal helps. For a visually disabled person a voice over and a screen reader in which a gesticulation communication, similarity and guidance are done by not able to see disable users according to structure reaction. Evaluation is done by the different participants with the disabilities under constraints conditions based on quantitative and qualitative measures.

A hybrid wearable device and name given is wearable deep learning (Wearable-DL) which has a combinational architecture encouraged by the human being nervous system, in which there is an option of junction of wearable technologies, deep learning & Internet of things. A three level architecture proposal given by (Dargazany, Stegagno, & Mankodiy, 2018; Smaradottir, Håland, & Martinez, 2018) where brain is analogous to deep learning for big data and cloud computing, the spinal string is analogous to Internet of things for smog computing and huge data transmit, peripheral sensory and motor nerves represent wearable technologies as boundary devices used for big data collection

Humanoid

Bots or also called robots are changing and revolutionizing the medical world. The requirement to progress therapeutic efficiency and decrease custom error increase the stipulate for healthcare support and computerized robots. The medicinal Humanoid promote is projected to reach trillions by the late 2050 will deploy humanoid on the way to handle time consuming tasks, reduce labour, and prevent errors thereby enhancing the sustainability of their business operations and improving patient safety. Robots can also be used for rehabilitation and physical therapy for example bionics, exoskeletons, nextgen wearable robots, elder-care assistance, autism to enhance social interaction skills and simplifying surgery. In fact, surgical robots comprise the largest component of the medical Humanoid market. By the year 2025, eighty percent of surgical procedures are likely to be performed by robots. A survey conducted assessment to identify people's acceptance of robots for delivering different types of healthcare services. They asked participants if they would be willing for a robot to perform a surgical procedure instead of a doctor. The results showed that close to half of all respondents would be willing to undergo minor surgery performed by a robot for example non-invasive or minimally all-encompassing surgery such as cataract surgery or laser eye surgery. Around forty five percent of respondents would be willing to undergo major surgery performed by a robot for example omnipresent surgery such as replacement of a knee or hip joint, removal of a tumor and heart surgery. The theory given by (Larburu et al., 2018) is the foremost compensation of using robots for delivering healthcare services were named but people have concern for robots replacing populace, artificial Intelligence and humanoid is the expectations of healthcare. (Larburu et al., 2018)

Wearables and Internet of Things

Sensors can be planned like electronic tattoos or directly printed onto human skin to enable long-standing physical condition observation. The chapter aims to offer a general idea of the up-and-coming inconspicuous and wearable technologies that are vital to the understanding of insidious health information achievement which includes:

- Unobtrusive sensing methods
- Smart textile technology
- Flexible-stretchable-printable electronics
- Sensor fusion, and then to identify some future directions of research.

Patients are reaching more involved in managing their own personal health. The wearable and associated devices lend a hand in creation of fit standard of living and address explicit diseases such as COPD, heart arrhythmia, asthma, pain management or much other variety of diseases

According to the previous researches the wearable technology market will grow around 30-40% in previous years with trillions of units sold out and such projects of the wearable market is reaching thousands to trillions units by 2023.The multiplicity of policy on the promotion actually astonishing.

Following are the largely accepted wearable medical device procedures are as follows:

- Smart watches for healthiness
- Continuous wearable glucose monitors (CGM)
- Pain management wearable devices
- Cardiovascular disease management wearable devices
- EEG Wearable monitors

Also additional budding areas given by the research of (Lightner, 2018; Gartner, 2015; Zheng et al., 2014) in which Internet of things and wearable be able to be functional to improve patient's health and overall lifestyle for example patient identification, smart hospitals, smart pills just like smart phones can be implemented.

Blockchain

In current computer-generated attack and figures breach only insert concern above the health statistics defense. More and more attention is being given to blockchain technology and it can be created as a fresh move toward and explanation for vulnerable tolerant patient's data storage and communication. Research from 2020's mostly the healthcare organization will force the pilot projects and to use blockchain for supply-chain management and long-suffering user characteristics. Various vendors are already exploring blockchain technology can be applied in medical chain arrangement. Leaders of the market like IBM, Intel, Microsoft, and Google contain still isolated units enthusiastic for increasing block chain goods which have a baseline for healthcare. Blockchain based health care systems bring the possibilities for an assortment of challenge as facts interoperability, veracity, refuge, portability. A qualitative and semi controlled version of discussions traverse the function of mechanized applications in healthiness concern surroundings can be conducted. By means of intended variety, it can be identified as a diverse range of stakeholders concerned in conceiving, procuring, developing and with the computerization in an assortment of nationwide and worldwide wellbeing requirements. Interviews can be recorded in binary forms, deciphered correctly which can be inspected using extremely technical software. This work (Dargazany, Stegagno, & Mankodiy, 2018) can be done to be informed by the socio technical perspective to make it understand that social and technical viewpoint are different and independent of each other.

How the Automation has Transformed the Medical Industry

Computerization has changed almost each manufacturing from business to shipping which makes industrialization easier, release resourceful, certification and reckoning easy and permitting additional citizens be alive high-quality existence. Furthermore, choices can be made and been low costs are the advantages come directly or indirectly from automation which is a contradiction to that the improved health will be given by an expensive healthcare. One of the expensive industries is the healthcare and it is making people believe that everything is going to be perfect. Most of the advancement is done in health care industry as physicians taking on new diagnostics or treatment methods. The healthcare industry is not integrated as compared to the automobile industry or computer industry did. The health industry is close enough to put into practice the accelerated changes because of the ground-breaking innovation and the consumer insist for a more charming and connected knowledge. Digital technologies can measure the new spectacle medicine in health and techniques are transportable applications, wearable devices, and predictive diagnostics and telemedicine devices. These are the innovative, easily available and efficiently available cheaper variety of health devices because of automation. Customary health care organizations be it a hospital, the drug industry is now in the line of realization the advantages of investment in this industry which will in return give quality of service, reduce in labor, reduction in waste along with higher ease of access and overstated patient. Many chief executive officers of health industry state the value reduction and effectiveness as prime priorities. Telemedicine has strong root in developing high quality applications to remove handwork from hospitalization. Although the idea of automation has gained popularity for the last few years because of advance devices, high speed communication internet and accuracy tools while it's been around for the last fifty years. Telemedicine have turn out to be an included service worn in hospitals, homes, private clinics and healthcare centers. The latest techniques like telegraphing radio, telephones, video calling, and live chatting have been replaced by the historical medical therapies. Automation has simply remodel telemedicine, but it has actually made it much more reasonably priced to the majority. By way of the progression in equipment enable actions are also attractively cheaper. Earlier it was impracticable to collect all the large data to predict diagnosis because it was a time-consuming task. Also attempts and efforts and ease of understanding was also difficult to gather at one place, but it is now possible as data can be digitized and algorithms available to do that. The remote diagnosis and treatment of patients by means of telecommunications technology is happened because of automation and community have started believing and opening up, keeping their trust in telemedicine because of many automation services like online shopping, net banking, money investing, keeping budgets and many more. Many more services like video or voice chatting, access to mobiles, point of sales are available in the market just because of their security and effectiveness. Many popular applications like skype, WhatsApp are making easy for the users to learn different languages, giving examinations and sometimes getting degrees over the internet believing that they may also see their doctors online and in front of their eyes online. Moreover, customers or patients can see the availability of beds and appointments of doctors online removing the burden. Today's patient is a modern patient who requires ease in his life, so he is making use of automation with open arms. The availability of staff 24*7 is no longer a worry for anybody as medical facility is available with just a click. Present day connected patient believe in not to waste time in getting checked or following up with the doctor. (May, 2017) suggested that such automation industry available in hospitals, skilled medical staff is giving a competition to freelancers in this competitive market.

Issues, Controversies, Problems

The record of health care of one patient is more divided as practitioners with their multi specialties mostly practice at various organizations. A committed person who has a authority of maintaining whole record might be having duplication of data, reiterating by numerous doctors by means of potential demo or transcription faults which changes the reliability of the whole in sequence. Such intrinsic shortcomings in the organization hamper the track quantifiable tribulations which offer conclusion in reproduction testing complicated to calculate outcome to trim down the expenditure of physical condition. There is a rise in complication of the health care whereas patient health check testimony has remained basically analogous. Earlier handwritten pages were achieved and stored in various warehouses or medical department by each health care department having some limitations. There is always pressure to change from different sources that the quality of the record may not be changed. diffidence to patients and health care providers, declining reimbursement, many more issues like rising medico legal and regulatory reporting matters. Each Clinic is maintaining patient records of well organized by repositories Henry Plummer, managing director of the Mayo Clinic stated that record is to be maintained of every patient in all spans of the life. According to (Sodhroa, Pirbhulalc, & Sangaiahe, 2017; Covell & Uman, 1985) this can be done by registering every client must be registered and assigned a unique sequential numeral.

Very important file consisting of a wrapping called a folder consisting to facilitate recognition numeral where patient's report is placed from arrival and later visit at clinic. After conclusion of all visits the record is cross-indexed in terms of ailment, surgical method, surgical outcome, and pathologic conclusion for the record archiving and data congregation for later stages. This practice resulted in proficiency in maintaining data and record of patients of millions of patient records making it as daily practice. Different colors codes more than 400 are given in different forms so that it can be identified by color. Huge number of people is involved for sorting, organizing and write down data to store the files and recover records. Before creation of charts clinical personnel physically transcribe laboratory and x-ray results. All records of laboratory and image check results are compiled in order to lessen the volume of records and to make it easier to use. Although long-suffering care which is quite economical and simple this simply enhances analytical activities by allowing fast access to necessary data. With the passage of time patient is also requiring the high level of service and neglecting the issues like reimbursements major reduction. In return to these services required by patients of the Mayo Clinic may has a chance to get better quality of the patients records by having automation along with rising effectiveness of the medical doctor who uses the opposite point in time, lessen in patient's in the making instant and decline in everyday expenditure. By automating the process it is supposed that with the achievement of medicinal information coordination can be enhanced next to by means of using the patient plan, order, bill, arrangement and result investigation along with the incorporation to put into practice by automating the processes .Theoretically there are some restrictions of computerized-based patient proceedings called CPRs, medical practitioner have restricted to use them. According to Barnett, experts have tried to with this organization information security, data retrieval and entry along with patient information should be clear. A recovery ought to give patient info in an exceedingly clear and sensitive format at the same time from any workstation to transform. It ought to transform the use of institutional resources. Focus is on that there must be single online locations available in types of electronic formats. Many physicians want machine-driven clinical measures which give duly ordered information of patients according to the format of their requirements. According to the publication in they also require relevant data trend and pattern to display the aptitude to systematize subsets of in order, bendable coverage necessities and entry ability. There is a larger drift from computerized patient report to electronic medical report to provide a good quality and patient satisfaction which is a combined model and it is an obligatory change ordered by authorities resulting in reduction of revenues when demand of such reports is increasing. According to the real restoration provides the device drive organization of an inclusive, longitudinal health record. For this purpose Electronic medical report is designed to meet such description. (Jin, Gubbi, Marusic, & Palaniswami, 2014; Xu, Da Xu, Cai et al., 2014; IOM, 1991; ASTM, 1991; Mayo Magazine, 1989) suggested that a widespread arrangement through a vital system EMR compasses the entire rudiments essential for a life span be concerned for each patient.

The major components are:

- Aural test, transcriptions, consultations, and hospital records
- Anamnesis
- Laboratory, surgery and pathology reports, radiology reports and radiology pictures

An easy to use graphical user interface along with the tools to customize it according to the needs of each and every patient to suit everyone lifestyle and priorities. Such user interface combines automated maintain services like ordering, arrangement, and organize activities of a business headquarters. Such factors quantify double which will be inflated and made to provide somewhere to stay depending where the health care desires. Because of electronic medical reports most of the boundaries are removed and will be well organized.. The order of any physician's as well as training requests are also measured doubled automatically processed by the personal computer where any patient to-do list is written instantaneously as a view on the view so that patient can quickly sent as his approach. Method of billing is maintained in an electronic billing display which in turn is all set to be sent to the customer. Clinics or organization will have the right to access present medical and monetary data immediately in order to make decisions instantly so that the records and data is validated, easy to get, reliable and more accurate. The fault rate is reduced since radiology in addition to laboratory coverage systems has undeviating data links with the Electronic medical report. As well as record is much more planned and organized via use of consistent transcription template contents which will vary according to the services used and makes billing, explanation for bill uncomplicated, clear and plain. It is to be believed that EMR will pave the way of growing towards the target of increasing potency and reducing cost. According to the (Jacksonville, Rochester, and Scottsdale) of mayo clinic stated that EMR should be realized at different levels because there is variation in the magnitude and intricacy of the organization. By applying more automation security can be assigned to different types of patients depending on the organization. Any individual with security access should be allowed to meet or given access to the data of the patient as well as of the hospital. With this move toward the system security has comforted physicians issue with reference to maintain the privacy of patient information. Because of no coordination between different medical organizations. Still there is a well-built aspiration to share data among the patients, differences in medical institutions and clinical methods along with there is a lack of practices, lack of common vocabularies and be short of regular statistics data, common clinical vocabulary and no proper format of keeping such data have hindered the, and data formatting have hampered the mobility and the required acquired knowledge for the final analysis of electronic medical reports..For the better evaluation of data a common vocabularies like SNOMED and XML formats are framed to meet up the difficulties faced devoid of compromise the required excellence and competence of the health botheration. All previous methods and policies are labor intensive and are expensive in terms of prices and other medical facilities along with maintaining record of patients. Our aim from the beginning was to get better enduring pleasure and the competence of patient concern delivery. After patients satisfaction general practitioner satisfaction will also be improved. When electronic medical reports are available immediate right of entry for patient proceedings, results of the laboratory, ordering as well as billing services has be converted to put into practice skill to which physicians have fervently responded. In the end on the other hand if acceptance has been elevated consequence will be better. The electronic medical report needed the noteworthy physician technical renewal which can fetch by changing the process and routine habits of doctors boast the urbanized methods after years of clinical exercise and perform. Such practitioners are at ease on paper work therefore adapting to their computerization of the same will take some time and contented and reliant in the lead of the dissertation documentation along with adapt to its deficiency require point in time and tolerance. A practitioner may require four to eight weeks of training after that workload will be reduced and practice data will return to the normality. In 1990's the institute of medicine gave conclusion that computerized patient reports are of prime importance for the health care information. It must include and arrange a person's longitudinal health record and bring monitor base structure supporting content along with graphics needs minimum training time and a sheltered figure which requires less time to transform on the paper. It has been established by (Sikorska et al, Standard, NEC, Kaleem Ullah et al, 2016) that most of the clinics are meeting these goals by building an expandable and an open architecture of the Computerized Patient Report for the future.

Table 1. Classification in global healthcare automation based on automation, use and geography

Based on Automation	Based on End Use	Based on by Geography
• Therapeutic Automation • Lab Pharmacy Automation • Logistics & Training • Automation • Diagnostics & Monitoring Automation	• Pharmacies • Research institutes • Home care • Labs • Others	• Italy, Rest of Europe, Asia Pacific, India, China • Japan, Rest of Asia Pacific, Middle East Africa • South Africa, U.A.E, Rest of Middle East • Africa, Latin America, Brazil • North America, U.S, Canada, Rest of North America • Europe, U.K, Germany, France

(Barnett GO, 1984; Clapesattle HB, 1954)

SOLUTIONS AND RECOMMENDATIONS

Major Trends and Opportunities in Global Healthcare Automation Market

With the accomplishment of computerization it is estimated that it will reduce the manual labor involving tasks like laboratory tests and clinical diagnostics and reducing the cost of the whole process by helping hospitals and clinics. Automation allows medical people to give away the chalk involving important tasks essential odd jobs as it will help in the removal of repetitive tasks and is predictable in moving the tasks efficiently. Such technologies surrounding area make use of different decisive tasks that may do with accuracy with the use of habitual machines indicating the lessening of operating cost decreasing the wastage of time compared to instruction booklet personnel. This issue is probably going to own a medium crash throughout the short-run amount. Growing administration venture is a significant issue moves world souk throughout the calculate amount. Making use of wise knowledge in the marketplace is propellant the command for the consideration of computerization. Higher management is also giving their support in implementing the automation process by providing money and financial investment to this industry. Let us take an example in Europe government agencies of pharmacy and healthcare related products authoritarian organization are supporting programmed system for pharmacies. Many government agencies region speculate funds in analysis and expansion and aid novelty for consciousness computerization sector. Day by day increase in issues of health is now a global concern and to overcome these issues latest automation technologies need to be demonstrating in the healthcare mechanization industry. Growing expansion in expertise is another pouring feature in this market. According to (Babu, Zhao, & Li, 2016; Jia, Lei, Lin, Zhou, & Lu, 2016) automation and technology will help in increasing power efficient technologies that will be helping in synchronized information compilation, uncontrollably monitor, forecast and alert the ever escalating risk of the severe strength issues with alerting the healthcare provider that intervention is essential.

In the previous year's medical automation was in use as mentioned in the table above.

FUTURE RESEARCH DIRECTIONS

Worldwide attentiveness is in automation market is alienated lying for process of relevance into remedial computerization laboratory and pharmaceutical mechanization, transportation, training computerization and investigation and monitor computerization. Previous history reverals restorative automation market resulted for the peak market income split. There is requirement of accurateness and growing prices of labor being the prime reasons bolster for the stipulation of this fragment internationally throughout estimate duration.

The idea given by (F. Yuan Jie, Y. Yue Hong, X. Li Da, Z. Yan et al., 2014) to finish make use of the marketplace is separated into pharmacopoeia; delve into experimentation organizations and labs, habitat concern and others. Fact finding places and workshops are in charge of the best market revenue globally all the way through the estimate the sum. The geological divide of the international marketplace encompass countries from Europe, Asia, Middle East and African.

Superlative marketplace split is given by North America which is adopted by Europe and Asia Pacific in previous years

FOOD AND DRUG REGULATION IMPEDE INNOVATION

Many innovators are designing medical equipment according to the requirement of food and drug regulations which leads to innovation in the clinical industry. For example some patients who are in pneumonic high blood pressure area unit usually captivated up to a breathing apparatus with flexible gas settings. The respirator is inches below the screen that indicates how much oxygen is in the blood. Problem is that two machines cannot converse with each other. If it can be done it will be easy to increase the flow of oxygen automatically the moment a emergency is detected. Engineers developed this kind of closed-loop respirator and introduced it in hospitals as a part of the achievability study. It blown up the point in time untimely babies used up at a secure gas level over two or more hours per day. But no biotechnology company has marketed the thought. There are different samples of appliance restricted systems with discontented potential to avoid wasting lives using the new intensive care units .Software that scans an ECG for faint heartbeat changeability can recognize pattern which are untraceable to the human eye that point out an prominent risk of heart attack. Beds in hospital that uses hearable feedback connect in tending crisis encourage simpler heart related revival. But the patients are not profitable because of the tools are commercial. The reason is which is still unknown is that these innovations have attracted commercialization of things. Getting approval for the innovative life sustainable devices from food and drug association is more complex in comparison of clearance of medicines. In publication of Journal of Public Economics Harvard Business School it was described that food and drug association intervene different companies from investing in innovation. Present scenario is that waiting for some to spend time and money to get consent for a new thing or product in market and then come in with same thing which will face less assessment. Such rigid regulations attach millions to the price of introducing new medical equipment. Supposing a corporation or a hospital is trying to develop a aid monitor will try to sell it an appropriate cost which should be avoided exorbitant. This result in that small companies having low turnover try to get permissions keeping on stake for the new inventions. According to Dr.Stern's who is the researcher wrote in his article that most of the newly device applications are coming from small organizations submitted to the government agencies. Previous research has shown that an unexpected significance is paid by the corporations for the introduction of medical device in comparison to Drug Company by the food and drug associations which increases the chances of motivation for drug companies to start up and follow innovative ideas. In peculiarity the present system discourage the major companies to join the same but their substitute devices are being approved. If some hospitals are able to afford these devices through some medical sites they lack in safety procedures despite of quality versions become available in larger time. Government agencies can extend a help by improving transportation companies to modernize. To maintain progress in the industry (D. E. Bloom, E. T. Cafiero, E. Jane-Llopis, S. Abrahams et al.,2011) can be done by reorganizing the passing of the new devices and contributing financial assistance to the new entrants will not intimidate dead set against authoritarian groups which will also help to the management to maintain progress in the health industry. Across the globe the countries must join hands in articulated interest expediting pharmaceutical approvals along with food and drug associations. This will also help in dislocation of jobs and careers means machines are not taking jobs of health professionals and it will be a commitment for making a better health for all. There will be many unreal fears from artificial intelligence X-ray understanding to the staff but human relationships can never be replaced from medical industry practice. Government and leaders should intervene for taking high level care of patients by release of automation into the medical wards and clinics.

CONCLUSION

Even though the attentiveness is on industry that reacts to change extremely gradually. In luminous dynamism it can be seen that accompanying and supplementary organization adopts new technology and advance to live to tell the tale in an outstandingly aggressive meadow. They are incoming to transfer to surrogate conclusion base heed draw near with a influential association sandwiched stuck between all participant of the take in asking price succession to form outlay effectual and consumer/patient paying attention awareness system. Socio technical challenges linked with the successful amalgamation of robotic application in wellbeing care are expected to be important especially for patient facing function. These need to be recognized and addressed for valuable innovation and acceptance.

REFERENCES

Alba, M. (2017). How the Internet of Things is Changing Product Lifecycle Management"

American Society for Testing and Materials (ASTM). (1991). Standard Guide for Description for Content and Structure of an automatic Primary Record of Care. Standard E, 1384-91.

Babu, G. S., Zhao, P., & Li, X. L. (2016, April). Deep convolutional neural network based regression approach for estimation of remaining useful life. In *Proceedings of the International conference on database systems for advanced applications* (pp. 214-228). Springer.

Barnett, G. O. (1984). The application of computer-based medical-record systems in mobile observe. *The New England Journal of Medicine, 310*(25), 1643–1650. doi:10.1056/NEJM198406213102506 PMID:6427610

Bloom, D. E., Cafiero, E. T., Jane-Llopis, E., Abrahams-Gessel, S., & Bloom, L.R. (2011). The Global Economic Burden of Non-Communicable Diseases. Geneva, Switzerland: World Economic Forum.

Boyi, X., Li Da, X., Hongming, C., Cheng, X., Jingyuan, H., & Fenglin, B. (2014). Ubiquitous Data Accessing Method in IoT-Based Information System for Emergency Medical Services. Industrial Informatics. *IEEE Transactions on, 10*(2), 1578–1586.

Cline, G. (2017). Integrated Product Lifecycle Management in the Era of IoT.

Covell, D. G., & Uman, G. C. (1985). Manning PR Information desires in workplace practice: Are they being met. *Annals of Internal Medicine, 103*(4), 596–599. doi:10.7326/0003-4819-103-4-596 PMID:4037559

Dargazany, A. R., Stegagno, P., & Mankodiy, K. (2018, November). WearableDL: Wearable Internet-of-Things and Deep Learning for Big Data Analytics—Concept, Literature, and Future, Mobile. *Information Systems*, (2), 1–20. doi:10.1155/2018/8125126

Dick, R. S., Steen, E. B., & Detmer, D. E. (Eds.). (1997). *The computer-based patient record: an essential technology for health care*. National Academies Press.

Gartner. (2015). Says 6.4 Billion Connected Things Will Be in Use in 2016. Retrieved from http://www.gartner.com/newsroom/id/3165317

Huang, M., & Chen, Y. (2018). Guest Editorial: Internet of things and intelligent devices and services. *CAAI Trans. Intell. Technol., 3*(2), 73–74.

IEEE. (2016). Standard for an Architectural Framework for the Internet of Things (IoT).

Jia, F., Lei, Y., Lin, J., Zhou, X., & Lu, N. (2016, May). Deep neural networks: A promising tool for fault characteristic mining and intelligent diagnosis of rotating machinery with massive data. *Mechanical Systems and Signal Processing, 72*, 303–315. doi:10.1016/j.ymssp.2015.10.025

Jin, J., Gubbi, J., Marusic, S., & Palaniswami, M. (2014). An information framework for creating a smart city through Internet of Things. *IEEE Internet of Things Journal, 1*(2), 112–121. doi:10.1109/JIOT.2013.2296516

Larburu, N., Artetxe, A., Escolar, V., Lozano, A., & Kerexeta, J. (2018). Artificial Intelligence to Prevent Mobile Heart Failure Patients Decompensation in Real Time: Monitoring-Based Predictive Model. Mobile Information Systems.

Lightner, N. J. (2018). Advances in Human Factors and Ergonomics in Healthcare and Medical Devices. *Proceedings of the AHFE 2018 International Conference on Human Factors and Ergonomics in Healthcare and Medical Devices*. Springer.

Mayo Magazine, . (1989). Old records never die: Medical records at the salad dressing clinic. *Mayo Magazine*.

Marsh, J. (2017). The Internet of Everything Manufacturing and Product Lifecycle Management.

NEC. (2016). NEC Helps Toshiba Machine Enhance Trouble Free Operations by Detecting Malfunctions of Machines before They Occur. Retrieved from http://www.nec.com/en/case/toshibamachine/index.html

NIDEC. (2016). Nidec and IBM Japan to Jointly Develop IoT Technology. Retrieved from http://www.nidec.com/enNA/product/news/2015/news0622-01/

Sannino, G., Bouguila, N., De Pietro, G., & Celesti, A. (2019). *Artificial intelligence for mobile health data analysis and processing*. Mobile Information Systems; doi:10.1155/2019/2673463

Sikorska, J., Hodkiewicz, M. R., De Cruz, A., Astfalck, L., & Keating, A. (2016). A collaborative data library for testing prognostic models. *Presented at the 3rd European Conference of Prognostics Health Management Society*. Academic Press.

Smaradottir, B. F., Håland, J. A., & Martinez, S. G. (2018). *User Evaluation of the Smartphone Screen Reader VoiceOver with Visually Disabled Participants*. Mobile Information Systems; doi:10.1155/2018/6941631

Sodhroa, A. H., Pirbhulalc, S., & Sangaiahe, A. K. (2017). Convergence of IoT and Product Lifecycle Management in Medical Health Care. VIT University.

Ullah, K., Shah, M. A., & Zhang, S. (2016). Effective Ways to Use Internet of Things in the Field of Medical and Smart Health Care. In *Proceedings of the 2016 International Conference on Intelligent Systems Engineering (ICISE)*. IEEE. doi:10.1109/INTELSE.2016.7475151

Winnig, L. (2016). GE's big bet on data and analytics. *MIT Sloan Management Review*, *57*(3).

Xu, B., Da Xu, L., Cai, H., Xie, C., Hu, J., & Bu, F. (2014). Ubiquitous data accessing method in IoT-based information system for emergency medical services. *IEEE Transactions on Industrial Informatics*, *10*(2), 1578–1586. doi:10.1109/TII.2014.2306382

Yuan Jie, F., Yue Hong, Y., Li Da, X., Yan, Z., & Fan, W. (2014). IoT-Based Smart Rehabilitation System. *IEEE Transactions on Industrial Informatics*, *10*(2), 1568–1577. doi:10.1109/TII.2014.2302583

Zheng, Y. L., Ding, X. R., Poon, C. C. Y., Lo, B. P. L., Zhang, H., Zhou, X. L., ... Zhang, Y. T. (2014). Unobtrusive sensing and wearable devices for health informatics. *IEEE Transactions on Biomedical Engineering*, *61*(5), 1538–1554.

Chapter 5
An Effective Diagnostic Model for Personalized Healthcare Using Deep Learning Techniques

Parul Agarwal
Jamia Hamdard, India

Syed Imtiyaz Hassan
https://orcid.org/0000-0003-2453-9580
Maulana Azad National Urdu University, India

Syed Khalid Mustafa
University of Tabuk, Saudi Arabia

Jawed Ahmad
Jamia Hamdard, India

ABSTRACT

This chapter discusses a deep learning and IoE (Internet of Everything) based analytical model for disease detection, prediction and correct treatment for the patient would be proposed. In the proposed model, all the stakeholders, namely doctors, patients, medical staff within a clinic, hospital or a medical institute, would be embedded with micro-sensors. The sensors would in turn sense and capture the information gathered from these sources and the surrounding environment and then send it to a single repository, a base or a server, where it would be stored for further processing. These sensors produce massive amounts of data, which needs to be encrypted as well. Then, in order to improve the effectiveness and accuracy of prediction from the data received from these sensors, deep learning methods are used. Further, the advantages of the proposed model would be explored. To conclude, the limitations, opportunities and future applications of deep learning techniques would be discussed in this chapter.

DOI: 10.4018/978-1-7998-2101-4.ch005

Table 1. Comparison of Machine learning and Deep learning approach

S. no./Approach used	Machine Learning	Deep Learning
1.	Works for small datasets	Requires large datasets
2.	Quickly, the model can be trained	Requires a lot of time to be trained
3.	The features need to be entered manually	Learns the features of the object automatically
4.	The classifiers need to be tried to obtain best results	Learns classifiers to be applied on the model automatically.
5.	Accuracy is limited	Accuracy is unlimited.

INTRODUCTION

Health-Care sector is one of the most prioritized sectors where technologies like Machine Learning, AI, and deep learning have the potential to bring about revolutionary changes.

Various types of data can be generated from the health care segment, which would include the health records in text form, images, sensor data and text which is complex, unstructured, poorly annotated and heterogeneous in nature. Traditional data mining (Kaur, 2014), machine learning statistical learning approaches has to first perform the feature engineering so as to get robust and effective features from the data, and build either prediction or clustering models on them. Due to the lack of sufficient domain knowledge, it poses a lot of challenges. Deep learning is a subtype of machine learning. With machine learning, you manually extract the relevant features of an image. With deep learning, you feed the raw images directly into a deep neural network that learns the features automatically. Deep learning needs lots of data to produce the best results, and is computationally intensive. Table 1 compares Machine learning and Deep Learning approach.

Neural networks (Macukow, 2016) have undoubtedly progressed and have found its applications in several industries (Szegedy, 2017). Deep neural networks are a network of several layers through which input passes to produce the output. This is carried out through transformations and by applying non-linear functions (Abadi, 2016). Data mining and artificial intelligence (Cun, 2014), are unable to solve the problems of deep learning. Deep learning during the training, has the ability to work upon unlabeled information, and can handle heterogeneous data and information for acquiring information and knowledge (Cun, 2015). As the data being generated today is generally massive or “Big Data”, so it can be applied for positive usage and it was understood that deep learning shall have broad applications in future (Chen, 2014) due to its ability to handle large datasets. Deep learning is capable to learn from data complex in nature as discussed in (Miotto, 2017; Wei, 2017), can be applied for image recognition (Shin, 2016) and for text categorization (Song, 2016), medical diagnosis (Lee, 2017; Suzuki, 2017), health informatics (Ravi, 2017), biomedicine (Mamoshina, 2016). Several other research papers also suggest the use of deep learning in healthcare (Jagannatha, 2016; Nie, 2017; Choi, 2016; Hauptmann, 2018; Litgens, 2017).

Thus, the latest deep learning technologies provide new and effective paradigms to obtain learning models (end to end) from this complex data. Deep learning solves the problems where machine learning fails in effectiveness. Through research, it has been established that deep learning techniques surpasses the machine learning techniques and can be used for the diagnosis and prediction of the learning and analytical system.

Healthcare using deep learning techniques, has several path-breaking applications. Deep learning collects massive data which could include the patient's history, reports, medical tests carried out in past, his personal information, symptoms etc. and applies its neural networks to obtain the best results. Currently, most of the deep learning tools are still struggling to identify relevant and important clinical elements, to establish meaningful relations between them and then for translating these relations into an actionable information for the end-user.

It is assisting doctors, professional practitioners and researchers in discovering hidden opportunities of data to analyze the disease and for making the medical diagnosis simpler and effective. This paper would be structured as follows. An extensive literature review on the use of deep learning techniques in health care would be done. Through this it would be established that these techniques serve as a catalyst in solving the problems of the health care sector. Then a model/architecture would be proposed for customized patient needs and for problem-solving of the diseases. Then, the limitations and opportunities followed by an insight into the future work would be explored. We would be using the features of deep learning in an effective analysis and prediction of diseases and their cure by proposing a deep learning-based architecture which is IoE based analytical model for disease detection, prediction and correct treatment for the patient. This would be supported by analyzing the advantages of using deep learning over the conventional methods for the health care.

This chapter shall also explain the applications, opportunities and challenges of using the deep learning methods/techniques in the Health Care sector.

The broad applications of Deep learning in health care include Drug discovery, Medical imaging, Insurance fraud and the most significant being disease diagnosis and its cure. Since, diagnosis is a complex task, and involves a myriad of factors, of which machines shall not be able to make sense and collate; but there's no doubt that a machine might help in supporting physicians to make an accurate diagnosis and treatment, as an extension of scientific knowledge.

Deep learning can assist in drug/ medicines discovery and its development. The patient's medical history would be analyzed and best suitable treatment would be provided for the same. The imaging techniques like the CT scans, ECG, MRI scans (Liu, 2018) are used to diagnose diseases like cancer, tumor, heart-related problems, etc. Deep learning techniques can help in the analysis of such diseases. Insurance fraud can be identified through predictive analysis of fraudulent insurance claims and would also benefit the insurance companies in providing discounts and other offers to the target patients.

LITERATURE REVIEW

In (Faust, 2018) the authors have discussed applications of deep learning techniques in the healthcare segment based upon the physiological signals. An extensive review has been carried out in this paper. Through this paper they have identified that it works best for large datasets, and some recent research exploits its benefits for physiological signals. In (Litjens, 2017), medical images-based survey of deep learning techniques especially using the CNN's has been carried out. The applications are analyzed particularly for datasets related to neural, retinal, pulmonary, breast, abdominal, cancer, and etc. Challenges and future directions in this field have been described. In (Schmidhuber, 2015), the deep Neural networks and their contents in Machine learning and pattern recognition has been discussed. Supervised/ unsupervised learning and evolutionary computations have been elaborated.

In (Shen, 2017), it has been identified that not only machine learning, but deep learning too plays a pivotal role in the identification, and classification of patterns in the medical images. Since deep learning learns the features automatically, so it provides a better analysis of the images for tissue segmentation, anatomical detection, and diseases diagnosis and image registration. Issues, challenges and opportunities are discussed too.

The authors perform an extensive survey of use of deep learning for image-based cancer detection and diagnosis (Hu, 2018). Several other papers are based on finding IoT based solutions for health care. A few of these papers are (Vippalapalli, 2016; Kinthada et al., 2017; Kirtana, 2017; Liu, 2017) and many others. A few of these propose a model based on wearable devices and others monitor the medicine intake by the patient. Some of the papers are based on monitoring heart, cardiovascular, diabetes and hypertension and provides solutions for them.

In (Kumar, 2016), the authors explore the usage of big data in the health-care domain using IoT based cloud solutions. Hadoop framework has been used for implementation and using IoT based cloud solutions, alerts are being generated to the doctor in real-time. In (Dhar et al., 2014), the paper proposes a solution so that the sensors used for monitoring the health of a patient work together. To achieve this, interference among the sensors and distortion of health care data. A prototype has been proposed and implemented. In (Hosseini et al., 2017), Brain-computer interface (BCI) is explored for identifying the characteristics for data collection. Epileptic Brain has been monitored, evaluated and regulated using edge computing. This ensures a timely and fast medical treatment.

Deep learning is also effective in predicting infectious diseases. As discussed in (Allen, 2016), influenza is a disease that is related to spatial and its temporal outbreaks. Social media platforms like Facebook, Whatsapp and Twitter can come helpful in this situation. In this paper, stress has been laid on using twitter for this purpose. The authors propose a framework that monitors influenza outbreaks and provides a platform where health officials in particular can handle the situation and suggest plans for examining the spread of this disease.

In (Volkova, 2017), the authors use the RNN for predicting influenza based on the social media data. They have analyzed the situation from 2011- 2014 influenza seasons whereby, the long short term memory units have been utilized for predicting in real-time and future of the disease spread. The study has then been evaluated using several measures. In addition, (Xu et al., 2017) predictive analysis is done to forecast Influenza about a week or two in advance, based upon covariates which include Met data, previously stored and recorded Influenza data like illness data, online social media-generated data, and the Google search queries data. This prediction has been carried out on patients of Hong Kong. The incidence of influenza in Nagasaki has been done in (He, 2017). Some other discussions of the applications of deep learning on the cancer data can also be found in (Esteva et al., 2017; Bychkov, 2018). Table 2 discusses some of the papers based upon the model used and the task performed.

Table 2. Comparison of several papers based upon the model used and features

Deep learning model/ feature	Disease detection and classification	Prediction of clinical events
RNN (Recurrent neural networks)	(Kam, 2017)	(Choi, 2016; Baor, 2016; Hang, 2017)
CNN (Convolutional neural networks)	(Acharya, 2017)	(Hao, 2017; Yang, 2017)
AE (Autoencoders)	(Suo, 2016; Yuan, 2017; Wang, 2017)	NA
GAN (Generative adversarial network)	NA	(Yahi, 2017)

PROPOSED MODEL/ARCHITECTURE OF IOE BASED ANALYTICAL MODEL FOR DISEASE DIAGNOSIS AND PREDICTION

In this proposed architecture, the stake-holders, (doctors, patients, staff of the clinic/ hospital, management, etc.) and other entities like lab-centers, clinic, hospital, etc. within the premises of the health system are embedded with various micro-chip based wire-less sensors, transponders and the actuators using either the wearable or the fixed devices. The sensors with their sense capability capture the information in its surroundings and then send the data collected to base sink) for processing. The amount of data produced is massive and travels from source to destination and again from destination to source by using a wireless medium. Since, this data relates to a patient's life, thus a strong security aspect needs to be incorporated. To ensure this, the Two-fish cryptographic algorithm (Schneier et al., 1998; Whiting and Schneider, 1998) would be used. In addition, for an optimal usage of bandwidth and a fast data exchange, the Software Defined Networking (SDN) (Braun & Menth, 2014; Kreutz et al., 2015) would be incorporated in the proposed model. Finally, the data collected from the sensors need to be accurately analyzed for predictions regarding the diseases, thus, deep learning techniques would be used.

TECHNICAL WORKFLOW OF THE PROPOSED ARCHITECTURE

Each stakeholder and entity of the proposed architecture is embedded with several sensors, which are used to capture the data. These sensors then transfer the data to the data encryption and standardization unit for processing. This unit then converts the collected unstructured data into a structured format and representation. The structured data is then passed to the encryption unit to obtain a secured form of data. Figure 1 contains the proposed analytical model. Various steps used for this process are listed below

- Data Source identification: Since, several sensors are used, thus the legitimate identification of the data from these sensors is an important aspect for ensuring security.
- Authentication Each sensor is assigned a unique id for its identification. So, authenticity can be established can be done at the Data Encryption and standardization unit.
- Data type and size: Since data collected, is heterogeneous in nature, so its type should be identified, again, this can be done at the data standardization unit. In addition, the data collected is massive and huge, so data size should be known.
- Choosing data Standards: owing to heterogeneity of data, a standardization of the data is an integral part for further processing.

- Each of the data in different formats has to be handled differently, thus storing and servicing the right type of request is essential.
- Data Cleaning: A process where noise and outliers are removed from the stored data.
- Normalization of data: Data is normalized to remove any anomalies and enhance data integrity.

Once, the data has been converted to a standard format, it is then converted to an accessible format to ensure secured data. This has been done using the Two-Fish cryptographic algorithm, asymmetric key cryptographic algorithm. Several advantages offered by this algorithm include its fast execution, highly secure in nature, a key size of variable length, and it is compatible with smart cards (micro-chip size). After the encryption of the data using the Two-Fish algorithm, the encrypted data is then sent to the sink maintained on the cloud so that decision by the system controller is taken. The system controller, with the help of the analytical unit, then analyses any requests from the user and then instructs the devices to take necessary operation in a learned and an intelligent manner. The SDN is responsible for governing the data transfer.

The SDN is responsible for dynamically selecting the best path for transfer of data based upon real-time traffic input. As discussed in (Braun & Menth, 2014; Xia et al., 2015; Kreutz et al., 2015), it also manages the traffic of the network, the network topologies and its bandwidth in a real-time manner. In any IoE based system, some requests may be user-centric or object/conditions centric as discussed in (Benson, 2016; Bagheri & Movahed, 2016; Bayani et al., 2017; Sethi & Sarangi, 2017). Deep learning tools and techniques play an important role in training the system to improve the device's precision in servicing these requests.

Role of Deep Learning Techniques for Developing this Analytical Model

Learning analytics is basically a repository of learning patterns, its retention and usage in order to improve and optimize the learning pattern, portraying intelligence and to enhance the retention capabilities. The short and the long-term memories define these capabilities. Thus, for achieving better retention, the short-term memory should be processed or converted into long term memory. This conversion is possible as synaptic proteins found in the human brain synthesize (Fioravante & Byrne, 2011). With Machine learning, gaining a deep insight into data cannot be achieved, but in contrast deep learning techniques make it possible to tune the learning as well as the behavioral patterns so as to improve the accuracy of results. These are helpful for enhancing the retention capabilities.

Steps for creating an analytical model:

- Take the input data from entities and devices. This data is then transformed into a structured format.
- Pre-process the data (remove noise).
- Feed this pre-processed data into the long-short term memory system for training.
- Identify the request from the users and feed it to the system.
- Recognize the key points in the data.
- Process the data.
- Provide the service to the user based upon the suggestions and feedback obtained from the patient. Note: d, e, and f form a part of the deep learning system. Figure 2 describes the same.

Figure 1. the proposed analytical model

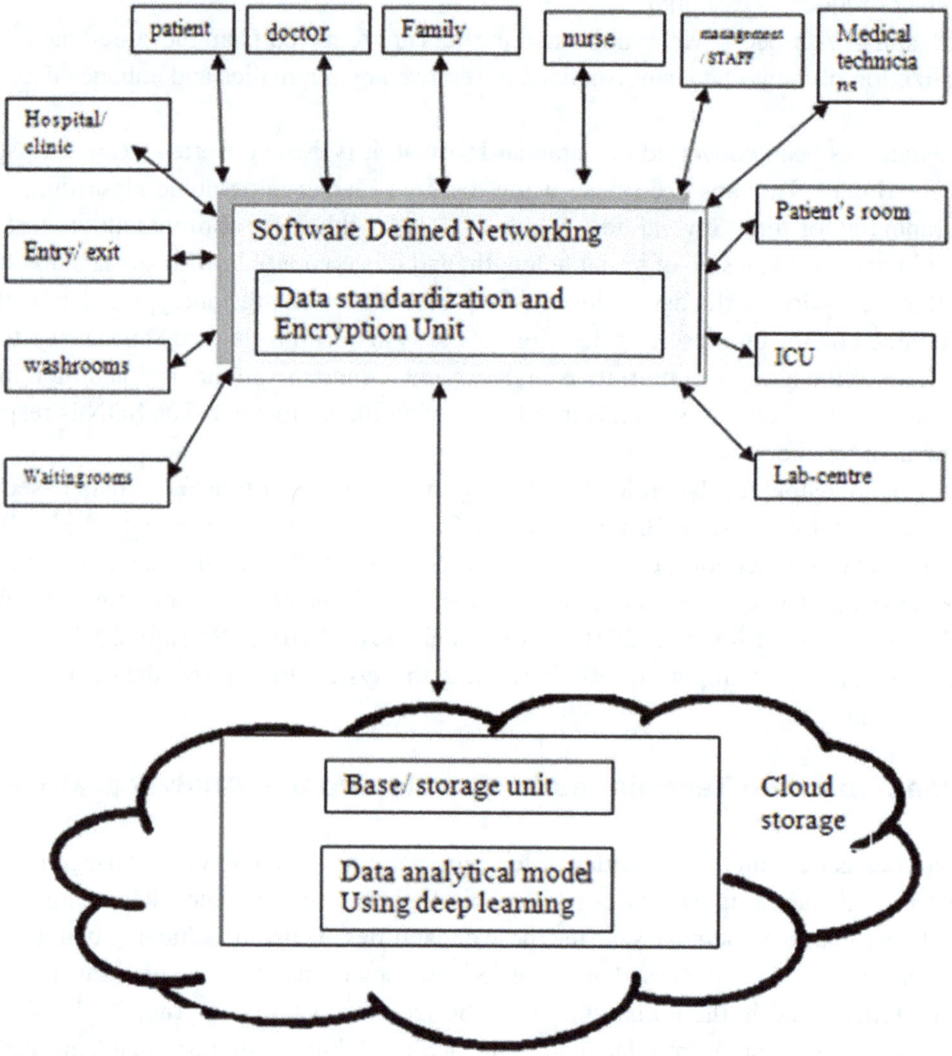

APPLICATIONS OF THE PROPOSED APPROACH

Several parameters serve as raw data which would be processed by the deep learning algorithms for a deep understanding of the disease and its cure. They are personal information of the patient, the demographies, Genetics/ family history (in case of hereditary diseases is an important input to the learning system), symptoms, lifestyle (working habits at home or workplace), environmental factors (Towers in surroundings as they are routed as major reason for causing several diseases), weather, climate, socio factors (intermingling with society/ police records), encounters with diseases (by through past prescriptions), checking the leave records if working, Social history of the patient (depression or ever attempted suicide etc.), past medications, procedures followed, past medical reports and examination tests, etc. In addition, data from the wearable devices and the sensors forms the input data to the deep learning system. The mentioned extensive raw data as input can result in various advantages as listed below:

Figure 2. The steps followed in the analytical model.

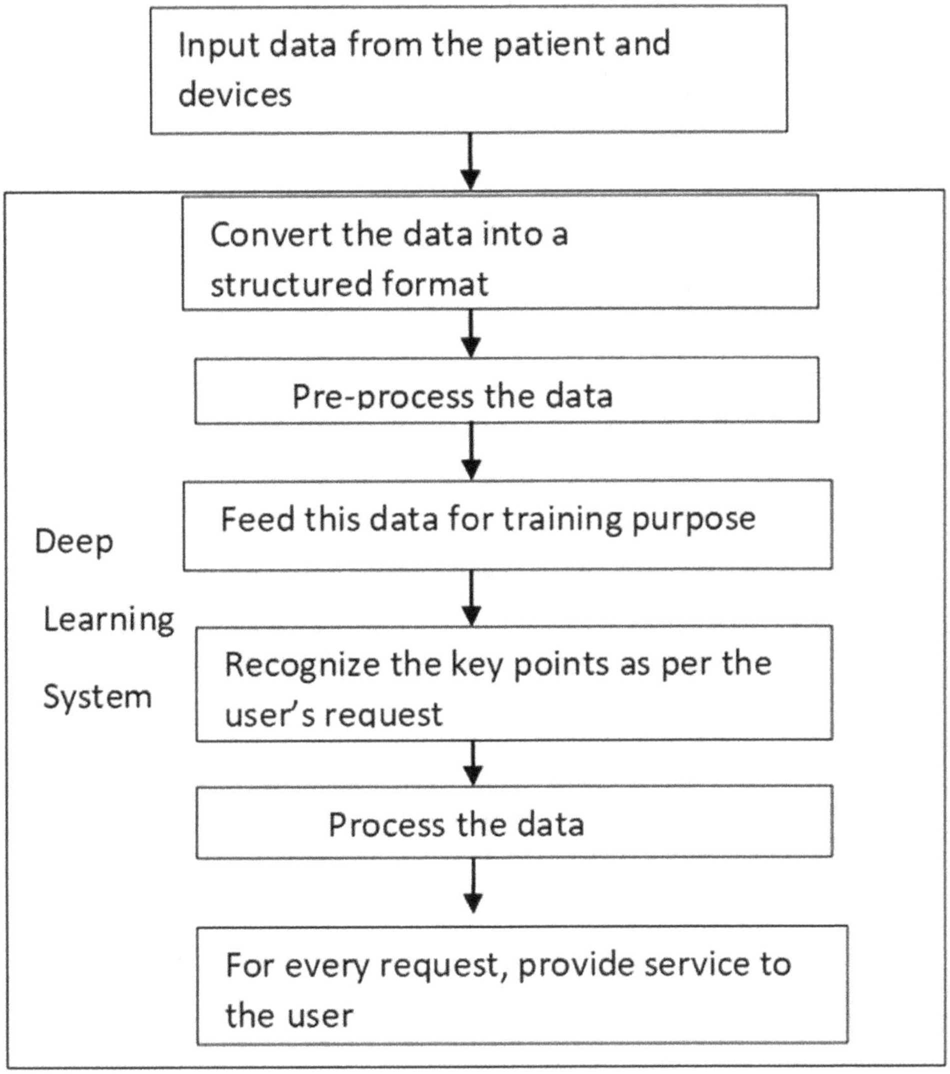

- Predictive in Nature
- Reduced cost incurred in health diagnosis and treatment
- Early identification can reduce the disease progression
- Helps in performing the prevention better from diseases
- Predicting the right medicine for cure
- Smart health monitoring.

Figure 3 describes major advantages.
Other advantages of the proposed approach:
Improved Security by access restricted to authorized persons:

Figure 3. Major advantages of the proposed approach achieved using Deep learning algorithms.

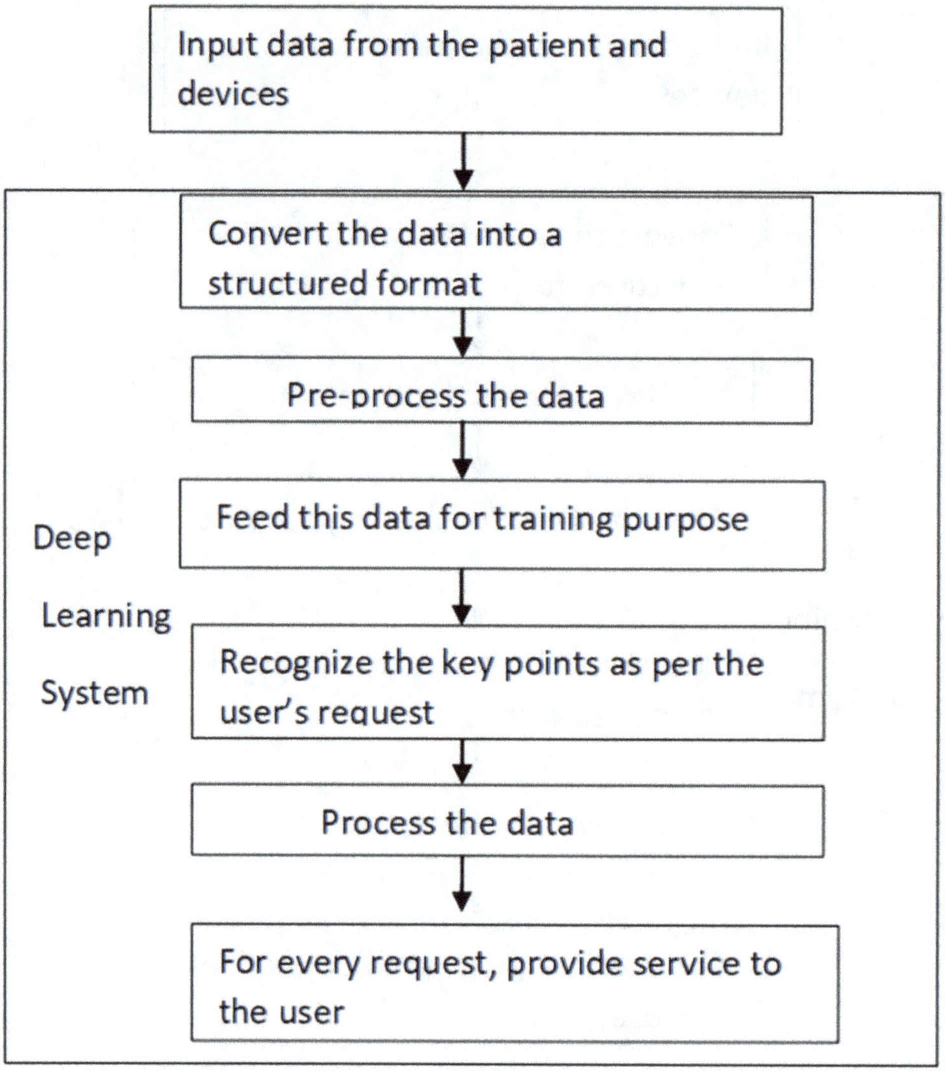

The hospital premises are embedded with micro-chip based which let the doors of personal rooms, operation theatres, ICU's, doctors chambers to be opened only by the authenticated doctors/ nurses/ patients, their restricted family members, hospital staff, thus preventing any trespassing attempts by an unauthorized user/ entity.

Reduced power consumption:

Since the hospital/ clinic premises shall be equipped with a smart electrical system for an optimal use of electricity, so reduced power consumption is incurred. In addition, the sensors shall have the capability to sense the temperature, pressure, and humidity, so they shall adjust dynamically to the surrounding conditions and regulate the devices accordingly. This will lessen the power usage and thus the carbon emission associated with the devices.

Attendance management:

The doctors are in a few cases found to be on a leave, thus making the patients suffer because of their callous attitude at times. In addition, the nurses and other hospital staff need to be monitored regularly.

Regular monitoring of the hospital

The patients as well as the doctors shall have a transparency in viewing the test reports, the medications, and patient's condition inside his room in-case of any accidental deterioration in health. This would ensure an effective and proper treatment and cure.

Health Monitoring

The hospital canteens shall be embedded with sensors to identify the eating habits of patients and customizing the menu plan for a patient if recommended by the doctor.

LIMITATIONS AND CHALLENGES

Though, past work demonstrates the potential that deep learning possesses in deriving insights of the clinical data, but the potential problems associated with neural networks pose major challenges in applying deep learning to the medical domain. Some of the major challenges are discussed below:

- Lack of Massive data: Deep learning delivers success only if the data are massive in nature with millions and billions of examples to work upon (Deng et al., 2009) but the data related to medical domain, is limited as it consists of mainly the electronic health records (Golderberg et al., 2000), which are about a few thousand cases. Though, medical images (Bodenreider, 2004) form a part but are not as massive to exploit the advantages of deep learning. Deep learning deals with extensive computational models working on massive data by using fully connected several layer neural networks, and requires hundreds of parameters as inputs for proper analysis, so medical care data lack this extensiveness in its volume. Primary Health Care is accessible to only hundreds of billions out of thousands of billions of people all over the world, so applying and training a deep learning model for such a number is not enough.
- Rare diseases and small clinics: Learning patterns of rare diseases, is another challenge currently being faced by the health sector. Small clinics with limited infrastructure and data are incapable to exploit the deep learning techniques for disease diagnosis.
- Data Quality: Data from multiple sources needs to be converted to a standard format.

Medical data is being received from multiple sources as highlighted in the proposed model. This data is in an unstructured form which needs to be converted to a structured format for usage and further processing. This data is ambiguous, noisy, heterogeneous and incomplete in several instances/records. Training the model with such varied data quality issues is a major challenge.

- Storage and processing: the medical data needs to be stored and processed using deep learning techniques. Both these aspects are a challenge by themselves.
- Possessing medical domain knowledge: a strong medical ontology needs to be built for prediction and diagnosis as discussed in (Che et al., 2015).

Medicine field is replete with several ontologies like UMLS (Bodenreider, 20014), SNOMED-CT (Cornet & Keizer, 2008) which have proved to be extremely useful for mining, and decision support

(Galiano, 2009). For deep learning, such sources serve as a means to accelerate the learning process. The structured knowledge needs to be combined with data-driven techniques (Machine Learning/ Deep Learning), and forms major challenge for medical data mining.

- Missing values in data:

Generally found in raw data, that is collected from the patient or through medical records. Due to no understanding of a typical problem, the medical reports might not be descriptive in nature. In addition, some reports like BP, heart Rate might have some missing values at a particular instant of time. Though, several methods exist for the replacement of missing values.

- Integration and transformation of subject-oriented knowledge for adaptation
- Improving the Deep Learning Algorithms
- Correct model selection and its optimization: Deep learning techniques are based on several models like the CNN (Convolutional Neural Networks), RNN (Recurrent Neural Networks), and the Feed Forward. Choosing the right model for right application in medical domain, is necessary for correct diagnosis and treatment.
- Choosing the appropriate Parametric Function approximation:

Several approximation methods like activation functions, initialization strategies, the architecture and learning techniques have to be carefully identified.

- Temporal nature of data: the non-deterministic manner in which the diseases are progressing, the change in symptoms and new diseases being observed, the volatile nature of the data are posing a challenge to apply deep learning methods. Since these models use static vector-based inputs, so handling the time and volatility is a challenging job.
- Domain complexity: A few diseases which have been observed in past years like Dengue, Chickenguinea, Nipah Virus causing calamities, etc., do not present a clear picture of the causes of these diseases and despite advance technological advances, medicines and cure are still a black box problem. Their progression and lack of proper infrastructure are the associated problems.

DISCUSSION

Though deep learning looks promising in the applications it offers particularly in the medical domain, but to prove that it would replace the role of doctors is not evident. Deep learning offers its wide use in several fields. Particularly, it finds its application in Transportation sector and for controlling the green-house gas emissions (Madu et al., 2017), Traffic Control (Fadlullah, 2017), Object detection (Zhou, 2017), speech detection (Badjatya, 2017; Deng, 2016), Text classification (Yousefi, 2017), translation (Singh, 2017) etc. The challenges introduce several opportunities and further research work in the area. It can be seen that they prove to be promising in the future that deep learning can provide in the health-care.

A few of notable opportunities are listed below:

- Feature enrichment: With a limited number of patients, the need of the hour is to capture as many features as possible so as to characterize the patient and find innovative and novel methods for processing this data. The data sources should not be limited to just EHR's but should also consider surveys, environment, genomics data, online communities, patient-related information to be made available on social media, and the likes. This data for privacy purpose might delete extremely personal details of the patient. Instead of combining the data source and then processing it, each data source should be processed separately with its specific deep model.
- Federated inference: As, privacy of the data is an important issue in the above-suggested opportunity, so, learning a deep model in this secure setting is an area which can be exploited. For this, encryption and several cryptographic algorithms can be suggested, developed and applied.
- Model privacy: Privacy becomes an important aspect, for scaling up the deep learning process. The amount of personal information which would be processed by the models in healthcare, calls for deploying care segment and risks associated with it need to be considered for implementation of a differential privacy standard (Miotto, 2018).
- Incorporating expert knowledge: Deep learning needs to be incorporated with expert knowledge for obtaining the best results. This arises as the data is limited and the quality issue discussed in the previous section. Several sources of information like online encyclopedias, PubMed Abstracts need to be mined for extracting reliable content.
- Temporal modeling: The medical data generated is time-series data. Thus, to understand the patient condition in an effective manner, and to provide a timely decision support, the need is to train deep learning models appropriately. To achieve this, coupling of RNN's and memory-based architectures is required.
- Interpretable modeling: Though deep learning models are being adopted by us, but adopting this system is tough. A trustworthy and a reliable system can only be built if the results generated by these models can be explained and made more understandable.

CONCLUSION

It can be concluded from the literature survey presented in this paper and the proposed Deep learning-based analytical model for disease diagnosis, treatment and effective/improved care that they have wide applications in the health care. As compared to Machine learning techniques, deep learning surely offers advantages over it. The deep learning network comprises of detection, segmentation, and prediction etc. As discussed in this paper, the raw data that goes as input to the deep learning model includes the patient's personal details, his socio-economic data, past data, socio-cultural data, demographies, environmental data, clinical examination data etc. But if this data is combined with other sources like the medical prescriptions, data obtained from feeds like Facebook, tweets, blogs, paper clinical notes, digital clinical notes and the like. Deep learning methods have a wide application in the medical field. In this case, medical application of the learning model would prove to be extremely predictive and effective in disease diagnosis and treatment. Through this it can also be established that Deep learning shall thrive to be exploited for the advantages it offers over any other learning model.

FUTURE RESEARCH

The need of the hour is to develop meaningful and holistic models/ architectures that would bridge the deep learning models and the human interoperability, especially in the health domain. In future Machine learning and deep learning shall find their applications not only for disease diagnosis or treatment and effective prediction also in bio-informatics. Deep learning algorithms can solve the issues related to sensor data, sensor text, electronic records, imaging, etc. this arises because the data generated from health domain is extremely heterogeneous, complex, and extremely high and multi-dimensional, thus because of these limitations, it actually offers future directions where solutions for such problems can be solved. Deep learning can make the unstructured data into a structured representation. The future technology can provide efficient paradigms to obtain learning models in handling complex data. It is time that healthcare of today, which comprises of importance as they offer a broad spectrum to reach a large section of society. Healthcare offers various advancements in several domains, but it holds its importance and priority in the health care.

Applications of deep learning range from prediction, to personalized services to the patients, its treatment and cure. Biomedical data have gained knowledge about several applications based on deep learning models/ techniques.

Data learning is recurrent and convolutional networks and algorithms have become a methodology by itself. Deep learning finds it applications in health care in areas like cancer, infectious diseases, neural, retinal, pathology, pulmonary sciences etc. But, in the near future, other domains of medicinal areas can be explored for exploiting the advantages that deep learning can offer.

REFERENCES

Abadi, M., Chu, A., Goodfellow, I., McMahan, H. B., Mironov, I., Talwar, K., & Zhang, L. (2016). Deep Learning with Differential Privacy. In *Proceedings of the 2016 ACM SIGSAC Conference on Computer and Communications Security* (pp. 308–318). ACM. 10.1145/2976749.2978318

Acharya, U. R., Oh, S. L., Hagiwara, Y., Tan, J. H., & Adeli, H. (2017). Deep convolutional neural network for the automated detection and diagnosis of seizure using EEG signals. *Computers in Biology and Medicine*. doi:10.1016/j.comp-Biomed.2017.09.017 PMID:28974302

Allen, C., Tsou, M., Aslam, A., Nagel, A., & Gawron, J. (2016). Applying GIS and Machine Learning Methods to Twitter Data for Multiscale Surveillance of Influenza. *PLoS One*, *11*(7), e0157734. doi:10.1371/journal.pone.0157734 PMID:27455108

Badjatiya, P., Gupta, S., Gupta, M., & Varma, V. (2017). Deep learning for hate speech detection in tweets. In *Proceedings of the 26th International Conference on World Wide Web Companion* (pp. 759–760). 10.1145/3041021.3054223

Bagheri, M., & Movahed, S. H. (2016). The Effect of the Internet of Things (IoT) on Education Business Model. In *Proceedings of the International Conference on Signal-Image Technology & Internet-Based Systems* (pp. 435-441). IEEE. 10.1109/SITIS.2016.74

Bajor, J. M., & Lasko, T. A. (2016). Predicting medications from diagnostic codes with recurrent neural networks. In *Proceedings of the International Conference on Learning Representations*. Academic Press.

Bayani, M., Leiton, K., & Loaiza, M. (2017). Internet of things (IoT) advantages on E-learning in the smart cities. *International Journal of Development Research*, *7*(12), 17747–17753.

Benson, C. (2016). The internet of things, IoT systems, and higher education. *EDUCAUSE Review*, *51*(4), 6.

Bodenreider, O. (2004). The Unified Medical Language System (UMLS): Integrating biomedical terminology. *Nucleic Acids Research*, *32*(Database issue), D267–D270. doi:10.1093/nar/gkh061 PMID:14681409

Braun, W., & Menth, M. (2014). Software-defined networking using OpenFlow: Protocols, applications and architectural design choices. *Future Internet*, *6*(2), 302–336. doi:10.3390/fi6020302

Bychkov, D., Linder, N., Turkki, R., Nordling, S., Kovanen, P. E., Verrill, C., ... Lundin, J. (2018). Deep learning-based tissue analysis predicts outcome in colorectal cancer. *Scientific Reports*, *8*(1), 3395. doi:10.103841598-018-21758-3 PMID:29467373

Che, C., Xiao, C., Liang, J., Jin, B., Zho, J., & Wang, F. (2017). An RNN architecture with dynamic temporal matching for personalized predictions of Parkinson's disease. In *Proceedings of the 2017 SIAM International Conference on Data Mining* (pp. 198–206). Academic Press. 10.1137/1.9781611974973.23

Che, Z., Kale, D., Li, W., Bahadori, M. T., & Yan, L. (2015). Computational Phenotyping. In *Proceedings of the 21st ACM SIGKDD Conference on Knowledge Discovery and Data Mining* (pp. 507-516). ACM Press. 10.1145/2783258.2783365

Chen, X.-W., & Lin, X. (2014). Big data deep learning: Challenges and perspectives. *IEEE Access*, *2*, 514–525. doi:10.1109/ACCESS.2014.2325029

Choi, E., Bahadori, M. T., Schuetz, A., Stewart, W. F., & Sun, J. (2016). Doctor AI: predict-ing clinical events via recurrent neural networks. In *JMLR Workshop Conference proceedings* (pp. 301-318). Academic Press.

Choi, E., Schuetz, A., Stewart, W., F., & Sun, J., (2016). Medical Concept Representation Learning from Electronic Health Records and its Application on Heart Failure Prediction.

Deng, J., Dong, W., Socher, R. L., Li, J., Li, K., & Fei, F. (2009). Imagenet: A large-scale hierarchical image database. In *Proceedings of the 2009 IEEE Conference on Computer Vision and Pattern Recognition*. IEEE. 10.1109/CVPR.2009.5206848

Deng, L. (2016). Deep learning: From speech recognition to language and multimodal processing. *APSIPA Transactions on Signal and Information Processing*, *5*, E1. doi:10.1017/ATSIP.2015.22

Dhar, S. K., Bhunia, S., & Mukherjee, N. (2014). Interference Aware Scheduling of Sensors in IoT Enabled Health Care Monitoring Systems. In *Proceedings of the Fourth International Conference of Emerging Applications of Information Technology* (pp. 152-157). Academic Press. 10.1109/EAIT.2014.50

Esteva, A., Kuprel, B., Novoa, R. A., Ko, J., Swetter, S. M., Blau, H. M., & Thrun, S. (2017). Dermatologist-level classification of skin cancer with deep neural networks. *Nature*, *542*(7639), 115–118. doi:10.1038/nature21056 PMID:28117445

Fadlullah, Z. M., Tang, F., Mao, B., Kato, N., Akashi, O., Inoue, T., & Mizutani, K. (2017). State-of-the-Art Deep Learning: Evolving Machine Intelligence towards Tomorrow's Intelligent Network Traffic Control Systems. *IEEE Communications Surveys and Tutorials*, *19*(4), 2432–2455. doi:10.1109/COMST.2017.2707140

Faust, O., Hagiwara, Y., Hong, T. J., Lih, O. S., & Acharya, U. R. (2018). Deep learning for healthcare applications based on physiological signals: A review. *Computer Methods and Programs in Biomedicine*, *161*, 1–13. doi:10.1016/j.cmpb.2018.04.005 PMID:29852952

Fioravante, D., & Byrne, J. H. (2011). Protein degradation and memory formation. *Brain Research Bulletin*, *85*(1–2), 14–20. doi:10.1016/j.brainresbull.2010.11.002 PMID:21078374

Galiano, M. C., Valdivia, M. T. M., & Lopez, U. (2009). Query expansion with a medical ontology to improve a multimodal information retrieval system. *Computers in Biology and Medicine*, *39*(4), 396–403. doi:10.1016/j.compbiomed.2009.01.012 PMID:19268924

Goldberger, A., Amaral, L. A. N., Glass, L., Hausdorff, J. M., Ivanov, P. C., Mark, R. G., ... Stanley, H. E. (2000, June 13). PhysioBank, PhysioToolkit, and PhysioNet: Components of a new research resource for complex physiologic signals. *Circulation*, *101*(23), E215–E220. doi:10.1161/01.CIR.101.23.e215 PMID:10851218

Hang, Y., Chen, R., Tang, J., Stewart, W. F., & Sun, J. (2017). LEAP: learning to prescribe effective and safe treatment combinations for multimorbidity. In *Proceedings of the 23rd ACM SIGKDD International Conference on Knowledge Discovery and Data Mining* (pp. 1315–1324). ACM.

Hauptmann, A., Arridge, S., R., Lucka, F., R., Muthurangu, V., & Steeden. J., A. (2018), Real-time Cardiovascular MR with Spatio-temporal De-aliasing using Deep Learning, Proof of Concept in Congenital Heart Disease.

He, F., Hu, Z., Zhang, W., Cai, L., Cai, G., & Aoyagi, K. (2017). Construction and evaluation of two computational models for predicting the incidence of influenza in Nagasaki Prefecture, Japan. *Scientific Reports*, *7*(1), 7192. doi:10.103841598-017-07475-3 PMID:28775299

Hosseini, M. P., Tuyen, X. T., Pompili, D., & Zadeh, H. (2017). Deep Learning with Edge Computing for Localization of Epileptogenicity using Multimodal rs-fMRI and EEG Big Data. In *Proceedings of the IEEE International Conference on Autonomic Computing* (pp. 83-92). 10.1109/ICAC.2017.41

Hu, Z., Tang, J., Wang, Z., Zhang, K., Zhang, L., & Sun, Q. (2018). Deep Learning for Image-based Cancer Detection and Diagnosis—A Survey. *Pattern Recognition*, *83*, 134–149. doi:10.1016/j.patcog.2018.05.014

Jagannatha, A.N. & Yu, H. (2016). Structured prediction models for RNN based sequence labeling in clinical text.

Jagannatha, A.N. & Yu, H. (2016). Bidirectional Recurrent Neural Networks for Medical Event Detection in Electronic Health Records.

Kam, H. J., & Kim, H. Y. (2019). Learning representations for the early detection of sepsis with deep neural networks. *Computers in Biology and Medicine*, *89*, 248–255. doi:10.1016/j.compbiomed.2017.08.015 PMID:28843829

Kaur, B., & Singh, W. (2014). Review on Heart Disease Prediction System using Data Mining Techniques. *International Journal on Recent and Innovation Trends in Computing and Communication*, *2*(10), 3003–3008.

Kinthada, M. R., Bodda, S., & Mande, S. B. K. (2016). EMedicare: MHealth solution for Patient Medication Guidance and Assistance. In *Proceedings of the International conference on Signal Processing, Communication, Power and Embedded System* (pp. 657-661). Academic Press. 10.1109/SCOPES.2016.7955523

Kirtana, R. N., & Lokeswari, Y. K. (2017). An IoT Based Remote HRV Monitoring System for Hypertensive Patients. In *Proceedings of the IEEE International Conference on Computer, Communication, and Signal Processing*. IEEE Press. 10.1109/ICCCSP.2017.7944086

Kreutz, D., Ramos, F. M., Verissimo, P. E., Rothenberg, C. E., Azodolmolky, S., & Uhlig, S. (1995). Software-defined networking: A comprehensive survey. *Proceedings of the IEEE*, *103*(1), 14–76.

Kumar, P. D., Kumar, R. S., Sujatha, K., Ponmagal, R. S., & Rajavarman, V. N. (2016). Big data Analytics of IoT based Health Care Monitoring System. In *Proceedings of the International Conference on Electrical, Computer and Electronics Engineering* (pp. 55-60). Academic Press.

LeCun, Y., Bengio, Y., & Hinton, G. (2015). Deep learning. *Nature*, *521*(7553), 436–444. doi:10.1038/nature14539 PMID:26017442

Lee, J. G., Jun, S., Cho, Y. W., Lee, H., Kim, G. B., Seo, J. B., & Kim, N. (2017). Deep Learning in Medical Imaging: General Overview. *Korean Journal of Radiology*, *18*(4), 570–584. doi:10.3348/kjr.2017.18.4.570 PMID:28670152

Litjens, G., Kooi, T., Bejnordi, B. E., Setio, A. A. A., Ciompi, F., Ghafoorian, M., ... Sánchez, C. I. (2017). A Survey on Deep Learning in Medical Image Analysis. *Medical Image Analysis*, *42*, 60–88.

Liu, S. (2017). Class-constrained Transfer LDA for Cross-view Action Recognition in Internet of Things. *IEEE Internet of things Journal, 5*(5), 3270-3277.

Macukow, B. (2016). *Neural Networks – State of Art, Brief History, Basic Models and Architecture* (pp. 3–14). Switzerland: Springer International Publishing. doi:10.1007/978-3-319-45378-1_1

Madu, C. N., Kuei, C. H., & Lee, P. (2017). Urban sustainability management: A deep learning perspective. *Sustainable Cities Society*, *30*, 1–17. doi:10.1016/j.scs.2016.12.012

Mamoshina, P., Vieira, A., Putin, E., & Zhavoronkov, A. (2016). Applications of Deep Learning in Biomedicine. *Molecular Pharmaceutics*, *13*(5), 1445–1454. doi:10.1021/acs.molpharmaceut.5b00982 PMID:27007977

Miotto, R., Wang, F., Wang, S., Jiang, X., & Dudley, J. T. (2017). Deep learning for healthcare: Review, opportunities and challenges. *Briefings in Bioinformatics*, *19*(6), 1236–1246. doi:10.1093/bib/bbx044 PMID:28481991

Nie, L., Wang, M., Zhang, L., Yan, S., Zhang, B., & Chua, T. S. (2017). Disease inference from health-related questions via sparsely connected deep learning, knowledge and data engineering. *IEEE Transactions*, *27*(87), 2107–2119.

Patel, R., Belousov, M., Jani, M., Dasgupta, N., Winokur, C., Nenadic, G., & Dixon, W. G. (2018). Frequent discussion of insomnia and weight gain with glucocorticoid therapy: An analysis of Twitter posts. *NPJ digital medicine, 1*, 20177. doi:10.103841746-017-0007-z

Ravì, D., Wong, C., Deligianni, F., Berthelot, M., Andreu-Perez, J., Lo, B., & Yang, G. Z. (2017). Deep learning for health informatics. *IEEE Journal of Biomedical and Health Informatics*, *21*(1), 4–21. doi:10.1109/JBHI.2016.2636665 PMID:28055930

Riccardo, M., Wang, F., Wang, S., Jiang, X., & Dudley, J. T. (2018). Deep learning for healthcare: Review, opportunities and challenges. *Briefings in Bioinformatics*, *19*(6), 1236–1246. doi:10.1093/bib/bbx044 PMID:28481991

Schmidhuber, J. (2015). Deep learning in neural networks: An overview. *Neural Networks*, *61*, 85–117. doi:10.1016/j.neunet.2014.09.003 PMID:25462637

Schneier, B., Kelsey, J., Whiting, D., Wagner, D., Hall, C., & Ferguson, N. (1998). Twofish: A 128-bit block cipher. *NIST AES Proposal*, *15*(1), 23–91.

Schneier, B., Kelsey, J., Whiting, D., Wagner, D., Hall, C., & Ferguson, N. (1999). *The Twofish encryption algorithm: a 128-bit block cipher*. John Wiley & Sons, Inc.

Sethi, P., & Sarangi, S. R. (2017). Internet of things: Architectures, protocols, and applications. *Journal of Electrical and Computer Engineering*, 25. doi:10.1155/2017/9324035

Shen, D., Wu, G., & Suk, H. I. (2017). Deep learning in medical image analysis. *Annual Review of Biomedical Engineering*, *19*(1), 221–248. doi:10.1146/annurev-bioeng-071516-044442 PMID:28301734

Shin, H. C., Roth, H. R., Gao, M., Lu, L., Xu, Z., Nogues, I., & Summers, R. M. (2016, May). Deep Convolutional Neural Networks for Computer-Aided Detection: CNN Architectures, Dataset Characteristics and Transfer Learning. *IEEE Transactions on Medical Imaging*, *35*(5), 1285–1298. doi:10.1109/TMI.2016.2528162 PMID:26886976

Simon, T., Goldberg, A., Daniel, A. L., Leykin, D., & Adini, B. (2014). Twitter in the CrossFire—The Use of Social Media in the Westgate Mall Terror Attack in Kenya. *PLoS One*, *9*(8), e104136. doi:10.1371/journal.pone.0104136

Singh, S. P., Kumar, A., Darbari, H., Singh, L., Rastogi, A., & Jain, S. (2017). Machine translation using deep learning: An overview. In *Proceedings of the 2017 International Conference on Computer, Communications and Electronics* (pp. 162–167). Academic Press. 10.1109/COMPTELIX.2017.8003957

Song, J., Qin, S., & Zhang, P. (2016). Chinese text categorization based on deep belief networks. In *Proceedings of the 2016 IEEE/ACIS 15th International Conference on Computer and Information Science Computer and Information Science*. IEEE.

Suzuki, K. (2017, September). Overview of deep learning in medical imaging. *Radiological Physics and Technology*, *10*(3), 257–273. doi:10.100712194-017-0406-5 PMID:28689314

Szegedy, C., Wei, L., Yang, J., Sermanet, P., Reed, S., Anguelov, D., . . . Rabinovich, A. (2015). Going deeper with convolutions. In *Proceedings of the IEEE Conference on Computer Vision and Pattern Recognition*. IEEE Press.

Tafti, A., Zotti, R., & Jank, W. (2016). Real-Time Diffusion of Information on Twitter and the Financial Markets. *PLoS One*, *11*(8), e0159226. doi:10.1371/journal.pone.0159226 PMID:27504639

Vippalapalli, V., & Ananthula, S. (2016). Internet of things (IoT) based smart health care System. In *Proceedings of the International Conference on Signal Processing, Communication, Power and Embedded System* (pp. 1229-1233). Academic Press. 10.1109/SCOPES.2016.7955637

Volkova, S., Ayton, E., Porterfield, K., & Corley, C. D. (2017). Forecasting influenza-like illness dynamics for military populations using neural networks and social media. *PLoS One*, 12. PMID:29244814

Wei, J., He, J., Chen, K., Zhou, Y., & Tang, Z. (2017). Collaborative filtering and deep learning-based recommendation system for cold start items. *Expert Systems with Applications*, *69*, 29–39. doi:10.1016/j.eswa.2016.09.040

Xia, F., Su, X., Wang, W., Zhang, C., Ning, Z., & Lee, I. (2016). Bibliographic Analysis of Nature-Based on Twitter and Facebook Altmetrics Data. *PLoS One*, *11*(12), e0165997. doi:10.1371/journal.pone.0165997 PMID:27906981

Xia, W., Wen, Y., Foh, C. H., Niyato, D., & Xie, H. (2015). A survey on software-defined networking. *IEEE Communications Surveys and Tutorials*, *17*(1), 27–51. doi:10.1109/COMST.2014.2330903

Xu, Q., Gel, Y. R., Ramirez, L. L., Nezafati, K., Zhang, Q., & Tsui, K. L. (2017). Forecasting influenza in Hong Kong with Google search Queries and statistical model fusion. *PLoS One*, 12. PMID:28464015

Yoon, H. J., Ramanathan, A., & Tourassi, G. (2016). Multi-task deep neural networks for automated extraction of primary site and laterality information from cancer pathology reports. In P. Angelov, Y. Manolopoulos, L. Iliadis, A. Roy, & M. Vellasco (Eds.), *Advances in Big Data* (pp. 195–204). Cham: Springer.

Yousefi, A. M., & Hamey, L. (2017). Text summarization using unsupervised deep learning. *Expert Systems with Applications*, *68*, 93–105. doi:10.1016/j.eswa.2016.10.017

Zhou, X., Gong, W., Fu, W., & Du, F. (2017). Application of deep learning in object detection. In *Proceedings of the 2017 IEEE/ACIS 16th International Conference on Computer and Information Science* (pp. 631-634). IEEE. 10.1109/ICIS.2017.7960069

Chapter 6
Real-Time Mental Health Monitoring:
The Indian Scenario

Ritika Wason
https://orcid.org/0000-0003-2836-6998
Bharati Vidyapeeth's Institute of Computer Applications and Management (BVICAM), India

Prashant Singh Rana
Thapar Institute of Engineering and Technology, India

Vishal Jain
Bharati Vidyapeeth's Institute of Computer Applications and Management (BVICAM), India

ABSTRACT

Mental disorders have been identified as one among the leading causes of the global disease burden. Despite being one of the first nations in the world to identify mental health as an important indicator of personal well-being and having adequate plans and policies for ensuring the same, one in every seven Indians is affected by mental disorders of varying severity. Through this manuscript we try to analyze how real-time mental health monitoring has helped improve productivity among the global workforce as well as prevented deterioration of individual mental health across the globe. Our main plan of this study is to identify the significant efforts in mental health monitoring across the globe and then chalk out a real-time mental health monitoring framework for India. We also propose a real-time mental health monitoring smartphone-based framework for India we name as SmartMHealth. We describe the basic components of this framework in this study itself.

INTRODUCTION

As per the World Health Organization estimations varied mental health issues cost the world economy approximately an annual $1 trillion loss in global productivity ("India is the most depressed country

DOI: 10.4018/978-1-7998-2101-4.ch006

in the world," 2018; James, 2019). About 450 million people globally experience some form of mental health disorders ("Augmented Mental Health," n.d.). $467 billion is the burden of mental disorders on the US economy annually. Given these startling estimates it is important to realize that a mentally healthy population is a key contributor in the success of any nation. Mental health is a key marker of the emotional, psychological and social well-being of an individual. As per World Health Organization (WHO) estimates, at least 6.5 per cent of the Indian inhabitants experiences some type of severe mental disorder, with no distinctive rural-urban discrepancy (World Health Organization, 2007). Positive mental health is a significant indicator of an individual's well-being at each stage of life (Vihan Sanyal, 2018). In fact, it is a fact that good mental health is one the underlying facets to prolonged and fruitful human life. Varied factors like stress, depression, social anxiety, drug addiction, obsessive compulsive disorder and other personality disorders may add to mental health issues leading to mental illness ("Mental health in India," 2017).

Hence, in the current times when competitive, technologically-driven social life is governing most people it has become imperative to verify the inception of mental illness to retain normal life balance. In an era when augmented mental health is emerging as the new paradigm in mental healthcare through data and digital therapeutics. Achieve early detection and prediction of human mental health is no longer a distant dream. Several machine learning algorithms and artificial intelligence have and can be applied for this realisation (Gurjit & Neena, 2006; Hillestad et al., 2005; Kumar & Hancke, 2015; Paul et al., 2018; Price et al., 2014). Such application when applied in real time shall profit the society at large by serving as a monitoring and control tool to identify onset of deviant or malicious behaviour among otherwise healthy and productive individuals.

The rest of the manuscript is structured as follows: Section I discusses the current scenario of world mental health. Section II highlights the need of effective mental health monitoring solutions. Section III stresses and analyzes the varied available mental health monitoring mechanisms. Section IV details the Indian state of affairs in mental health monitoring. Section V proposes SmartMHealth framework for real-time mental health monitoring. Section VI concludes the discussion.

Need of Mental Health Monitoring

As per global statistics (Kamdar & Wu, 2017), Neuropsychiatric or mental disorders along with cardiovascular diseases, cancer and other communicable diseases are a major contributor to the global burden of diseases and disease-related mortality. Table 1 below lists certain major neuropsychiatric disorders that are currently daunting the human race.

Though these disorder types contribute more than 10% to the prevalent disorders and diseases, however, research in monitoring or control of these disorders is still lagging behind (Kamdar & Wu, 2017). As per WHO estimates many developing and developed nations across the world are bearing the burden of mental disorders. Outcome based monitoring and feedback systems on therapeutic mechanisms have become popular in recent times and have been implemented by several health care providers all over the world. However, these don't seem to be implemented widely in mental health care ("India is the most depressed country in the world," 2018) (Birla, 2019). Mental healthcare as opposed to other non-communicable diseases requires continuous monitoring on a regular basis. Patients with psychiatric disorders may suffer behavioral symptom on a relapsing basis. Hence, to provide optimal care to such patients it is important to have some low-cost, widely available, real-time monitoring mechanisms in

Table 1. Classification of Neuropsychiatric Disorders(Garcia-Ceja et al., 2018).

S. No.	Disorder Class	Signs & Symptoms
1	Mood Disorders like depression, unipolar and bipolar disorders	Hypoactive Electrodermal Response, Reduced Motor Activity (Chang et al., 2014; Sarchiapone et al., 2018; Todder, Caliskan, & Baune, 2007; Volkers et al., 2003), Cardiac Autonomy Disregulation (Chang et al., 2014)
2	Anxiety-Related Disorder (Anorexia, Eating Disorders, OCD (Obsessive Compulsive Disorder), Panic Disorder, Post-Traumatic Stress Syndrome)	Sleep Problems, Heart Palpitations, Unable to stay calm and still
3	Schizophrenia	Reduced Motor Activity (Winograd-Gurvich, Fitzgerald, Georgiou-Karistianis, Bradshaw, & White, 2006)
4	Dementia	Memory Problems, Depression, loss of ability to do everyday tasks
5	Substance Use Disorder	Disorientations

place. Table 1 above establishes that there are direct relations between physiological/behavioral and mood states. Wearable sensors are hence, suitable mechanisms to continuously monitor mental conditions in an unassuming mode (Garcia-Ceja et al., 2018).

As clear from table1 there are multiple neuropsychiatric disorders plaguing humans. However, detection and monitoring of these disorders majorly rely on descriptive criteria. Limited clinical tests or medical devices are available for mental health monitoring (Kamdar & Wu, 2017). Information used by physicians in treating such patients is episodic relying on patient's visit. Tools and mechanisms for continuous, real-time data collection are desirable for such patients. EEG and video monitoring-based mechanisms though effective are insidious and do not allow incessant data collection. Further, output of these methods may not always be easy to interpret. Hence, more robust and patient-friendly mechanisms are desirable to improve the state of mental health monitoring as well as care.

Mental Health Monitoring Mechanisms

Globally current mechanisms to supervise mental health engage the prolific use of wearable technologies (Kamdar & Wu, 2017). Advances in EEG and video monitoring have lagged far behind due to the difficulty involved in their widespread use (Pantelopoulos & Bourbakis, 2009). Wearable technologies have surfaced as an emerging, omnipresent mechanism for providing uninterrupted, quantitative data about an individual (Pantelopoulos & Bourbakis, 2009). These mechanisms allow for easy, passive accumulation of quantitative data enabling proactive mental health management and better treatment. The wearable devices market has grown exceptionally in the last few years. As per Transparency Market Research, "the global wearable technology market is expected to grow from US$750 million in 2012 to US$5.8 billion in 2018" (Wei, 2014). This expansion and growth in the hardware device market forecasts creation and implementation of efficient mechanisms for wearable devices-based mechanisms for real-time mental health monitoring. It is important to note that these products can be easily empowered to measure varied attributes related to the surrounding environment, human physiology and activity. Hence, data can be easily collected passively without interfering the day-to-day activities of the user. Sentiment analysis on such data streams provides more accurate results as compared to surveys. Development and implementation of wearable-device based mental health monitoring frameworks shall enable early diagnosis of unidentified users providing chances for preventive care as well as better diagnosis and treatment for diagnosed patients. Table 2 below details some notable mental health monitoring mechanisms applied in different perspectives.

Real-Time Mental Health Monitoring for India

As per WHO estimates, India was the initial nation globally, to identify the need for incorporation of separate mental health services along with general health services at the primary level (Agarwal, Goel, Ichhpujani, Salhan, & Shrivastava, 1946). The National Mental Health Programme (NMHP) was launched as early as 1982, to treat mental disorders among the community with the available care services. However, as a nation we somehow lagged behind in proper mental health monitoring and treatment of our mental disorder affected population. These mentally ill patients are seen more as a social stigma and are abandoned by their family and community. Our policy and community failure was highlighted in 2001, when an asylum fire in Ramanathapuram district of Tamil Nadu killed 26 mentally ill patients residents of this asylum (Agarwal et al., 1946). Following this incident, the Directorate General of Health Services in May 2001 undertook a Current Situation Analysis (CSA) survey in order to evolve a inclusive plan of action to reenergize the NMHP. As a result, the NMHP was re-reviewed and reoriented at district level also known as District Mental health Programme (DMHP) with an outlay of approximately 190crore in the 10th Five Year plan. The DMHP plan now aims to cover every district across the country to reorient mental colleges and hospitals to establish high standards of care and treatment. The plan receives a huge grant in each of the five year plans and is to be re-reviewed in 2020, as NMHP 2020 (Agarwal et al., 1946). However, despite the long presence of this national policy framework, India as a nation has failed to eliminate the stigma of mental disorders from its society. As per records, Kerala one of the most literate and high life quality states in the country reports rising incidence of suicide cases amongst its population (Agarwal et al., 1946; Bachani & Srivastava, 2012; Manoranjitham et al., 2010). Such is the state of affairs despite the fact that India has a well-laid policy framework for mental health in the form of NMHP and the plan is well-aided financially. It is notable to mention here that it costs Rs. 500/day to maintain a patient in a mental hospital whereas the per capita national expenditure on health is only Rs. 200/year. Gujarat spends more than Rs. 37.2 million on its 4 mental hospitals with a total bed strength of only 680(Agarwal et al., 1946). These facts bring to light certain important observations, which we list below:

- Mental disorders in India are associated with unwarranted social stigmas and superstitions resulting in abandonment of mentally ill patients by immediate family and community. As a result, cost of maintenance of such patients goes up. Destigmatisation of mental disorders is important.
- India should realize that mental health is not related to the purse but to the mind.
- It's time to call for a spirit of invention of practical solutions empowered with available technical skills to accomplish real-time mental health monitoring and care. IoT enabled services and smart devices can be used as a basis to design a framework for continuous mental health monitoring of our able population as well as mentally-ill patients to enable early identification of disorders and ensure their proper prevention and treatment.

Globally lot of notable work has already been conducted in smart health monitoring through m-Health applications as well as through wearable biosensors (Berrouiguet et al., 2018; Chandrashekar, 2018; Chen, Ma, Song, Lai, & Hu, 2016; Pantelopoulos & Bourbakis, 2009)

Some of these applications also monitor the varied mental disorders of patients providing them a close loop monitoring and interaction with their physicians. However, recognizable volume of this work especially in general mental health assessment and analysis of seemingly normal population but on risk of mental health disorders is missing especially in India ("Mental health in India," 2017). As per

Table 2. Notable Mental Health Monitoring Mechanisms

S. No.	Title	Ref.	Description	Achievements
1.	PRISM: A Data-Driven Platform for Monitoring Mental Health	(Kamdar & Wu, 2017)	Recapitulates user-reported ratings of their emotional state through applying supervised and unsupervised learning to PRISM — Passive, Real-time Information for Sensing Mental Health. Integrates motion, light and heart rate data obtained from smart watch application along with user interactions and text obtained from a web application.	Platform enables collection of incessant streams of passive data for near the beginning diagnosis or regular monitoring of patients with mental disorders.
2.	A Zigbee-Based Animal Health Monitoring System	(Kumar & Hancke, 2015)	An animal health monitoring system (AHMS) for checking the physiological parameters like rumination, body temperature, and heart rate with neighboring temperature and humidity has been developed. The system can also analyze the stress level corresponding to the thermal humidity index (THI).	The device has proved to be helpful in low-cost health care of livestock.
3.	Consume: A Privacy-preserving authorization and authentication service for connecting with health and wellbeing APIs	(Wetzels et al., 2018)	Current proliferation of Internet of things (IoT) enabled devices in health and well-being domain empowers individuals to monitor their health. However, the variety of devices leads to complexity of data aggregation and scattered overviews. Consume facilitates the integration of these APIs and data aggregation over a common platform.	Consume promises to aid researchers in development of personalized healthcare systems. It has provided the base for a universal data aggregation system for varied APIs. Thus, it shall accelerate development of new health monitoring as well data collection devices.
4.	Mental Health Monitoring with multimodal sensing and machine learning: A survey	(Garcia-Ceja et al., 2018)	Surveys research work in mental health monitoring systems through the use of ubiquitous sensing technologies for data collection and machine learning to predict the related user contextual information.	The papers surveys all research works on mental state monitoring through sensors that gather wearable data. The classification given is helpful in understanding the basics.
5.	Complexity Index from a Personalized Wearable Monitoring System for Assessing Remission in Mental Health	(Lanata, Valenza, Nardelli, Gentili, & Scilingo, 2015)	Introduces PSYCHE, a t-shirt with embedded sensors for monitoring electrocardiogram heart rate variability (HRV) series, respiration activity and activity recognition for patients suffering with mental disorders.	Continuous interface between clinicians and patients advances the quality of life of patients aiding the clinicians in the analysis and preventing relapses.
6.	Ginger.io Commercial app (The Ginger App)	(Matheson, 2014)	The app passively analyzes mobile data to detect if a patient with mental illness is acting symptomatic. The symptoms may vary from lethargy to infrequent texts. On detecting an unusual pattern the app sends messages to the patient as well as their health care provider.	The app is currently being used by thousands of patients at more than 25 health care institutions and academic centers across the United States. The app has also been applied for research at a number of universities across the globe.

WHO, "Vigilant monitoring and assessment of a nation's mental health policy and plan are essential for improving services, healing and care and for guiding future policy directions"(World Health Organization, 2007).WHO under its Mental Health Policy and Service Guidance Package has laid down clear guidelines to assist nation's in laying down policies and plans to assist nation's in improving the mental health of their populations. Mental health remains the elephant in the room in the formidable corridors of corporate India. Of the country's 1.1 million active registered companies, only 1,000 are estimated to have a structured employee assistance programme (EAP) for mental health (James, 2019). Notable studies have already been conducted on varied aspects related to mental well-being of Indian population (Hasumi, Ahsan, Couper, Aguayo, & Jacobsen, 2012). However, practically efficient solutions are still a distant dream.

SmartMHealth: Real-Time Mental Health Monitoring Framework for India

Our SmartMHealth framework aims at the development of a low-cost smartphone based, unobtrusive solution for continuous mental, emotional and activity status monitoring of individuals. The proposed system shall provide real-time feedback about an individual's mental health. This continuous data when shared with a central monitoring unit (node) or self-checked by individuals can alarm in case of possible imminent mental health threatening conditions like stress, increased cardiac activity etc.

The proposed SmartMHealth App shall be a smart phone-based app to monitor physiological, emotional signals as well as physical activity rate of its user. Figure 1. depicts the major components of the proposed SmartMHealth framework.

Figure 1 visualizes the concept of a possible SmartMHealth app that could passively monitor the user's usage patterns and send alarm signals to the central monitoring node in case of any deviation. However, this should not be considered as standard system design, as actual implementation may vary significantly. As can be seen from Fig.1 of all possible smart wearable devices we have chosen SmartMHealth as a smartphone enabled app. It can be argued that any other low-cost smart device can also be used, however smartphone was a natural choice as almost 94% of the world population are cell phone subscribers and Internet users irrespective of external factors like place of residence, level of education, etc. (Chan, Estève, Fourniols, Escriba, & Campo, 2012; Vashist, Schneider, & Luong, 2014). Further, behavioral health analytics startup Ginger.io has also identified smartphones as "automated diaries" that can provide valuable insight into the mental well-being of any individual including mentally ill patients (Matheson, 2014). Smartphones inherently produce significant behavioral data regarding an individual in the form of location, calling and texting records as well as app usage history. This data can be easily used to map a user's daily patterns. A deviation in this pattern is enough to raise an alarm. The alarm can be transmitted to the individual under observation as well as their health care provider as well as the central monitoring node. The central monitoring node with the help of appropriate machine learning algorithms can help analyze the humongous passive health data collected to usable information for passive health care monitoring of healthy individuals. The details of the smartphone-based apps, required resources for creation of the central monitoring unit as well as the machine learning algorithms are being worked out at the time of this writing and shall soon be discussed and implemented. This tool would be effective in realizing the world of augmented mental health.

Figure 1. Architecture of Smartphone based SmartMHealth App

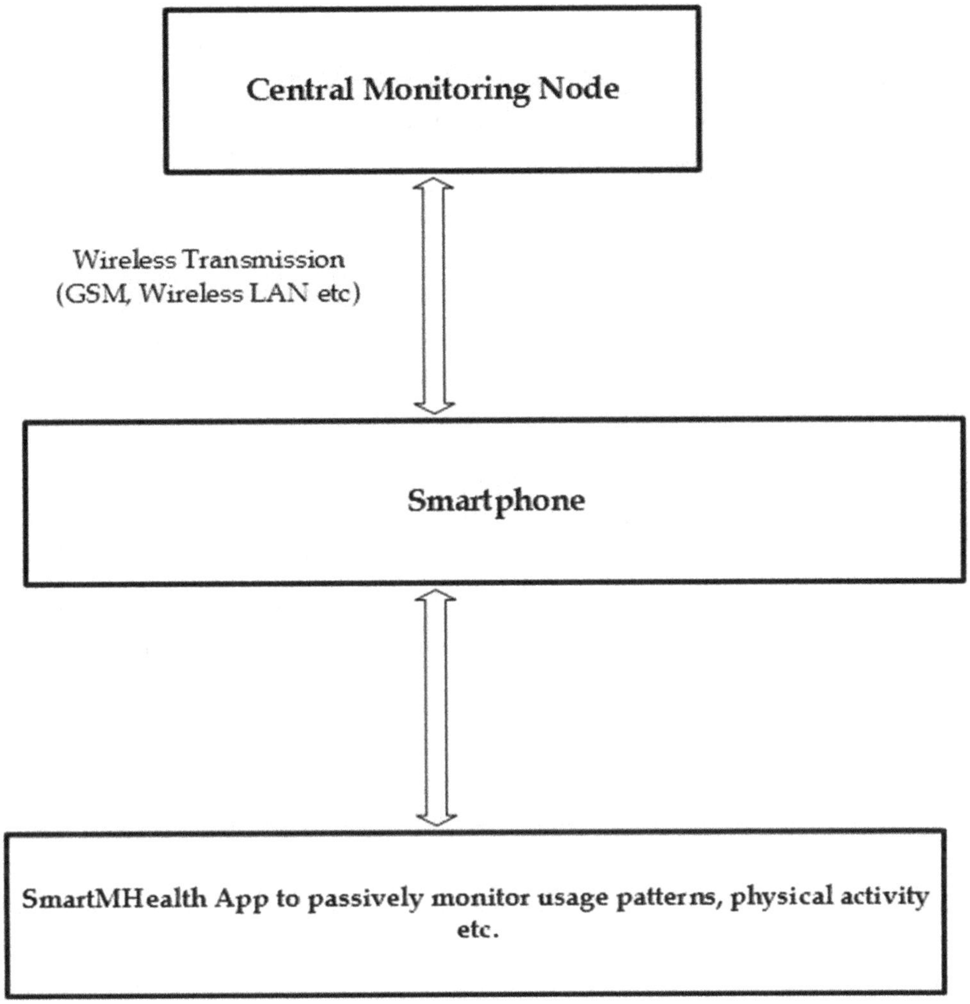

CONCLUSION AND FUTURE SCOPE

As per our analysis, for effective solution of mental disorders India actually requires a paradigm shift from the hospital care to community care. This also calls for an early diagnosis of alarming mental conditions and thus shifting from treatment to prevention. As a country, we need to rise and realize that mental health is not a social stigma, it is not a government policy initiative and neither just a personal initiative. Instead mental well-being and health is more of community care and monitoring.

REFERENCES

Agarwal, S. P., Goel, D. S., Ichhpujani, R. L., Salhan, R. N., & Shrivastava, S. (1946). *Mental Health An Indian Perspective Directorate General of Health Services Ministry of Health and Family Welfare New Delhi*. Retrieved from https://s3.amazonaws.com/academia.edu.documents/38096568/MENTAL_HEALTH_-INDIA.pdf?AWSAccessKeyId=AKIAIWOWYYGZ2Y53UL3A&Expires=1557355752&Signature=gmg4Gum%2Fh5cENamksdHfPZpuii8%3D&response-content-disposition=inline%3Bfilename%3DPostgraduate_psychiatric_

Augmented Mental Health. (n.d.). Retrieved from https://www.augmentedmentalhealth.com/

Bachani, D., & Srivastava, R. (2012). Burden of NCDs, Policies and Programme for Prevention and Control of NCDs in India. *Indian Journal of Community Medicine*, *36*(5), 7. doi:10.4103/0970-0218.94703 PMID:22628916

Berrouiguet, S., Perez-Rodriguez, M. M., Larsen, M., Baca-García, E., Courtet, P., & Oquendo, M. (2018). From eHealth to iHealth: Transition to participatory and personalized medicine in mental health. *Journal of Medical Internet Research*, *20*(1), 1–8. doi:10.2196/jmir.7412 PMID:29298748

Birla, N. (2019). Mental health in India: 7.5% of country affected; less than 4,000 experts available. The Economic Times. Retrieved from https://economictimes.indiatimes.com/magazines/panache/mental-health-in-india-7-5-of-country-affected-less-than-4000-experts-available/articleshow/71500130.cms?from=mdr

Chan, M., Estève, D., Fourniols, J.-Y., Escriba, C., & Campo, E. (2012). Smart wearable systems: Current status and future challenges. *Artificial Intelligence in Medicine*, *56*(3), 137–156. doi:10.1016/j.artmed.2012.09.003 PMID:23122689

Chandrashekar, P. (2018). Do mental health mobile apps work: Evidence and recommendations for designing high-efficacy mental health mobile apps. *mHealth*, *4*, 6–6. doi:10.21037/mhealth.2018.03.02 PMID:29682510

Chang, H. A., Chang, C. C., Tzeng, N. S., Kuo, T. B. J., Lu, R. B., & Huang, S. Y. (2014). Heart rate variability in unmedicated patients with bipolar disorder in the manic phase. *Psychiatry and Clinical Neurosciences*, *68*(9), 674–682. doi:10.1111/pcn.12178 PMID:24612182

Chen, M., Ma, Y., Song, J., Lai, C. F., & Hu, B. (2016). Smart Clothing: Connecting Human with Clouds and Big Data for Sustainable Health Monitoring. *Mobile Networks and Applications*, *21*(5), 825–845. doi:10.100711036-016-0745-1

Garcia-Ceja, E., Riegler, M., Nordgreen, T., Jakobsen, P., Oedegaard, K. J., & Tørresen, J. (2018). Mental health monitoring with multimodal sensing and machine learning: A survey. *Pervasive and Mobile Computing*, *51*, 1–26. doi:10.1016/j.pmcj.2018.09.003

Gurjit, K., & Neena, G. (2006). E-health: A New Perspective on Global Health (india). *Journal of Evolution and Tenhnology*, *15*(1), 23–35.

Hasumi, T., Ahsan, F., Couper, C. M., Aguayo, J. L., & Jacobsen, K. H. (2012). Parental involvement and mental well-being of Indian adolescents. *Indian Pediatrics*, *49*(11), 915–918. doi:10.100713312-012-0218-y PMID:22728626

Hillestad, R., Bigelow, J., Bower, A., Girosi, F., Meili, R., Scoville, R., & Taylor, R. (2005). Can electronic medical record systems transform health care? Potential health benefits, savings, and costs. *Health Affairs*, *24*(5), 1103–1117. doi:10.1377/hlthaff.24.5.1103 PMID:16162551

India is the most depressed country in the world. (2018). India Today. Retrieved from https://www.indiatoday.in/education-today/gk-current-affairs/story/india-is-the-most-depressed-country-in-the-world-mental-health-day-2018-1360096-2018-10-10

James, N. (2019). Mental health is the elephant in the rooms of corporate India. The Hindu Business Line. Retrieved from https://www.thehindubusinessline.com/blink/cover/mental-health-the-elephant-in-the-rooms-of-corporate-india/article30211327.ece

Kamdar, M., & Wu, M. (2017). PRISM: A data-driven platform for monitoring mental health. *Physiology & Behavior*, *176*(1), 139–148. doi:10.1016/j.physbeh.2017.03.040 PMID:28363838

Kumar, A., & Hancke, G. P. (2015). A zigbee-based animal health monitoring system. *IEEE Sensors Journal*, *15*(1), 610–617. doi:10.1109/JSEN.2014.2349073

Lanata, A., Valenza, G., Nardelli, M., Gentili, C., & Scilingo, E. P. (2015). Complexity index from a personalized wearable monitoring system for assessing remission in mental health. *IEEE Journal of Biomedical and Health Informatics*, *19*(1), 132–139. doi:10.1109/JBHI.2014.2360711 PMID:25291802

Manoranjitham, S. D., Rajkumar, A. P., Thangadurai, P., Prasad, J., Jayakaran, R., & Jacob, K. S. (2010). Risk factors for suicide in rural south India. *The British Journal of Psychiatry*, *196*(1), 26–30. doi:10.1192/bjp.bp.108.063347 PMID:20044655

Matheson, R. (2014). Mental-health monitoring goes mobile. MIT News. Retrieved from http://news.mit.edu/2014/mental-health-monitoring-goes-mobile-0716

Pantelopoulos, A., & Bourbakis, N. (2008, August). A survey on wearable biosensor systems for health monitoring. In *Proceedings of the 2008 30th Annual International Conference of the IEEE Engineering in Medicine and Biology Society* (pp. 4887-4890). IEEE. doi:10.1109/iembs.2008.4650309

Paul, Y., Hickok, E., Sinha, A., Tiwari, U., Mohandas, S., Ray, S. … Bidare, P.M. (2018). *Artificial Intelligence in the Healthcare Industry in India*. Retrieved from https://cis-india.org/internet-governance/files/ai-and-healtchare-report

Price, M., Yuen, E. K., Goetter, E. M., Herbert, J. D., Forman, E. M., Acierno, R., & Ruggiero, K. J. (2014). mHealth: A mechanism to deliver more accessible, more effective mental health care. *Clinical Psychology & Psychotherapy*, *21*(5), 427–436. doi:10.1002/cpp.1855 PMID:23918764

Sanyal, V. (2018). Why India needs to focus on mental health and wellbeing. Yourstory. Retrieved from https://yourstory.com/2018/10/india-needs-focus-mental-health-wellbeing

Sarchiapone, M., Gramaglia, C., Iosue, M., Carli, V., Mandelli, L., Serretti, A., ... Zeppegno, P. (2018). The association between electrodermal activity (EDA), depression and suicidal behaviour: A systematic review and narrative synthesis. *BMC Psychiatry*, *18*(1), 22. doi:10.118612888-017-1551-4 PMID:29370787

Todder, D., Caliskan, S., & Baune, B. T. (2007). Longitudinal changes of day-time and night-time gross motor activity in clinical responders and non-responders of major depression. *The World Journal of Biological Psychiatry*, 1–9. doi:10.1080/15622970701403081 PMID:19921969

Vashist, S., Schneider, E., & Luong, J. (2014). Commercial Smartphone-Based Devices and Smart Applications for Personalized Healthcare Monitoring and Management. *Diagnostics (Basel)*, *4*(3), 104–128. doi:10.3390/diagnostics4030104 PMID:26852680

Volkers, A. C., Tulen, J. H. M., Van Den Broek, W. W., Bruijn, J. A., Passchier, J., & Pepplinkhuizen, L. (2003). Motor activity and autonomic cardiac functioning in major depressive disorder. *Journal of Affective Disorders*, *76*(1–3), 23–30. doi:10.1016/S0165-0327(02)00066-6 PMID:12943930

Wei, J. (2014). How wearables intersect with the cloud and the internet of things: Considerations for the developers of wearables. *IEEE Consumer Electronics Magazine*, *3*(3), 53–56. doi:10.1109/MCE.2014.2317895

Wetzels, M., Ayoola, I., Bogers, S., Peters, P., Chen, W., & Feijs, L. (2018). Consume: A privacy-preserving authorisation and authentication service for connecting with health and wellbeing APIs. *Pervasive and Mobile Computing*, *43*, 20–26. doi:10.1016/j.pmcj.2017.11.002

Winograd-Gurvich, C., Fitzgerald, P. B., Georgiou-Karistianis, N., Bradshaw, J. L., & White, O. B. (2006). Negative symptoms: A review of schizophrenia, melancholic depression and Parkinson's disease. *Brain Research Bulletin*, *70*(4–6), 312–321. doi:10.1016/j.brainresbull.2006.06.007 PMID:17027767

World Health Organization. (2007). *Monitoring and evaluation of mental health policies and plans*. Retrieved from http://www.who.int/mental_health/policy/services/14-monitoringevaluation_HKprinter.pdf

World Health Organization. (2017). Mental health in India. Retrieved from http://www.searo.who.int/india/topics/mental_health/about_mentalhealth/en/

Chapter 7
Disease Diagnosis and Treatment Using Deep Learning Algorithms for the Healthcare System

Nirbhay Kumar Chaubey
https://orcid.org/0000-0001-6575-7723
Ganpat University, India

Prisilla Jayanthi
https://orcid.org/0000-0002-4961-9010
K. G. Reddy College of Engineering and Technology, India

ABSTRACT

This chapter explicates deep learning algorithms for healthcare opportunities. Deep Learning is a group of neural network algorithms and learns from various levels of representation and abstraction to aid in the data interpretation. Since the datasets get bigger, computers become more powerful, and the training of the datasets (images or numeric) gets much easier and the results achieved using deep learning are better. In contrast to machine-learning algorithms that rely on large amounts of labelled data, human cognition can find structure in unlabeled data, a technique known as unsupervised learning. It was noted that using deep learning algorithms on the dataset will reduce the number of unnecessary biopsies in future. In this chapter, the authors study deep learning algorithms to diagnose diabetic retinopathy retinal images and training a convolution neural network (CNN) algorithm to identify object tumors from a large set of brain tumor images.

INTRODUCTION

In this study, the authors' throw light on the algorithms of the artificial neural networks (ANN) and convolution neural network (CNN) which is implemented for the diagnosis of the various diseases in

DOI: 10.4018/978-1-7998-2101-4.ch007

the healthcare. Diagnosing the disease early and providing the treatment is key principle of the health care. Artificial Intelligence is used for healthcare services and the major areas of AI are early detections, diagnoses, and treatment followed with results of prediction and evaluation of prognosis. The prediction of any diseases is carried out by ANN and CNN algorithm. In this chapter, the algorithms of machine learning (ML) namely regressions have proved to analyses the logistic and confidential interval for the disease. ML algorithms basically need some data, to use as training set (Granville, 2017). For prediction and treatment analysis of disease were carried out using ML (Jiang, 2017). ANN is used to predict diseases of known and unknown symptoms. The study on Diabetic Retinopathy (DR) using Inception and CNN is highlighted in this chapter. A case of tumor detection using CNN is also implemented. DL techniques were implemented for bio-signal analyses and classification of growing number of applications (Ganapathy, 2018). DL techniques are used in healthcare, industries, and research perspectives (Goodfellow, 2016); and are used for classification of images, detection of various objects, segmentation, registration, and other tasks (Litjens, 2017). The study includes application area like neuro, retinal, pulmonary, digital pathology, breast, cardiac, abdominal, and musculoskeletal.

REGRESSION

Regression is machine learning approach which helps to determine the strength of the relationship between one response variable with a series of predictor variables.

SUPPORT VECTOR MACHINE (SVM) DECISION TREES - LOGISTICS REGRESSION – PREDICTION OF HEART DISEASE

The rule-based framework provided by (Mythili, 2013) shown in the figure 1 for predicting the heart disease using SVM decision tree and Logistic Regression. The method is based on six modules involving preprocessing, training, testing with individual models, rules for application, and comparison of results for the prediction of heart disease. The database was collected from Cleveland Heart Disease Dataset UCI repository with 13 features such as age, sex, chest pain type, resting blood pressure, serum cholesterol in mg/dl, fasting blood sugar > 120 mg/dl, resting electrocardiographic result, maximum heart rate achieved, exercise induced angina, ST depression induced by exercise relative to rest, the slope of the peak exercise ST segment, and number of major vessels (0-3) colored by fluoroscopy. All these feature helps in predicting the disease and trains the required model, here regression model and decision tree model is built. The results proved that there is a need for more complex models and combinations among the models to improve the performance and to increase the accuracy of predicting the heart disease. The system will be known to be intelligent with huge amount of data fed into the system database.

Regression –Confidential Interval- Thyroid – Gynec Case

In this case study of regression, few cases were obtained from Gandhi Hospital Secunderabad, India which indicates gynec cases that includes thyroid cases leading to abortion, and healthy cases. The data analysis was carried out on a licensed Stata IC 12.1.

Figure 1. Framework for predicting heart disease (Mythili, 2013)

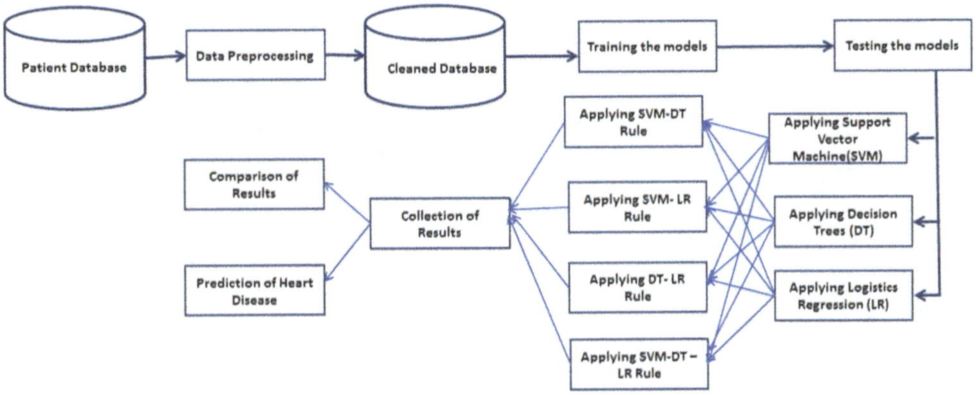

The dataset of abortion cases and healthy cases were considered as study-1 with attributes like systolic pressure, diastolic pressure, hemoglobin, red blood cell, and pulse rate as shown in Table 1 and Table 2. The thyroid hormone dataset (study-2) shown in table 3 and table 4 included T2, T3 and Tsh apart from all the attributes included for the study-1. The regression was calculated in two cases which imply that R-square should be in between 0 and 1. The statistical measure, R-squared supports to understand how close the data gets fit into the regression line and also known as the coefficient of determination. The percentage of response variable variation which is explained by a linear model; R-squared is represented as Explained variation / Total variation. In table 2, the calculated value of the R-squared for study -1 is calculated as 0.0825 between Hb vs BP_U, BP_L, PR which is close to 1 this includes all the parameters except RBC and WBC. In table 4, the calculated value of the R-squared for study-2 is found to be 0.7475 which is very near to 1. It proves that the R-squared value obtained is suitable and lies between 0 and 1.

LOGISTICS REGRESSION – ANALYSIS OF ELECTROMAGNETIC RADIATION- ENVIRONMENTAL POLLUTION

A case study of environmental pollution; the electromagnetic radiation emitted by the mobile, causes various health diseases. Logistics regression was calculated on the data obtained from www.tarangsanchar.

Table 1. Regression for healthy case with HB, WBC, RBC as attributes

	SS	df	ms	No. of Obs. = 35 F (2, 32) = 0.10 Pb > F = 0.905 R-sq = 0.0062 Ad Sq = -0.0559 RMSE = 1.2886	
Model	0.3323	2	0.166		
Res.	53.13	32	1.66		
Total	53.46	34	1.57		
HB	Co-ef	SE	t	p > t	95% CI
WBC	-0.067	0.161	-0.41	0.68	- 0.39 to 0.262
RBC	0.033	0.121	0.28	0.78	- 0.213 to 0.280
Cons	10.42	1.259	8.28	0.00	7.85 to 12.98

Table 2. Regression for Healthy patient with attributes- HB BP_U BP_L PR

	SS	df	ms	No. of Obs. = 35 F (2, 31) = 0.93 Pb > F = 0.4384 R-sq = 0.0825 Ad Sq = -0.0063 RMSE = 1.2579	
Model	4.41	3	1.470		
Res.	49.05	31	1.582		
Total	53.46	34	1.572		
HB	Co-ef	SE	t	p > t	95% CI
BP_U	-0.0114	0.0143	-0.80	0.428	- 0.0406 to 0.0176
BP_L	0.0151	0.0124	1.22	0.233	- 0.0102 to 0.0405
PR	0.0160	0.0165	0.97	0.339	-0.0176 to 0.0498
cons	10.42	1.259	8.28	0.00	4.59 to 13.09

Table 3. Regress with HB RBC WBC of thyroid patient

	SS	df	ms	No of Ob. = 9 F (2, 6) = 6.45 Pb > F = 0.0320 R-sq = 0.6824 Ad Sq = 0.5766 RMSE = 0.83266	
Model	8.940	2	4.470		
Res.	4.159	6	0.693		
Total	13.1	8	1.637		
HB	Co-ef	SE	t	p > t	95% CI
RBC	0.270	0.415	0.65	0.539	- 0.746 to 1.287
WBC	-1.361	0.656	-2.07	0.0.83	- 2.967 to 0.2447
Cons	20.756	3.195	6.50	0.001	12.937 to 28.575

Table 4. Regress Hb BPU BPL PR T3 T4 Tsh -of Thyroid patient dataset

	SS	df	ms	No. of Obs. = 9 F (6, 2) = 0.99 Pb > F = 0.5824 R-sq = 0.7475 Ad sq = -0.0101 RMSE = 1.2861	
Model	9.791	6	1.631		
Res.	3.308	2	1.654		
Total	13.1	8	1.637		
HB	Co-ef	SE	t	p > t	95% CI
BPU	0.0083	0.0482	0.17	0.878	-0.1991 to 0.2158
BPL	0.0104	0.0985	0.11	0.925	-0.4134 to 0.4343
PR	0.0843	0.0644	1.31	0.321	-0.1929 to 0.3616
T3	6.329	3.6048	1.76	0.221	-9.181 to 21.839
T4	-1.658	1.532	-1.08	0.392	-8.253 to 4.936
Tsh	0.150	0.346	0.46	0.706	-1.341 to 1.642
Cons	12.107	9.449	1.28	0.329	-28.550 to 52.765

Figure 2. Mobile towers in city near to residential areas

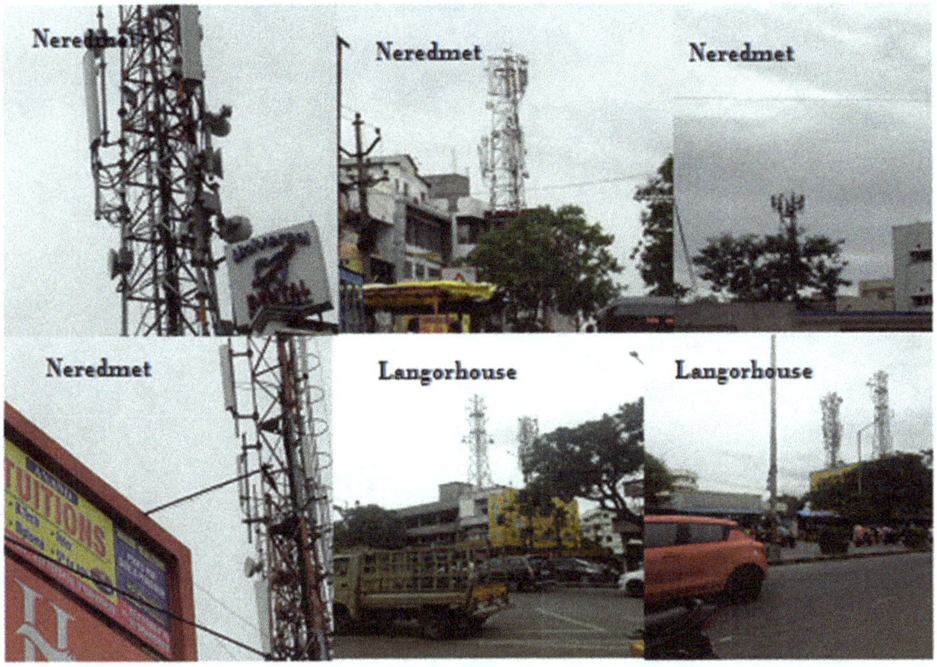

gov.in from 2018 to 2020. Geographic Information System (GIS) mapping of the mobile towers in the year 2017 -2018 and 2018-2019 in Telangana (TS) and 2018-2019 and 2019-2020 in Andhra Pradesh (AP) shown in figure 3 respectively. The people living near the mobile towers in figure 2 were unknowingly associated with health risk in the long-term.

From the data collected for AP state, the logistic regression (LR) was calculated for the year 2018-2020 as shown in table 5. In three iterations (I), the log likelihood (LL) was -12.476 in the first and the remaining it was zero for the number of observations equal to 18. The confidence interval (CI) calculated between Measured-value-Watt-per-meter (MWP) as the dependent and DoT-Prescribed-Limit (DPL) as independent variable and poisson exposure variable is DPL was shown in table 6.

I0: LL = -12.476
I1: LL = 0
I2: LL = 0

In TS state for the year 2018- 2020, LR was calculated shown in table 7. In three iterations LL was -12.4766 in the first and the remaining it was zero for the number of observations equal to 18.

I0: LL = -12.4766
I1: LL = 0
I2: LL = 0

Figure 3. mobile mapping in Telangana and Andhra Pradesh

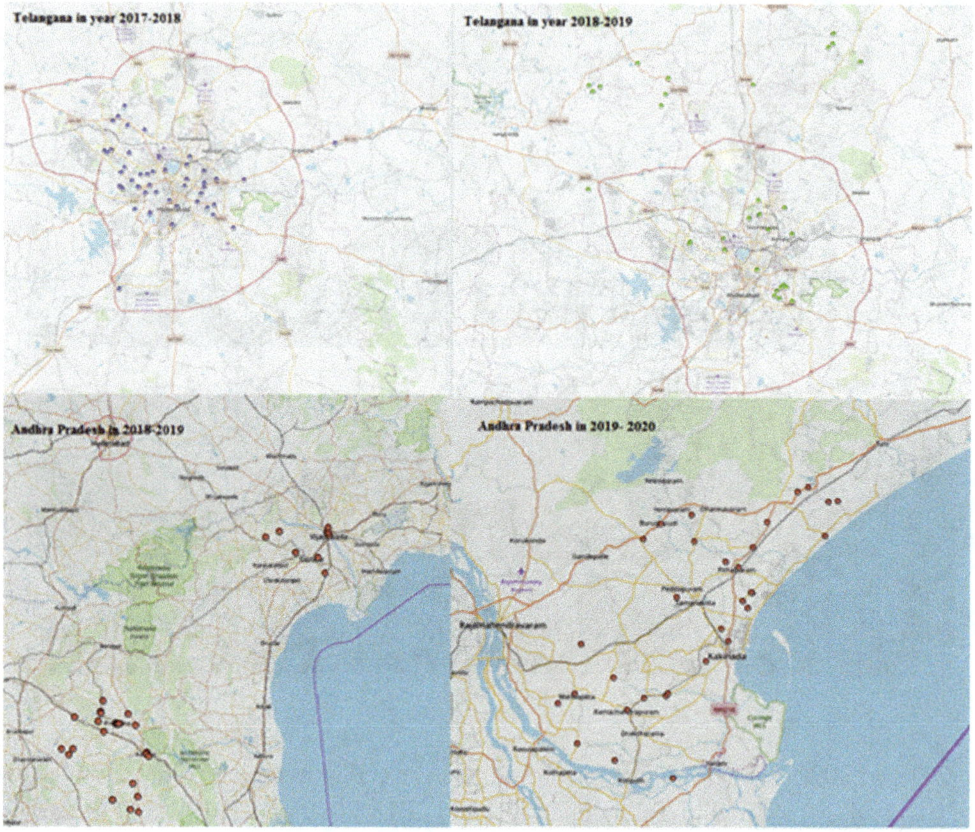

Table 5. Logistics regression (in AP)

LR LL= 0	Obs. = 18 Wald chi2 (0) = . Pr > chi2 = .
MWP DPL: 73.327	Coef. S E z P>lzl [95% Cl] - - - - -

Table 6. Confidence Interval (AP)

Var.	Exp	Mean	SE	95% CI
MWP	47473.38	0	0	0 to 0.00007

Table 7. Logistics regression (TS)

LR LL = 0	Obs. = 18 Wald chi2 (0) = . Prob > chi2 = .
MWP DPL: 74.0445	Coef. S E z P>|z| [95% CI] - - - - -

The confidence interval calculated between the dependent (MWP) and independent variable (DPL) and poisson exposure variable is DPL was shown in table 8. From the above calculation it showed that people living very near to the mobile towers were at risk for health diseases.

ARTIFICIAL NEURAL NETWORK

ANN is nonlinear statistical data modeling tool with the various complex relationships between inputs and outputs. In this model, several inputs are passed into the number of hidden layers to get the predicted outcome in the output layer. The hidden layer depends on the user requirement. ANN is and was successful in diagnosing the various diseases and predicts the disease faster.

ANN FOR PREDICTING DISEASES

(Weng, 2016) discusses about neural network that have been successful in assisting the diagnosis of various diseases. The significant improvement through training a finite number of neural networks for the generalization ability of learning systems and the results obtained. (Dakappa, 2018) in their case study implemented ML algorithm named ANN classifier that classified infectious and non-infectious diseases from 24 hour continuous recording of patient tympanic temperature. A study was carried out on 103 patients who suffered with undifferentiated fever. ANN classifier was able to give the accuracy of 91.31. Mantzaris (2008) in their case study explored ANN models for classification efficiency in an orthopedic disease. Multilayer perceptrons (MLPs) and probabilistic neural networks (PNNs) were used for the osteoporosis risk factor prediction. MLPs and PNNs are feed-forward networks; and PNN assist specialists in osteoporosis prediction, avoiding unneeded further testing with bone densitometry. (Selvi, 2000) in their work implemented ANN model called BIONET for diagnosis of diseases. BIONET is a multilayer feedforward neural network with number of hidden nodes. Designing and developing a model, diagnosing diseases and solution strategy for solving XOR problem. (Wahyunggoro, 2013) discussed about the use of NN for predicting the tuberculosis disease in US, based on the historical data.

Table 8. Confidence Interval (TS)

Var.	Exp	Mean	S E	95% CI
MWP	19.2096	0.0520	0.0520	0.0013 to 0.2900

Table 9. Network Simulation Parameters

Arch.	Train. Algo.	Corr.	R-sq	Avg RE
9-4-1	QP	0.98	0.95	0.02
9-4-1	QN	0.95	0.87	0.04
9-4-1	LM	0.95	0.38	0.08

The datasets were obtained from the summary of notifiable diseases from the Morbidity and Mortality Weekly Report published by Centers for Disease Control and Prevention (CDC). Different NN models were tested to select the most appropriate model. The results were obtained with three layers of multi-layer perceptron with inputs of 9 nodes, hidden layers of 4 nodes, and output as 1 node as the best model. The three different training algorithms applied were: Quick Propagation (QP), Quasi-Newton (QN) and Lavemberg-Marquardt (LM). QP is the most accurate algorithm since the value of correlation and R-square was near to 1. Average RE value of 0.029 indicates a good correlation between the targets and predicted outputs shown in table 9.

CONVOLUTION NEURAL NETWORK

(Abiyev, 2018) discussed about CNNs for diagnosis of chest diseases. For this case study back-propagation neural networks (BPNNs) with supervised learning and CpNNs with unsupervised learning are built for diagnosis chest diseases. (Sharif, 2019) implemented VGG16 and VGG19 deep convolutional (CNN) supported on Euclidean Fisher Vector for detecting gastrointestinal tract (GIT) infections such as ulcers, bleeding, polyps, Crohn's disease and cancer. Geometric features are extracted from segmented disease region. The challenges exist in this domain, such as lesion shape, colour, texture, size and irregularity. (Prajapati, 2017) experimented CNN performance for diagnosis the datasets of labeled dental data. Accuracies improvement was implemented by transfer learning. Labeled dataset consists of 251 Radio Visiography (RVG) x-ray images of 3 different classes that are used for classification. DL is applied for MRI processing chain, retrieval of image (Shen, 2017), segmentation and disease prediction (Lundervold, 2019).

Deep Learning for Diabetic Eye Disease Detection (Diabetic Retinopathy)

In a case study of diabetic retinopathy (DR), Varun Gulshan (2016) used an optimization algorithm called back-propagation, deep learning algorithm to detect DR (Yalçin, 2018). This disease is known to be one of the fastest growing blindness among the diabetic patients. Almost 415 million diabetic patients are suffering throughout the world. This disease can be treated; else it can also lead to irreversible blindness. The authors have obtained 128,000 images from different hospital database as dataset, evaluated by 3-7 ophthalmologists (OP) from a panel of 54 OP. This dataset was used to train a deep NN algorithm to detect referable DR. The validation sets images were graded by OP for the presence of DR, diabetic macular edema, and image quality using an annotation tool. Based on the International Clinical Diabetic Retinopathy scale, DR severities were graded as none, mild, moderate, severe, or proliferative as shown in table 10. US board-certified OP with the highest rate of self-consistency were

Figure 4. Diabetic Retinopathy

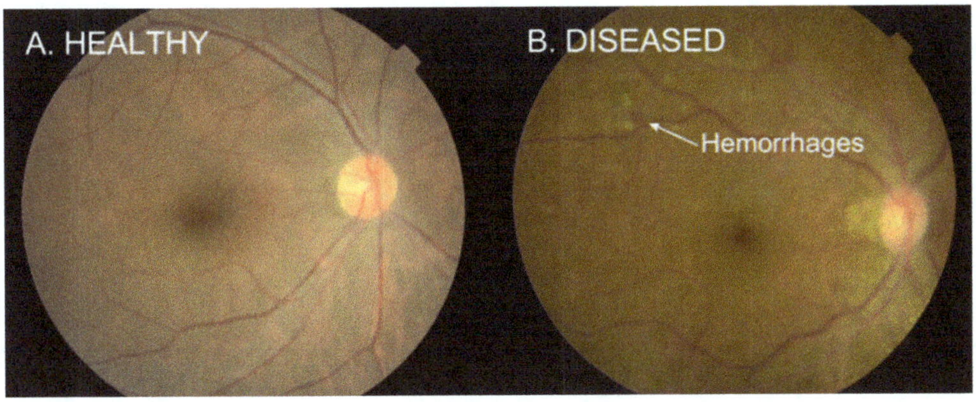

invited to grade the clinical validation sets, EyePACS-1 (n = 8) and Messidor-2 (n = 7). The decision of an image was classified as referable if ≥ 50% of OP graded served as the reference standard for both refer-ability and grade-ability.

Deep learning (DL) neural network processes a large mathematical function with millions of parameters to perform a given task. For training this function, it requires a large set of images for which DR severity is known as training set.

Each image is given by a function with the severity grade and is compared with the known grade from the training set, and parameters of the function are modified to decrease the error on that image. The process is repeated for every image in the training set over many times, and the function learns to compute accurately severity of DR from the pixel intensities of the image for all images in the training set.

The continuous number between 0 and 1 for DR and other DR classifications are generated by trained NN. Plotting receiver operating curves by varying the operating threshold and development set and 2 operating points for the algorithm were selected. The first operating point estimates the OP specificity from the set derivation for detecting referable DR (approximately 98%) and algorithm's performances was found to give better results. The second operating point corresponded to a sensitivity of 97% for detecting referable DR because a high sensitivity is a prerequisite in a potential screening tool. In evaluation, an algorithm is based on deep Machine Learning that produced high sensitivity and specificity for detecting referable DR.

In other case study (Masood, 2017), the performance of Convolutional Neural Networks (CNNs) has been exceptional for the recognizing of various real objects. The pre-trained models perform object classification from an image of the object which is given as an input. However, the pre-trained models are retrained for the set of classes; the model retains to measure the severity of DR in eye images the scale of 0-5. A CNN classifier designed from Inception V3 network is trained for ImageNet, for 5-class severity (Table 11) classification performed best with an accuracy of 48.2%. The procedure consists of two main steps namely Image preprocessing and retraining the Inception V3 (figure 5).

Image preprocessing can be carried out using three major subtasks-

1. The images are down sampled to a specific radius.
2. Removal of Local Average Color from the images.
3. The borders of image are cropped.

Inception V3 model was been used to achieve the outputs as shown in the table 11; because of its deepest architecture and the increased size in terms of both width and height, it was used for DR. The table 12 describes the architecture layers of the Inception with output size, parameters, and strides. In simple terms the complete outcome of the Inception model with the parameter.

Table 10. The dataset with number of images available (Masood, 2017)

Class	Number
0 (no DR)	25810
1 (mild)	2443
2 (average)	5292
3 (extreme)	873
4 (proliferate DR)	708

Figure 5. Inception V3 model

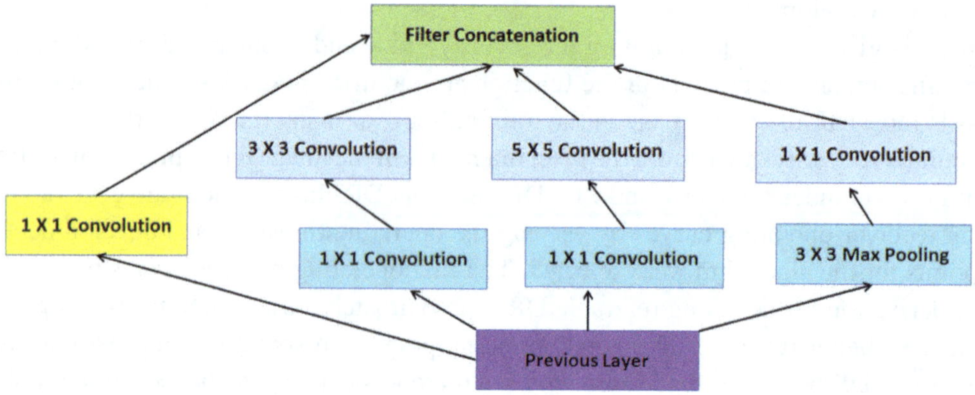

Table 11. Results (Masood, 2017)

	E1	E2	E3	E4
No. of class	5	4	5	4
Img /class	500	500	800	800
Img radi (px)	200	200	500	500
Train steps	500	4000	500	500
Acc. of Training (%)	61	63	58	58
Acc. of Validation (%)	36	55	50	59
Final test acc. (%)	37.6	47.2	48.2	48.8

Table 12. Instances of GoogLeNet derived from Inception architecture (Szegedy, 2014)

Type	Pat_size Stride	O/P Size	Dep	1_1	3_3 Reduce	3_3	5_5 Reduce	5_5	Pool	Params	ops
Conv	7 X 7 / 2	112 X 112 X 64	1							27 K	34 M
Max-pool	3 X 3 / 2	56 X 56 X 64	0								
Conv	3 X 3 / 1	56 X 56 X 192	2		64	192				112 K	360 M
Max-pool	3 X 3 / 2	28 X 28 X 192	0								
Incep 3-a		28 X 28 X 256	2	64	96	128	16	32	32	159 K	128 M
Incep 3-b		28 X 28 X 480	2	128	128	192	32	96	64	380 K	304 M
Max-pool	3 X 3 / 2	14 X 14 X 480	0								
Incep 4-a		14 X 14 X 512	2	192	96	208	16	48	64	364 K	73 M
Incep 4-b		14 X 14 X 512	2	160	112	224	24	64	64	437 K	88 M
Incep 4-c		14 X 14 X 512	2	128	128	256	24	64	64	463 K	100 M
Incep 4-d		14 X 14 X 528	2	112	144	288	32	64	64	580 K	119 M
Incep 4-e		14 X 14 X 832	2	256	160	320	32	128	128	840 K	170 M
Max-pool	3 X 3 / 2	7 X 7 X 832	0								
Incep 5-a		7 X 7 X 832	2	256	160	320	32	128	128	1072 K	54 M
Incep 5-b		7 X 7 X 1024	2	384	192	384	48	128	128	1388 K	71 M
Avg-pool	7 X 7 / 1	1 X 1X 1024	0								
Drop-40%		1 X 1 X 1024	0								
Linear		1 X 1 X 1000	1							1000 K	1 M
Softmax		1 X 1 X 1000	0								

CNN FOR DETECTING BRAIN TUMORS

The brain tumor case study was carried out based on CNN algorithm for object detection. The CNN model generated is shown in the figure 6 and the results obtained are shown in the figure 7. The table shows the details of all the parameters computed during each layer. The results achieved were 99.9% and calculations are shown the figure 8. In this study, the filters taken were 32 and the filter size is 3x3 and

Figure 6. Convolution Neural Network layers for detecting tumor

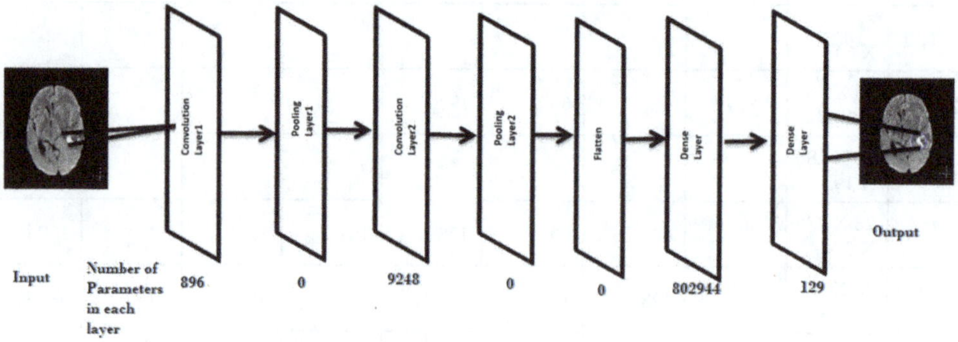

Figure 7. Input and output Images of Brain Tumors

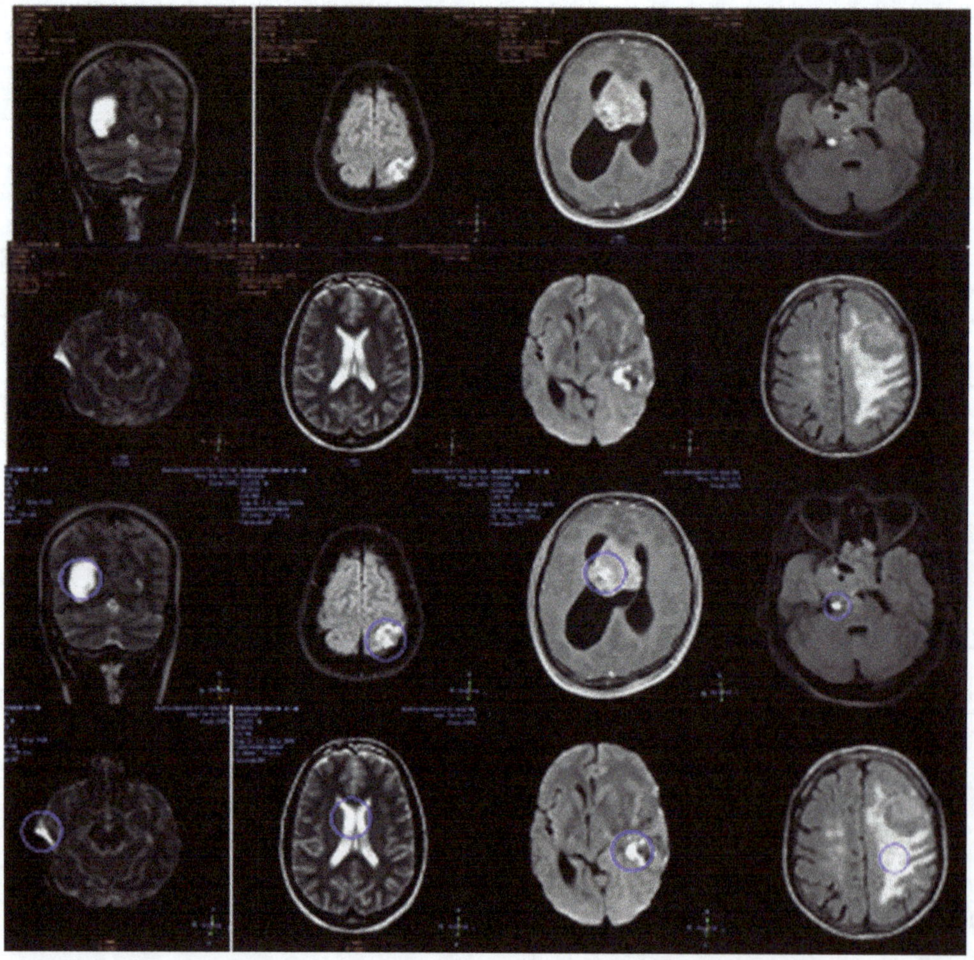

layers are conv2d, pooling, flatten and dense. The size of activation map result is given by the equation (N +2P - F)/stride +1, where N is the input size, P is padding, F is the filter size and the stride applied on the image.

Summary of parameters is the parameter summation of all the layers = 896 + 0 + 9248 + 0 + 0 + 802944 + 129 = 813217.

Table 13. Total number of CNN Layers

Type	output shape	parameters
Conv	62 x 62x 32	896
Max-pool	31 x 31 x 32	0
Conv	29 x 29 x 32	9248
Max-pool	14 x 14x 32	0
Flatten	6272	0
Dense	128	802944
Dense	1	129
Total		813217

Figure 8. CNN parameters calculations layout

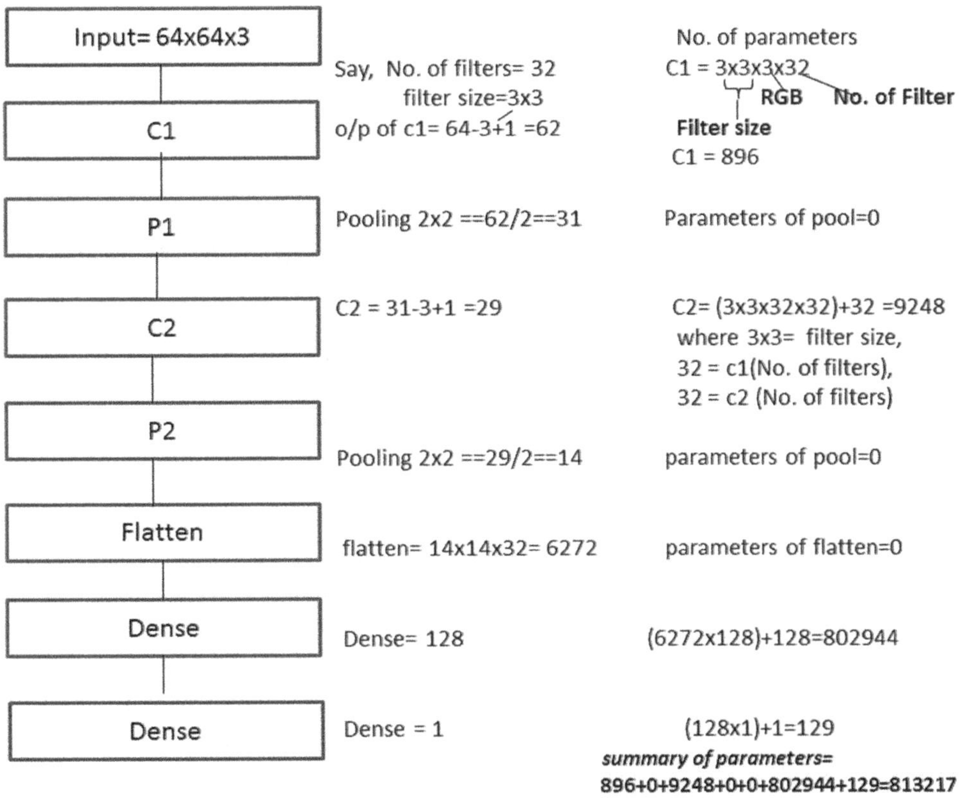

Figure 9. Thresholding HSV extraction of the disease in DR

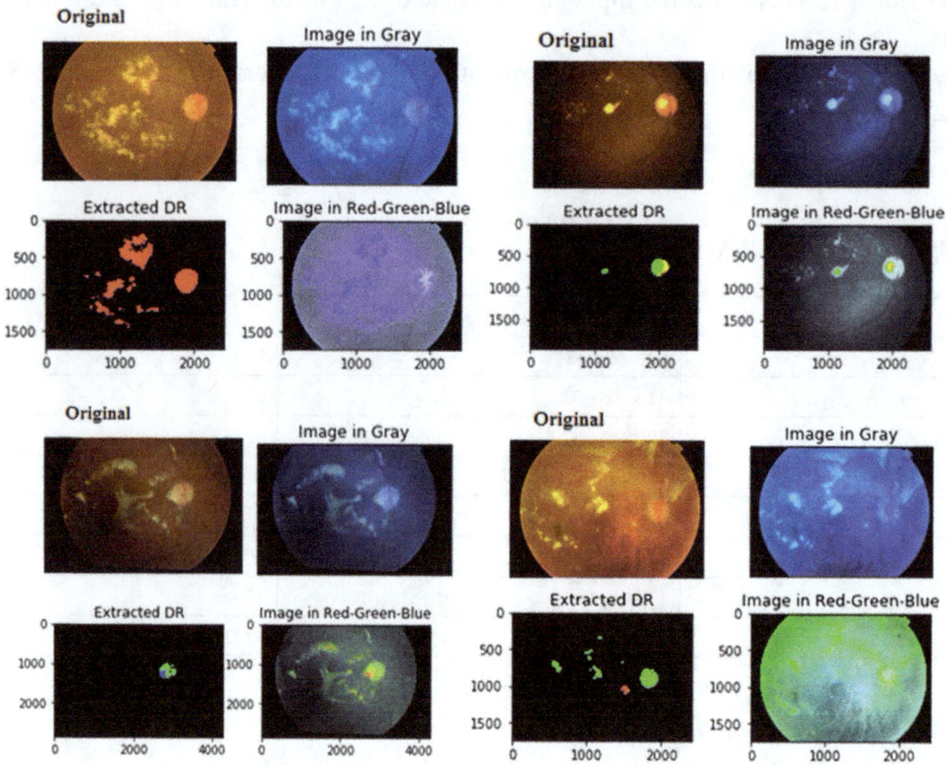

CNN USING DIABETIC RETINOPATHY

The images are obtained from kaggle and the thresholding Hue-Saturation-Value (HSV) was applied for them. The figure 9 shows the results of the gray color images where the images undergoes blurrness and eroded with boundaries and this was carried out using python code. The images in RED-Green-Blue shows the diseases in Retinopathy and are extracted in third image in the figure 9.

Using HSV color space one can obtain the disease or tumor in the DR, which helps in extracting only the part of disease shown in the figure 9 in second row to the left. Which in-turn helps to understand the size and shape of the tumor (disease).

CONCLUSION

The prediction of various diseases can be carried out by ANN algorithm and CNN algorithm. Diabetic Retinopathy and Tumors are easily detected by the Convolution neural network. These techniques are popular in the healthcare and play a key role in analysis of various diseases and assist the medical specialist in diagnoses. Authors conclude that the regression models are built to understand the R-Squared, Probability of F, and the p-value of any diseases in the healthcare. ANN can predict and diagnose the disease faster, further, ANN analyzes whether the input data fits in the line of regression model.

CNN predicts the various diseases and assist the physicians at the health care and CNN can also extract the tumor or the part of the disease in the human. Thus, machine learning and deep learning algorithms plays a significant role in the healthcare and carries out the early prediction, detection and diagnoses of any disease.

REFERCENCES

Abiyev, R. H. & Ma'aitah, M. K.S. (2018). Deep Convolutional Neural Networks for Chest Diseases Detection. *Journal of Healthcare Engineering.*

Dakappa, P. H., Prasad, K., Rao, S. B., Bolumbu, G., Bhat, G. K., & Mahabala, C. (2018). Classification of infectious and noninfectious diseases using artificial neural networks from 24-hour continuous tympanic temperature data of patients with undifferentiated fever. *Critical Reviews in Biomedical Engineering*, *46*(2).

Ganapathy, N., Swaminathan, R., & Deserno, T. (2018). Deep Learning on 1-D Biosignals: A Taxonomy-based Survey. *IMIA Yearbook of Medical Informatics*, *27*(1), 98–109. doi:10.1055-0038-1667083 PMID:30157512

Goodfellow, I., Bengio, Y. & Courville, A. (2016). Deep Learning (1st ed.). Cambridge, MA: The MIT Press.

Granville, V. (n.d.). Difference Between Machine Learning, Data Science, AI, Deep Learning, and Statistics. Data science central. Retrieved from https://www.datasciencecentral.com/profiles/blogs/difference-between-machine-learning-data-science-ai-deep-learning.

Gulshan, V., Peng, L., Coram, M., Stumpe, M.C., Wu, D., Narayanaswamy, A., … Webster, D.R. (2016). Development and validation of a deep learning algorithm for detection of diabetic retinopathy in retinal fundus photographs. In Innovations In Health Care Delivery. American Medical Association.

Jiang, F., Jiang, Y., Zhi, H., Dong, Y., Li, H., Ma, S., ... Wang, Y. (2017). Artificial intelligence in healthcare: Past, present and future. *Stroke and Vascular Neurology.*, *2*(4). doi:10.1136vn-2017-000101 PMID:29507784

Litjens, G., Kooi, T., Bejnordi, B. E., Setio, A. A. A., Ciompi, F., Ghafoorian, M., ... Sánchez, C. I. (2017). A Survey on Deep Learning in Medical Image Analysis. *Medical Image Analysis*, *42*, 60–88. doi:10.1016/j.media.2017.07.005 PMID:28778026

Lundervold, A. S., & Lundervold, A. (2019). An Overview of Deep Learning in Medical Imaging Focusing on MRI. *Zeitschrift fur Medizinische Physik*, *29*(2), 102–127. doi:10.1016/j.zemedi.2018.11.002 PMID:30553609

Mantzaris, D. H., Anastassopoulos, G. C., & Lymberopoulos, D. K. (2008). Medical disease prediction using Artificial Neural Networks. In *Proceedings of the IEEE International Conference on BioInformatics and BioEngineering*. IEEE Press. . 8-10.10.1109/BIBE.2008.4696782

Masood, S., Luthra, T., Sundriyal, H., & Ahmed, M. (2017). Identification of Diabetic Retinopathy in Eye Images Using Transfer Learning. In *Proceedings of the International Conference on Computing, Communication and Automation (ICCCA)*. Academic Press. 10.1109/CCAA.2017.8229977

Mythili, T. Mukherji, D. Padalia, N. & Naidu, A. (2013). A Heart Disease Prediction Model using SVM-Decision Trees-Logistic Regression (SDL). *International Journal of Computer Applications,* 68(16).

Prajapati, S. A., Nagaraj, R., & Mitra, S. (2017). Classification of dental diseases using CNN and transfer learning. In *Proceedings of the IEEE 5th International Symposium on Computational and Business Intelligence (ISCBI)*. IEEE Press. doi:10.1109/ISCBI.2017.8053547

Selvi, S. T., Arumugam, S., & Ganesan, L. (2000). BIONET: An Artificial Neural Network model for diagnosis of diseases. *Pattern Recognition Letters*, *21*(8), 721–740. doi:10.1016/S0167-8655(00)00027-1

Sharif, M., Khan, M. A., Rashid, M., Yasmin, M., Afza, F., & Tanik, U. J. (2018). Deep CNN and geometric features-based gastrointestinal tract diseases detection and classification from wireless capsule endoscopy images. *Journal of Experimental & Theoretical Artificial Intelligence*. doi:10.1080/0952813X.2019.1572657

Shen, D., Wu, G., & Suk, H. I. (2017). Deep Learning in Medical Image Analysis. *Annual Review of Biomedical Engineering*, *19*(1), 221–248. doi:10.1146/annurev-bioeng-071516-044442 PMID:28301734

Szegedy, C., Liu, W., Jia, Y., Sermanet, P., Reed, S., Anguelov, D., Erhan, D., Vanhoucke, V., & Rabinovich, A. (2014). Going deeper with convolutions.

Wahyunggoro, O., Permanasari, A. E., & Chamsudin, A. (2013). Utilization of Neural Network for Disease Forecasting. In *Proceedings 59th ISI World Statistics Congress* (pp. 549- 554). Academic Press.

Weng, C., Huang, T. C.-K., & Han, R.-P. (2016). Disease prediction with different types of neural network classifiers. *Telematics and Informatics*, *33*(2), 277–292. doi:10.1016/j.tele.2015.08.006

Yalçin, N., Alver, S., & Uluhatun, N. (2018). Classification of retinal images with deep learning for early detection of diabetic retinopathy disease. In *Proceedings of the 26th Signal Processing and Communications Applications Conference (SIU)*. Academic Press. 10.1109/SIU.2018.8404369

Chapter 8
Elderly Behavior Prediction Using a Deep Learning Model in Smart Homes

Sridevi U. K.
PSG College of Technology, India

Sophia Sudhir
Sri Krishna College of Engineering and Technology, India

Shanthi Palaniappan
https://orcid.org/0000-0001-7721-8305
Sri Krishna College of Engineering and Technology, India

ABSTRACT

The goal of a smart home is to keep track of the behaviors of the older adults with disabilities within the home, and then anticipate their activity to help with other actions. Elderly and disabled people have problems with their daily lives, while most other people are unaware of their difficulties. Helping the elderly to live independently allows them to lead their daily lives in a better manner. The implementation of analytics and machine learning algorithms leads to a predictive approach to health care services. In this chapter, a learning model in a smart home concept focuses on making it possible for the elderly to remain safe and comfortable at home. The transformative home security device learning architecture of the smart home platform is a valuable solution to studying mobility patterns at home, with the ability to identify behavioral changes related to issues of wellbeing. A predictive learning system can effectively recognize and identify the behavior of the elderly. A learning model, a recurrent neural network (RNN) is proposed to evaluate the people's activity. The focus of the present study is to forecast the deterioration in mental function and give warnings for the benefit of seniors.

DOI: 10.4018/978-1-7998-2101-4.ch008

INTRODUCTION

The elderly who live independently are the main issue and the control of daily living practices helps assess their ability to care for them and ensure better living life. In the case of elderly patients, there is always a need for constant monitoring and rapid diagnosis. Daily living tasks, also known as physical daily activity of living (ADL) include essential skills normally required to manage their daily activities. These responsible abilities are learned at the start of life and are generally retained in contrast to higher-level tasks in the face of deteriorating cognitive functioning. Specific ADLs are typically classified separately from Daily Living Instrumental Activities (IADLs), which include more specific task depends on the cognitive ability of the brain. IADL task is prone to early neuro degeneration in comparison to regular activity is often an important driver of core ADL skills. IADL deficiency shows slight cognitive decline and Alzheimer's can indeed develop, although simple ADL changes often do not occur until later stage of dementia. Regular Living Ability Evaluation Instrumental Training helps to assess independent living. The assessment of ADL, IADL, relies on psychological variables and forecasting helps to assess the independent living. Successful longevity, autonomy and on-site aging capability include sustaining and preserving the physical, mental and social well-being of individuals. ADLs are used to describe a situation that may or may not be critical to the capacity of a person to live comfortably. The cognitive impairment has different impact on ADL and IADL activity. The low cognitive persons will have difficulty in performing the ADL activities. As the old people segment grows, the method to identify the cognitive decline is essential. Smart homes are capable of tracking and supporting people by monitoring their activities. The health care services can be improved by proving better living environment.

ADLs could include the dressing, getting up in the morning, drug administration, self-clean, and their related activities. A common concern amongst older people, especially loved ones becomes a responsibility on everyone else. Changes in activity will estimate further depressive symptoms with important implications for probable treatment arrangements. Rising reliance can imply the need of a care conversation among doctors, the patient and their family to explain the wishes of the patient. The alert message is needed if they are unable to meet their basic needs. Elderly people need to retain the potential for both day-to-day living and day-to-day living practices. In recent decades, medical advancements and technology, education and healthcare welfare, combined with increased knowledge of nutrition have paved the way for a significant increase in global lifespan. The monitoring devices in the home technology system is capable of tracking people's well-being and everyday behaviors and smart alert system enhance their standard of living.

Developing easy and inexpensive healthcare solution is essential to meet the increasing need for medical services for the old people. Elderly people may need medical care regularly, immediately, which otherwise could have fatal consequences. Continuous monitoring of older people's medical parameters and activities may avoid such emergencies conditions. Smart homes will allow older people to stay in safer home rather than expensive and restricted health facilities. Medical care professionals can also track older people's general health status in real time and even provide support and advice from remote services. Miniaturized and low-cost monitoring systems, embedded systems and wireless networking technology have been introduced. Remote health monitoring allows inoffensive, pervasive and real activities of person. Able to monitor everyday living habits and recognizing shifts in past trends is important to assess an elderly individual's ability to live habits and recognizing shifts in past trends is important to assess an elderly individual's ability to live in freedom in their environment and identify potential important situations earlier on.

The willingness of an older adult to manage everyday self-care tasks also is impaired by self-neglect. Elderly people who ignore themselves may have inadequate supplementation, bad personal grooming. They may not satisfy their basic needs. It was shown that self-neglect is related to general neurodegeneration. Elderly people's quality of life can be determined in terms of their health and lifestyle. Park and Lee (2017) discussed the need of individual and health services professionals wants to know more about to survive of safely. Daily living (ADLs) behaviors include cleanliness, weaning dress, using bathroom, shopping, and dining. The daily tasks will decrease relative due to cognitive functioning and issues are discussed by Michelle et al. (2016).

In order to recognize mid- or later stages of dementia, Ran et al. (2017) has updated the diagnosis of ADL ability. The executive functional potential is assessed using the capacity to function the daily tasks. Deep Learning and Machine Learning System developed Zhu et al. (2018) to learn about the regular routine of older adults by using motion and environmental sensors. Vepakomma et al. (2015) represented the ADL's basic self-care activities and complex IADL tasks can define a senior's independent living. The senior's physical capacity can be associated with the activities of the ADLs. Decisions and behavioral features can be analyzed using IADLs activities. When IADL activities are reviewed, the identifying of cognitive decline can be challenging. IADL and class reviews can assist with the type of medical care needed for older adults.

Elderly people face problems in their daily lives, and when they are at home alone, their basic need is to continue their daily activities. The primary objective given by Qin et al. (2015) discussed about the need of monitoring helps the individual lives of the aged is to make their own lives safe and comfortable at home. The regular daily habits of the elderly people are needed to be monitored. If there is any shift in regular activities, the preventive measures can be scheduled. The work done by Suryadevara et al. (2013) proposed home automation system that earlier detecting sick older people would help avoids future health care costs. One of the biggest desires and wishes of the elderly is to continue their day-to-day tasks when they are at home alone and no one is there to help them. There are many reports on the network of smart houses aimed at helping elderly people and people with disabilities. Studies in elderly living and well-being has been directed at health research and promoting the independent living of elderly people with the increasing elderly population. Some studies seek to improve the lives of people with medical problems, such as diabetes and cognitive impairments, by studying resident activities in sensor-based settings. This study proposed to identify and recognize ADLs as a deep learning model. The primary goal of this research is to assess the physical, mental and cognitive state of the elderly person and to connect with caregivers effectively. The research proposed a learning model that focused on activity. This system forecast the behavior and recognizes abnormal actions of the elder people. The actions of older adults at different time are considered as their behavior. The data generated at the time series based identifies the possible number of different actions. The mathematical predictive model is essential to identify the next action of the elders.

Literature Review

The movement of senior citizen needs to be deduced by tracking the physical activities. By applying the learning algorithm to identify patterns in actions, captured behaviors could be further examined. Learning algorithms detect alterations in behavioral patterns of older adults. The irregular trend can alert caretakers or emergencies. People's well-being can be concluded by tracking daily living practices and IADL operations. Recognition of human activity is a wide field of study that focuses primarily on identifying the actual motion or behavior of an individual based on statistical data. Typical behaviors may include working, resting, dining, or more oriented behaviors such as driving and studying. Mobile internet connectivity and computational learning with the advent of connected devices, the detection and recognition of daily human activity has become increasingly interested in areas such as Intelligent assistive technologies for sectors where manual work remains predominant and mental health facilities where human movement tracking is needed.

Human monitoring is generally accepted as a major component for the ongoing analysis of human activities in the field of smart automation system. Taking advantage of the potential of wearable devices combined with deep learning capabilities is introduced with the goal of identifying a person's most common daily activities at home. In this context, smart controls can be used in different ways, from the smallest emergency button to the active monitoring of the user's medical parameter. A convergence of machine learning technologies as well as the development of robust sensors and actuators has brought interest in the design of intelligent environments to emerge and serve useful capable functions in daily living activities.

Gokalp et al. (2013) conceived a telemonitoring study to identify the value of older people's health. By monitoring the ADL, their health care will benefit. Regular monitoring results predict people's behavior. The main advantages of tracking are recognizing and predicting changes in physiology in an earlier stage. The smart home project defined utilizes a wide range of technologies which serve different objectives. Blue tooth and Wi-Fi software incorporation in home appliance control will benefit and improve the lifestyle of all user groups in terms of safety and comfort, particularly for the disabled and the elderly. Smart homes that integrate environmentally friendly and portable medical detectors and modern communication will enable constant remote tracking of the wellness of elderly people at low cost. Advances in Smart Home technology are increasingly capable of providing instant, regular and longitudinal assessments of the functional ability of a person in his / her home. The types of smart devices used for behavior analysis vary from wearable sensor technology to sensors mounted inside a resident's home. When ubiquitous computing technologies have become more available, the use of off - the-shelf sensor equipment now allows for continuous monitoring at home. Maybe the smart home is the one most associated with IoT, a system where a house has many sensors appliances to provide an interconnected living environment. IoT based health care devices are innovations in smart health care services. A continuous glucose monitor (CGM) is announced on the world diabetes day. The remote care monitoring of the glucose level can be done for the patients suffering from the mobility issues. The smart pills are used for drug management. The technology advances like Pillcam takes photos of the bowel and transmits the image to a recorder. The study on recorded images is made for further analysis. mHealth is a remote monitoring health care device and also serve as the daily care wellness monitoring system. Wearable healthcare devices are updating the health care tracking features. There have been many applications developed to record health statuses and medicine management systems. The body activity and sleeping patterns are recorded in the applications and dashboard reports are sent to the care takers.

Sedentary has become one of the greatest threats to public health in the world. Experts tell us that a minimum amount of daily physical activity is needed to avoid chronic illness risks such as hypertension, cardiovascular diseases. Elderly people can stay with friends and relatives in their comfortable home setting and maintain their healthy lives while tracking and evaluating their wellbeing from a remote center based on the behavioral data gathered by different on-body sensors. The model can carry out trend analysis based on the history of health condition, identify abnormalities and produce signals in emergency situations. The measurement scales used by Che-Yang and Hsu (2012) had identifies the functional autonomy that assesses the ability to function. The extent of illness can be determined from the elderly independent living. It makes it easier to identify individual self-care needs. Through monitoring the daily routine of the older population, this will assess their health and wellbeing. Awais et al. (2019) discussed the wellbeing movements such as lying, moving, walking and sleeping. Using support vector machine, the living condition is classified. Michelle et al. (2016) examined the elderly person's movement by diagnosing the ADL test. This investigated the mental abilities relationship between the ADLs. The factors that influence the ADL's quality are established. The service providers must provide guidelines for patient capability enhancement. The level of cognitive condition can be used to identify the treatment. Monitoring can capture the eight characteristics. Graf (2008) given a scale for further analysis and assessment and will be a warning signal. The common index of evaluation using the model of health care is the ADL scaling index given by Katz (1983). The index indicates the level of cognitive decline of the older people. The cognitive decline is measured by Hartigan et al. (2007) and the degree of autonomy can be identified using the index.

Artificial intelligence technologies dominate human interaction and it starts to serve humanity's day-to-day needs, and particularly our elderly people. Assistive social robots can be used to monitor elderly people's safety and mental well-being, a particular type of assistive robotics developed for human social interaction. Such robots are supposed to serve as a technology for older generations by offering support to improve the standard of living. AI system consists of lightweight sensors and wearable designed for seniors to collect rich data sets about senior activity and behavior patterns unobtrusively and autonomously. Such behaviors include feeding, drinking, walking, shaving, sleeping, bathing, and toileting, but are not limited to. Ercolano et al. (2017) proposed the RDG-D Camera based a deep learning model that tracks the elderly lives. The model uses long-term memory learning architectures. Deep learning network model was used by Welhenge et al. (2018) to predict the activity of older individuals which aims to include preventive health care.

According to Alshammari et al. (2018) automatic learning algorithms are primarily used to study the behavior pattern of everyday lives of the older adults. Unmonitored methods are used when the ADLs do not have ground truth names. It is possible to organize related ADLs into clusters. Smart homes provide network tracking, home security tools, medical alert devices, and analytical reports. Health care workers must carefully analyze the health condition and provide services when needed. Data gathered provide vital information about the elderly everyday activities, which can be used to detect the medical problems. Different monitoring systems based on sensors provide information about the movements inside the home. These sensors include a huge amount of interdependent input data that needs to be processed, analyzed and incorporated in order to collect the most valuable information's activities of daily living. Data analytics technologies coupled with deep learning strategies include the infrastructure for massive amounts of sensor data storage and processing. The framework can be used by health services to recognize the pattern of the senior and variations from this pattern in addition to identifying the daily activities performed by an elder.

The problem of wandering people was addressed by Qiang et al. (2014) and discussed the need to protect them. Habits of older adults such as repeated wandering often it can result in bad outcomes like getting lost. The elderly conduct must be controlled. As people age, cognition is critical to functional independence, including whether someone can live independently, manage finances, take medicines properly and drive safely. Aitor et al. (2018) used the information produced from sensor-based surveillance is taken as the data series and is generally processed for activity recognition through statistical and machine learning methods.

The large amounts of information's are produced by sensors and machine learning algorithm can be applied to infer the results. This can promote threat identification, tracking, prediction, and risk determination. Forbes et al. (2019) discussed the increasing value of collected data, the assessment evaluates the chance of slipping. Sensor-based methods are oriented on the use for behavior and activity tracking of evolving sensor network techniques. Murman et al. (2015) has discussed the essential to know what kinds of cognition modifications are anticipated as part of ordinary aging and could suggest the occurrence of a brain disease. Using machine learning, smart wearable, and advanced kinematics to measure the daily activities of older adults and predict health conditions including elevated risk of falling, anxiety, and urinary tract infections.

The need for care rises with era, thus endangering the sustainability of the present social and health care system was discussed by Mora et al. (2018). Monitoring of daily living tasks (ADL), classifying them and recognizing daily routine trends. Smart devices support is one of the main requirements used to obtain automated home for seniors in their home environment were suggested by Vanus et al. (2017). Activity daily living capability can be cognitive capacity, which is the ability to complete the job, motor and perceptual capability. ADLs can be framed through sensors based on self-reporting, caregiver and automatic information observation. Correct behavior analysis is important as it recognizes behaviors and choice-making in healthcare analysis. It is possible to recognize actions with simple binary sensors. User movement viewing can be identified by the sensor data changes. Self-reports are convenient to administer if individuals are relatively cognitively intact, but data is valid if the individuals do not have awareness on their functional impairments. Anomalous behavior can be detected first by developing routine patterns of behavior, mapping ADLs to standard and other day-to-day behaviors. For most elderly people in-house monitoring, anomalous activity may be marked as risky if the agreed sequence of events is disrupted for some way. Debes et al. (2017) works indicated the need to track daily living behaviors and recognize deviations from previous habits is essential. This determines the willingness of the elderly to remain in their society peacefully and to consider essential circumstances in the near future. Deep learning models can be implemented to the volume of data produced by sensors. This can foster awareness of behavior, identification, prediction, and acceptance of threat. The increasing difficulty of collecting sensor data, correct analysis and applying machine learning techniques are very important to identify the risk of falling. Research study will be discussed against the use of intelligence collection of data at home. This is done by taking into account the viability of continuous monitoring using perception based and wearable devices.

The main objective is to design smart home that guides, assists and alerts the house mates to help and support elders and differently-abled people to be in safe, secure and empowering environment and revolutionize the assistive independent living. The indicators of assistance free ADL activities like meal preparation, personal hygiene, bathing, and dressing without help from a caregiver. Advanced machine learning algorithms would evaluate the inmates ' health status based on walking pace, sleep time, and other activity collected from the unique sensor information. Since daily activities are cyclic, its evaluation helps in modeling the behavior of a person.

The major challenges of automatic recognition are that it is complex and has human interaction also. Concurrent multiple tasks, activity done in different style activities executed i.e. varying time slots orders etc. should also be taken into account. This will have an impact on the labeling of the training set in the execution of statistical machine learning techniques. Rapid adaptation to change in internal behavior and routine change in the home environment needs to be tracked. If this adaptation is not done it could lead to abnormal alarm notifications and increases the chance of wrong detection. This work combines classification algorithms to detect the routine of a elders regular activities and identifies the irregular patterns.

The proposed system can be used for early diagnosis of cognitive diseases as decision support systems (DSSs). Presenting DSSs can be used to screen for further evaluation suspected cases of cognitive disease. Large numbers of patients and healthy subjects may lead to more accurate cognitive disease study. It also seems to be possible to reduce the diagnostic error by using other different classifiers. ADL showed significant orderly correlations with expected wellbeing, serious sufficient depression to include predictor usage, and neurological history. Techniques could be easily applied to such a wide variety of information and activity assessment obtained by remote monitors. Practical life statistical analysis permitted the application to really be evaluated in both dimensions of architecture and technology. An IOT based approach was proposed by Mora et al. (2019) implemented unsupervised segmentation methods to test multiple regular cognitive samples.

Predicting Behavioral Model

Older people face challenges in the daily lives, whereas most others do not understand the challenges. The main challenge is to perform the day-to-day tasks at their house without any support. There are several researches on the framework of intelligent home designed to help aged people. Predictive Intelligence environment collects information from sensors from different places in house. The movements are captured from sensors and predict the behavior of daily activity. ADLs can be viewed as abstract sensor data information with context in sensor data analysis and behavior recognition. The smart home system built in without affecting or contemplating the subjects, passive in-house sensors apply. Typically, these devices are designed to detect the effects of user behavior at residence, like sensing gate flapping, activity in a room and usage of electrical appliances. The behavioral data is analyzed and statistical methods are used to detect changes in the activities detected by the sensor. Household activity is gathered at various times and utilizing forecasting methods to analyze the extracted pattern. The activity classification based on the daily task can be grouped as regular or irregular period. A novel model of prediction of actions has been planned and developed for everyday activity and monitoring analysis. Real-time analysis of daily living information activities is important to identify the actions of the activity and to predict unusual circumstances of the elderly. The model contains components for discovering, modeling and recognizing the patterns of activity such as

- Tracking the daily activity using the sensor data
- Using Sensor data, the information about ADLs (Activity of daily living) and environment contexts are derived, analyzed and controlled
- Monitor the behavior of people and sending alert to the caretaker when abnormal situations are detected
- Deep learning is used to analyze activities that are sufficiently rich to show behavioral variations
- Enhancing detection and prediction rates in non-trivial situations

The data generated from the different activities is helpful in modeling the behavior and further predicting abnormal behavior of the inmates. Based on the features extracted upon comparison with the available set of library data cumulative study on each activity, the behavior can be classified as the normal and abnormal conditions. The different response level of the person can also be classified as

Figure 1.

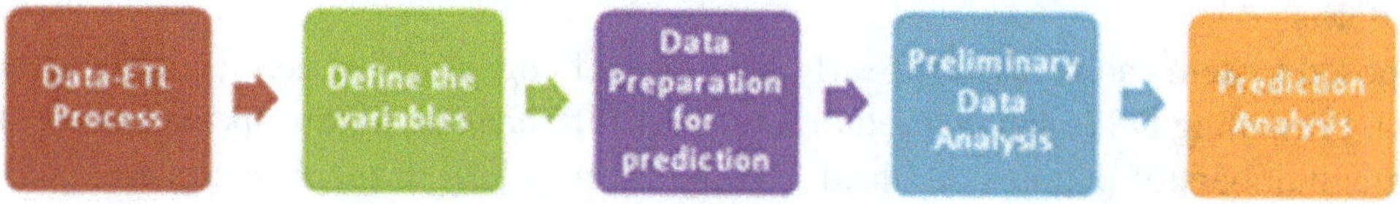
Data-ETL Process
Define the variables
Data Preparation for prediction
Preliminary Data Analysis
Prediction Analysis

activity level, mobility level, and non- responsive level. The severity level is considered as low, medium and severe. Different ADL activities are the variables of prediction. Various stages of prediction are shown as in Figure 1.

The system collects the following information:

1. Sensing and collecting data, along with temporal information, for various events. For further storage, the data is stored in archives.
2. Activities are noted through the application of a conditional probabilistic method.

The main features used in Prediction are:

- Time of sleep and time to getup
- Number of times to bathroom during sleep and duration spent in bathroom
- Movement in bed during sleep and the total static time during sleeping
- Door usage
- Electrical appliances usage
- Count of pills available in the box from time to time
- Time taken to turn the pages of the book
- Time duration in which the TV is on
- Walking pattern like start, taking a turn or stopping, etc.

The system gathers Activities Daily Life (ADL), Analyze and Disseminate for Decision Making

(i) Sensor enabled solutions for simple activity detection along with machine learning based adaptation and identification of the behavior pattern
(ii) Regular monitoring and real time behavior assessment helps in detection of impairment through parameters like walking, sleeping reading etc.
(iii) Decision Making, Automatic reminder and Alert Systems critically dependent on timely availability of the sound data under lonely and non- assistance condition.

The forecasting model requires the elderly person to assess the independent living state and their ability to carry out tasks without support from anyone. Measuring functional capacity uses the scale of the assessment and forecasts the patient category. Senior care analytics was applied to calculate the amount of value to individuals such as sleeping patterns, use of toilets, etc. The user's normal pattern is established and if changes are observed then it is important to activate s reporting to the health center or care taker. In a given time series, the trends can be analyzed. Seeing repeated trends of user behaviors

Figure 2.

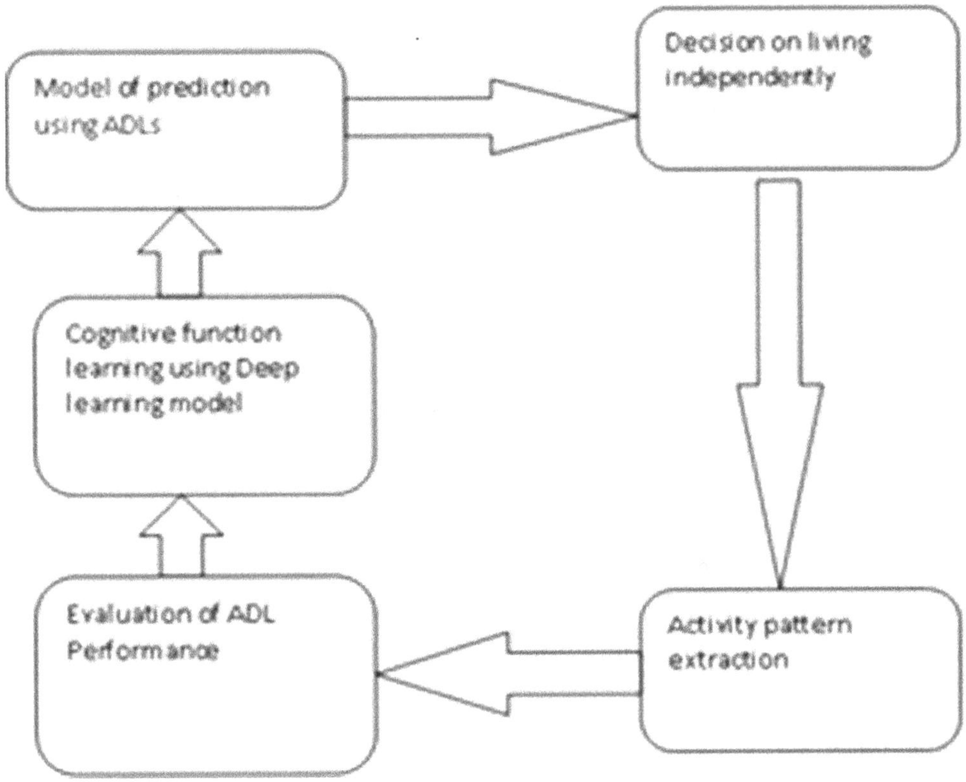

is useful and reveals persistent user information patterns. Effective detection of functional and mental disabilities may support recovery practitioner. The care providers identify to detect the medical problems and the statistically significant abnormalities in older individuals. Daily activity habits include detail about the person's specific health and the well-being. Assessing the information being tracked constantly will contribute to anticipate the individual person behaviors. It is possible to predict behaviors and habits based on learning patterns. These tasks are identified as follows:

- Collection of activity data. The behavior patterns are predicted and classified. Time and duration of user tasks are recorded on different slots. The series of different activities is dependent on social behaviors.
- The features needed to introduce into the model are selected in the extraction layer.
- In the learning, the features are given as input to the framework and learned to predict. Figure 2 displays the architecture of learning model.

Behavioral Analysis Model

One of the most common architectures of Recurrent Neural Networks (RNN) based Long Short-Term memory is capable of learning prediction problem. The human activity recognition problem can be addressed using deep learning architecture. Yu et al. (2018) proposed LSTM method to enhance the human activity recognition rate. LSTM uses position memory cells or secret layers of neurons. The architecture collects information with high predictive ability dynamically. The architecture of LSTMs can be separated into the source module, pattern extraction and the predictive model. Based on the work suggested by Zhang et al. (2015), LSTM design takes the input features that are extracted. Based on the batch size the learning models generalize various input data. If the sample volume is less value the learning frequency will be reduced. The objective function needs iteration steps. The predictive analytical model takes the older adult's past data at different intervals and the analysis was done on behavior supported with the features. The prediction model suggested by Wang et al. (2018) identified the task mapping with the ADL and IADL task. The output variable depends on the performance of activity of older adults and the time-based activity function is used to identify the movement in the learning algorithm. The feature extraction filters the related features and seeks to prevent collinear problems. Feature extraction is done in CNN layer. The feature map is generated from the input data. The Deep learning used in a multilayer information processing is equipped with probabilistic regression method using two hidden layers of back propagation network model. The main objective is to forecast success and the correct prediction depends on accuracy. The predictions can be used to test multi-class prediction system results. Evaluate if the patient may gain with knowledge, and services on health promotion, early identification and search for resources to help them. The statistical analysis identifies the changes in the activity between time periods. The complex decision patterns of the elder person can be observed by monitoring daily. The score determines the dependence or autonomous residing status of the senior person. The classification of functional addiction classes the senior as seriously affected and non serious people.

Experimental Results

Healthy, independent living environment determines the quality of life. Public involvement of elder people is related to be highly dependent on health and quality of life. Cognitive decline in older people will lead to a lack of social communication and inability to care them self. Senior health care services are needed for the elders with limitation in mobility. The application's accuracy is tested using the ADL UCI machine learning data set and City's Aging and Disability Services client level data set. The individual's daily activities are registered. Table 1 and Table 2 list the operation of the ADL measure evaluation given by Ran et al. (2017).

Dwolatzky et al. (2010) has suggested that depending on the assessment of mild cognitive decline and dementia, it is possible to assess the everyday lives of older people. Based on Lawton et al. (1969), the Instrumental activities of Daily Living (IADL) were used as the main tool for measuring elderly people's behavior. The IADL tasks identify the cognitive health. There is also an important distinction

Table. 1 Index Scale proposed by Katz (1983)

Item	Description
Food	Food eating habit
Self-cleaning	Cleanliness
Self-Care	Self-grooming
Dressing	Trying to wear shoes and clothes without support
Using toilet	Use of restroom as well as the time spend in the toilet

Table 2. Activity description based on IADL Scale proposed by Lawton and Brody (1969)

Item	Description
Phone usage	It involves how a person uses a telephone
Purchase	Shopping
Kitchen activity	Food preparation
House Maintenance	House cleaning
Washing	Handling washing machine
Transportation	Using public transport facility
Medicines	Taking medicines by self
Finances	Ability to handle finance

between the capacity of the person to complete the task and the ability to recognize the task without prompting. During the mid-and later phases of dementia, ADL ability assessment is often needed but may also occur in care for a serious case such as a stroke.

ADL abilities assessment guide can include a question of mental, psychological or behavioral variables that may connect within the operation of these essential skills as well as how to address these obstacles to improve elderly care. The senior is graded on the basis of the IADL operation without any challenge, medium challenges and extreme challenges. The data sets are being tested with deep learning networks and support vector machines. This model is designed to empower people with cognitive decline to retain their stability at their house. Communicating with caretaker is itself a difficult for them. The system will send automatic alert message to the caretaker based on the elder person movement. The proposed model could be used to monitor the people's everyday lives of older people. Behavioral surveillance is intended to recognize clusters of human behavior events, reinforcing conclusions and findings of recurrent patterns and trends in behavior. The system can identify the behavioral disorder by monitoring the movements using deep learning model in the smart home environment. The more precise study on predictive cognitive disorders can be made by using deep learning algorithm. The system enables the cake taker to monitor the elder adult activities daily and behavior weekly trends and act promptly if abnormality is predicted, and alerts about risk conditions based on the severity level to the caretaker.

According to Brown et al. (2013), the IADL activity threshold was classified as 0 to no difficulties involved, 1 in moderate discomfort, 2 in progressive difficulty and 3 in acute difficulty and 4 in high complexity. Table 3 shows the activity classification of IADL.

Daily Living Activities are daily activities done in everyday life and the aim is to classify them as standard sequences of different sensor activations using passive sensors in-house. Identifying ADLs, their frequency and time shifts may help to understand risky behavior. Figure 3 show the performance of the learning module by defining the normal and abnormal actions of the child.

The forecasting efficiency of a method is evaluated based on the activities in order to determine the consistency of the events. In addition to using trained identifying attributes, incorporating attribute interpretations allow decisions to be made about both the similarities among activities. The classification identifies the boundaries between the activities.

The logistic regression is applied to identify the relationship between the variable and outcome category. Ordinal logistic regression is a type of logistic regression in which the categorical outcome parameter is grouped in even more than two classes. The table 4 shows the model estimation and identifies the health and mental conditions are significant.

Table 3. Classification based on IADL activity

Daily activity recorded	Stage	Level
Normal Activity	0	No problem
Purchasing difficulty	1	Mild problems
Not able to do household activities	2	Moderate problems
Capable of performing simple tasks	3	Severe problems
Required help to perform simple tasks	4	Complete problems

Figure 3.

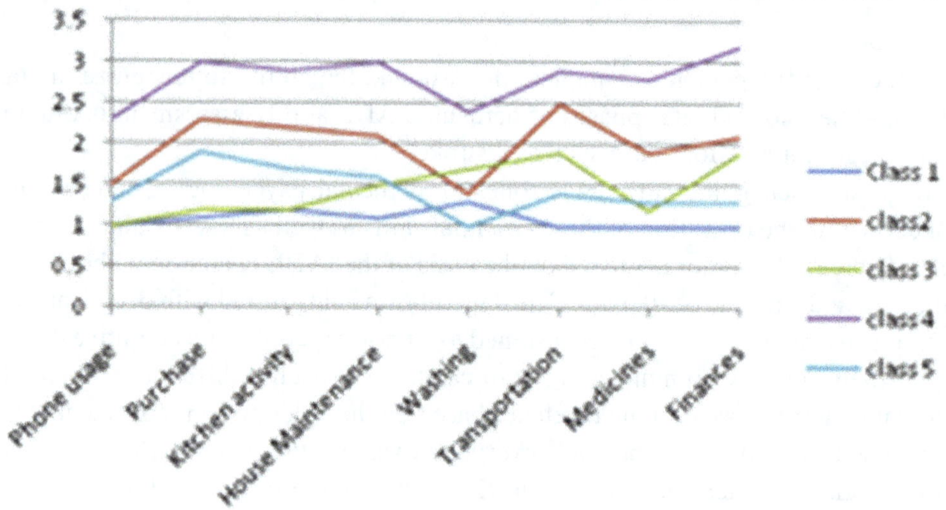

Table 4. Model estimation

Variables	Coefficient	Standard error	Odds Ratio	Confidence interval	
				Lower Limit	Upper Limit
Health condition	3.4	0.44	1.8	0.95	3.3
Mental Health	1.6	0.4	4.8	2.3	10.7

Table 5. Performance evaluation of activity

Activity	Accuracy (Precision)	Recall (R)	F-Score
A1-Kitchen	95.10%	97.60%	96.90%
A2-Living	95.30%	94.00%	94.70%
A3-Bathroom	95.50%	96.00%	95.70%
A4-Door	92.80%	90.40%	91.60%
A5-Moving out	88.80%	91.50%	90.20%
A6- Bedroom	100.00%	99.10%	99.60%

The features are extracted based on the correlation analysis. We used all 6 training topics to retrain the SVM classifier using the earlier chosen characteristics to achieve a final forecast model. The activity and non-active day of elder people can be obtained using the system. The root mean square error metric is used for the residual analysis on predicted values and given as follows:

$$RMSE = \sqrt{\frac{1}{n}\sum_{i=1}^{n}\left(y_i - \hat{y}_i\right)^2}$$

Where n is the number of datasets, the observed and predicted values are y_i and $\hat{y}_i$.

Regular machine learning methods were used to identify, showing the slight advantage of the SVM. Table 5 shows the daily activities gives F-score results ranging from 95.6% to 97.9%.

Deep learning model combined with SVM performs better in accuracy and results accurately identify datasets with an accuracy of 87.20%. The learning model comparison is given in Table 6. The classification results show that behavioral changes can be detected on a daily basis. The work is to estimate the elder's risk based on their movement pattern. The behavior modification can be identified and earlier identification of their health can be recorded and it also help reduce overall healthcare costs. Personalized daily activity monitoring can provide for a more effective treatment based on the individual health data combined with paired with predictive analytics. The statistical technique suggested by Max et al. (2013) was used to determine the model efficiency. By holding the gradients steep enough, model solves the problems of falling gradients. This makes the quality of the short practice high. The model input selected based on features strongly associated with the output prediction. The 80% of the data is taken as training data and remaining as testing data. The residual analysis is performed and finds the difference between the observed and predicted values. Based on learning algorithm training and testing are performed. The error rate decreases with the anticipated increase in data volume and convergence of about 200 iterations. The figure 4 shows the activity classification.

Figure 4.

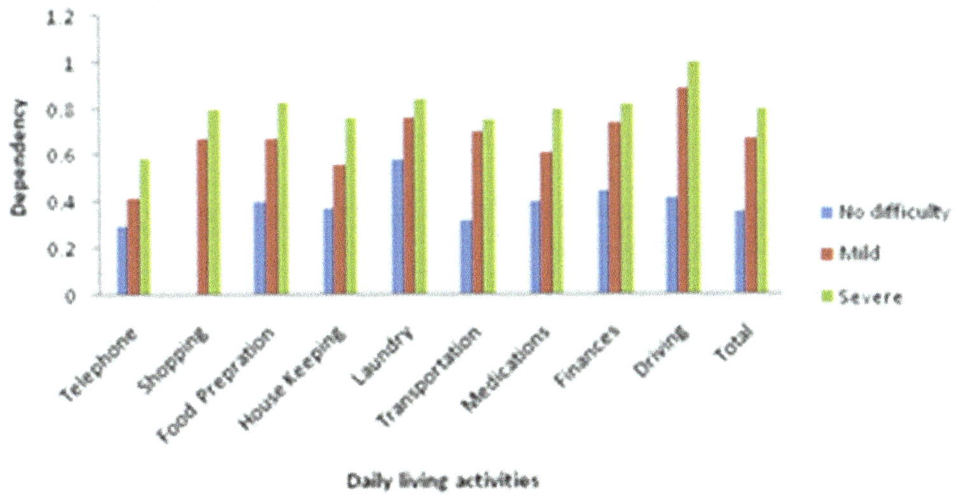

Table 6. Learning Model Comparison

Learning methods	Performance
LSTM –RNN	97%
Singular value decomposition	75%
Logistic Regression Model	80%

The table 6 shows the comparison of the logistic regression with the RNN-LSTM model and about 20% performance improvement is achieved. The multilevel classification is better in RNN-LSTM for sequential learning. The deeper architecture will be good predictive model but the care needs to taken with the issue of local minimum. The logistic regression applied on the small dataset will produce better results. The findings inform strategies for user-centered functional evaluation and the design and implementation of assistive technology, including data collection, assessment at home with the potential to support elder people. Time series for the activity prediction can be combined to improve the results. For a given time activity the system predicts the activity sequence. The deviation can be identified and health care analysis can be performed on time series data.

CONCLUSION

The research work discussed the application of learning algorithm to identify the cognitive decline of elderly people. The biggest benefit of software training is that elderly people can discover behavioral changes. A solution to support older people's independent living by equipping their homes with an easy sensor network to monitor their behavior. The studies in this review show that the use of passive in-home sensors can effectively model behavior. Thus, the conclusion is that the findings of the deep learning technique are better in identifying the ADLs. The behavioral analysis will assist in early detection of cognitive disorders. Understanding the daily lives of the elderly will allow them to have a healthy living and care climate. Predictive analysis performed will help the geriatric centers for monitoring the older adults. The statistical inference compared with the deep learning model. The method learns the patterns of the activity and helps to take care the needs of the older adults. The results shows the behavior changes by observed and predicted outcome of activity of adults.

REFERENCES

Aitor, A., & Gorka, A. (2018). Predicting human behavior with recurrent neural networks. *Applied Sciences Journal*, *8*(2), 305. doi:10.3390/app8020305

Alshammari, T., Alshammari, N., & Sedky, M. (2018). Evaluating machine learning techniques for activity classification in smart home environments. *International Journal of Information and Communication Engineering*, *12*, 2.

Awais, M., Chiari, L., Ihlen, E. A. F., Helbostad, J., & Palmerini, L. (2019). Physical activity classification for elderly people in free-living conditions. *IEEE Journal of Biomedical and Health Informatics*, *23*(1), 197–207. doi:10.1109/JBHI.2018.2820179 PMID:29994291

Brown, J., Kurichi, J. E., Xie, D., Pan, Q., & Stineman, M. G. (2013). Instrumental activities of daily living staging as a possible clinical tool for falls risk assessment in physical medicine and rehabilitation. *PM & R*, *6*(4), 316–323. doi:10.1016/j.pmrj.2013.10.007 PMID:24140738

Debes, C., Merentitis, A. S., Sukhanov, S., Niessen, M., Frangiadakis, N., & Bauer, A. (2016). Monitoring activities of daily living in smart homes: Understanding human behavior. *IEEE Signal Processing Magazine*, *33*(2), 81–94. doi:10.1109/MSP.2015.2503881

Dwolatzky, T., Dimant, L., Simon, E., & Doniger, G. (2010). Validity of a short computerized assessment battery for moderate cognitive impairment and dementia. *International Psychogeriatrics*, *22*(5), 795–803. doi:10.1017/S1041610210000621 PMID:20519066

Ercolano, G., Riccio, D., & Rossi, S. (2017). Two deep approaches for ADL recognition: A multi-scale LSTM and a CNN-LSTM with a 3D matrix skeleton representation. In *Proceedings of the IEEE International Symposium on Robot and Human Interactive Communication (RO-MAN)* (pp. 877-882). IEEE Press. 10.1109/ROMAN.2017.8172406

Forbes, G., Massie, S., & Craw, S. (2019). Fall prediction using behavioral modeling from sensor data in smart homes. *Artificial Intelligence Review*, 1–21.

Gokalp, H., & Clarke, M. (2013). Monitoring activities of daily living of the elderly and the potential for its use in telecare and telehealth. *Telemedicine Journal and e-Health*, *19*(12), 910–923. doi:10.1089/tmj.2013.0109 PMID:24102101

Graf, C. (2008). The Lawton instrumental activities of daily living scale. *The American Journal of Nursing*, *108*(4), 52–62. doi:10.1097/01.NAJ.0000314810.46029.74 PMID:18367931

Hartigan, I. (2007). A Comparative review of the Katz ADL and the Barthel Index in assessing the activities of daily living of older people. *International Journal of Older People Nursing*, *2*(3), 204–212. doi:10.1111/j.1748-3743.2007.00074.x PMID:20925877

Katz, S. (1983). Assessing self-maintenance: Activities of daily living, mobility and instruments of daily living. *Journal of the American Geriatrics Society*, *31*(12), 721–726. doi:10.1111/j.1532-5415.1983.tb03391.x PMID:6418786

Lawton, P. M., & Brody, E. M. (1969). Assessment of older people: Self-maintaining and instrumental activities of daily living. *The Gerontologist*, *9*(3), 179–18. doi:10.1093/geront/9.3_Part_1.179 PMID:5349366

Max, K., & Kjell, J. (2013). Applied predictive modeling. Springer.

Michelle, E. M., & Michelle, C. F. (2016). Assessment of activities of daily living, self-care, and independence. *Archives of Clinical Neuropsychology*, *31*(6), 506–516. doi:10.1093/arclin/acw049 PMID:27475282

Mora, N., Grossi, F., Russo, D., Barsocchi, P., Hu, R., Brunschwiler, T., & Ciampolini, P. (2019). IoT-based home monitoring: supporting practitioner's assessment by behavioral analysis. *Sensors, 19*(14), 3238.

Mora, N., Matrella, G., & Ciampolini, P. (2018). Cloud-based behavioral monitoring in smart homes. *Sensors, 18*(6), 1951.

Murman, D. L. (2015). The impact of age on cognition. *Seminars in Hearing, 36*(3), 111–121. doi:10.1055-0035-1555115 PMID:27516712

Park, J., & Lee, Y. J. (2017). Patterns of instrumental activities of daily living and association with predictors among community-dwelling older women: A latent class analysis. *BMC Geriatrics, 17*(1), 158. doi:10.118612877-017-0557-6 PMID:28732473

Qiang, L., Daqing, Z., Liming, C., Hongbo, N., & Xingshe, Z. (2014). Managing elders wandering behavior using sensors-based solutions: A survey. *International Journal of Gerontology, 8*(2), 49–55. doi:10.1016/j.ijge.2013.08.007

Qin, N., Ana, B., Garcia, H., & Ivan, P. (2015). The elderly's independent living in smart homes: A characterization of activities and sensing infrastructure survey to facilitate services development. *Sensors (Basel), 15*(5), 11312–11362. doi:10.3390150511312 PMID:26007717

Ran, L., Jiang, X., Li, B., Kong, H., Du, M., Wang, X., ... Liuf, Q. (2017). Association among activities of daily living, instrumental activities of daily living and health-related quality of life in elderly ethnic minority. *BMC Geriatrics, 17*(1), 74. doi:10.118612877-017-0455-y PMID:28330442

Suryadevara, N. K., Mukhopadhya, S. C., Wang, R., & Rayudu, R. K. (2013). Forecasting the behavior of an elderly using wireless sensors data in a Smart Home. *Engineering Applications of Artificial Intelligence, 26*(10), 2641–2652. doi:10.1016/j.engappai.2013.08.004

Vanus, J., Belesova, J., Martinek, R., Nedoma, J., Fajkus, M., Bilik, P., & Zidek, J. (2017). Monitoring of the daily living activities in smart home care. *Human Centric Computing and Information Sciences, 7*(1), 30. doi:10.118613673-017-0113-6

Vepakomma, P., De, D., Das, S. K., & Bhansali, S. (2015). A-Wristocracy: Deep learning on wrist-worn sensing for recognition of user complex activities. In *Proceedings of the IEEE/SICE International Conference on Wearable and Implantable Body Sensor Networks (BSN)*. IEEE Press. 10.1109/BSN.2015.7299406

Wang, T., Qiu, R. G., & Yu, M. (2018). Predictive modeling of the progression of Alzheimer's disease with recurrent neural networks. *Scientific Reports, 8*(1), 9161. doi:10.103841598-018-27337-w PMID:29907747

Welhenge, A., & Taparugssanagorn, A. (2018). Human activity classification using long short-term memory network. *Signal, Image and Video Processing, 13*, 11.

Yang, C., & Hsu, Y. (2012). Remote monitoring and assessment of daily activities in the home environment. *Journal of Clinical Gerontology and Geriatrics, 3*(3), 97–104. doi:10.1016/j.jcgg.2012.06.002

Yu, Z., Rennong, Y., Guillaume, C., Ximeng, X., & Zhenxing, Z. (2018). Deep residual bidir-LSTM for human activity recognition using wearable sensors. *Mathematical Problems in Engineering*.

Zhang, S., Zheng, D., Hu, X., & Yang, M. (2015). Bidirectional long short-term memory networks for relation classification. In *Proceedings of the 29th Pacific Asia Conference on Language, Information and Computation (PACLIC)* (pp. 73-78). Academic Press.

Zhu, H., Chen, H., & Brown, R. (2018). A sequence-to-sequence model-based deep learning approach for recognizing activity of daily living for senior care. *Journal of Biomedical Informatics*, *84*, 148–158. doi:10.1016/j.jbi.2018.07.006 PMID:30004019

Chapter 9
A Surrogate Data-Based Approach for Validating Deep Learning Model Used in Healthcare

Meenakshi Srivastava
https://orcid.org/0000-0002-5202-1183
Amity University Uttar Pradesh, Lucknow, India

ABSTRACT

IoT-based communication between medical devices has encouraged the healthcare industry to use automated systems which provide effective insight from the massive amount of gathered data. AI and machine learning have played a major role in the design of such systems. Accuracy and validation are considered, since copious training data is required in a neural network (NN)-based deep learning model. This is hardly feasible in medical research, because the size of data sets is constrained by complexity and high cost experiments. The availability of limited sample data validation of NN remains a concern. The prediction of outcomes on a NN trained on a smaller data set cannot guarantee performance and exhibits unstable behaviors. Surrogate data-based validation of NN can be viewed as a solution. In the current chapter, the classification of breast tissue data by a NN model has been detailed. In the absence of a huge data set, a surrogate data-based validation approach has been applied. The discussed study can be applied for predictive modelling for applications described by small data sets.

INTRODUCTION

Pathological reports are one of the most significant sources for diagnosis of diseases, but it depends on human interpretation. With the growth in various digital medium generating diverse electronic reports/ data the need for specialists who can interpret these reports/ data has drastically increased specially for the rural areas. Automated diagnosis from available reports through machine learning, specifically the deep learning, may well address this problem. IoT based communication between medical devices has

DOI: 10.4018/978-1-7998-2101-4.ch009

encouraged the healthcare industry to use automated systems which provide effective insight from the massive amount of gathered data. AI and deep learning have played a major role in the design of such systems. Deep learning enables analysis of information to improve and optimize decisions and performance. Deep learning-based models have also transformed computer vision and significantly improved machine translation. It is now being used to guide and enhance all sorts of key processes in medicine, finance, marketing and beyond.

In the past decade Deep learning has been used by many researchers for designing computational system which can analyze this massive amount of data in time efficient manner. These deep learning based computational systems were not only able to diagnose the disease, but their performance were identical or surpassing the human's diagnostic also. This success has produced significant excitement and enthusiasm in the community of researchers. These systems provide a foundation for evidence-based clinical diagnosis. With the help of evidence based diagnostic systems physicians can easily monitor and forecast patient diagnoses as well as these systems are able to improve outcomes in terms of optimized pricing, streamlining the claim process, control costs and improve operational efficiency.

One of the major issues why deep learning is gaining popularity over other machine learning algorithms is its ability to perform self-feature engineering. Unlike other supervised and un-supervised machine learning algorithms, deep learning algorithm scan the data set by its own, for corelated feature. Once the corelated features are identified, the algorithm combines them so that fast learning is enabled. Valuable insights that are suitable for the training deep learning model can be drawn from the dataset even if the dataset is in a different format.

Besides being so robust and efficient at delivering high quality results performance of neural network is constrained by few factors. The most stated challenges in the literature, for neural network based deep learning may be summarized as-

- Firstly, the requirement of high volume of data set to train the model
- Second, sequence of input of trained data may result in different speed of learning
- Third, no clarity about how the neural network has predicted a result
- Finally, a neural network cannot provide solution to a problem for which it was not trained

In the present study first two issues, mentioned above i.e. requirement of huge volume of data set to train the network and effect of change in sequence of input of trained data speed of learning have been addressed.

BACKGROUND OF STUDY

In order, the objective of a classification algorithm is to foresee the objective class by investigation the preparation dataset. This should be possible by finding legitimate limits for each objective class. By and large of saying, Use the training dataset to show signs of correlation between the fields of data set as well as to limit the conditions which could be utilized to decide each objective class (Jiawei & Micheline, 2016). When the limit conditions are decided, the next step is to foresee the objective class. This entire procedure is known as classification. Classification algorithm presents a clear picture of boundary levels by which a data set falls under a specific class/ label. Classification algorithms have its use in many areas like art and science, medicine, education, information retrieval, bioinformatics, etc. In bioinformatics, the investigation of quality expression information from DNA-microarrays is of extraordinary enthusiasm, since it enables us to break down expression levels in countless qualities in a living organism sample (Rong et al., 2009). This element makes quality articulation investigation a key instrument of research for human wellbeing (Bazi & Melgani, 2006). It gives recognizable proof of new genes playing key role in the beginning of a disease.

Deep learning offers significant potential for medical diagnostics. The presented chapter aimed to evaluate and provide the diagnostic accuracy of deep learning algorithms in classifying health informatics which, is constrained due to availability of limited training sample data. Generally, for predictive modelling on small datasets linear regression models are used. The linear regression models follow the tradition of linearity between dependent and independent variables, statistical impartiality of the input variables, normality of the residuals, and the absence of variables which are determined by their relationship with other variables within the model (Foody, 2006). Theses conventions are moreover become despoiled in many applications, specifically if the applications involve complex limitations (Hsu & Lin, 2002). Therefore, more intelligent models are required, which are basically based on regression but also apply the machine learning algorithms. Artificial Neural Networks based on feedforward backpropagation (NNs) are example of such sophisticated intelligent approach. Artificial neural networks systems are computing systems resembling biological neural networks that constitute animal brains. Such systems "learn" to perform tasks by considering examples, generally without being programmed with task-specific rules. Just like animal brain Neural System based computational systems learns by responding to the ecosystem. Neural Network based learning systems have been implemented in many fields like image recognition, speech recognition, machine translation etc. and have achieved good accuracy. Available literature on Neural network doesn't constrain the success of Neural Network by any factor (Jossinet, 1998). Neural networks based on multilayer feedforward can approximate any measurable function in a dataset.

In many previous studies which were based on deep learning, were constrained with limitations such as such as inefficiency, and being uncomfortable and time-consuming because of the use of only few variables related to the particular domain of health informatics or because of lack of big data use (Bowden, 2002; Wasserman, 1989; Cunningham et al., 2000). Therefore, research is needed to develop a predictive model using the deep learning method based on big data for the small sized datasets. Most of the previous methods have the advantage of being relatively accurate and specific to the type of diseases because of their limited sized dataset. Regardless of their superior performance, accuracy and versatility, of Neural Networks are considered with the presence of copious training data. Since the size of datasets is medical domain is constrained by the complexity and high cost of large-scale experiments, hence abundant dataset is rarely feasible in the field of medical research. Applications of NNs for regression analysis and outcome prediction based on small datasets remain infrequent and thus require further exploration (Forman & Cohen, 2004; Hudson & Cohen, 2000; Grossi & Suzuki, 2011).

PROPOSED METHODOLOGY

Unstable performance and irregular variations are experienced by neural network which are trained with small datasets. The reason for asymmetry in performance of neural network is that NNs are primarily affected by the order of input of training data as well as to the initial values of parameter values (Khovanova et al., 2015; LeBaron & Weigend, 1998; Bowden, 2002). In order to improve convergence to the global minimum of the correlated cost function, an intentional degree of randomness is introduced at the time of initialization of Neural Network and while training NN using backpropagation algorithms (Haykin, 1999; Hudson & Cohen, 2000; LeBaron & Weigend, 1998; Wasserman, 1989). The level of convergence of neural network is influenced by the order of input of training data to the NN hence can and generate inconsistent results (LeBaron & Weigend, 1998; Bowden, 2002). The reliability of the outcome and the actual comparison between various NN designs for potential optimization and validation are limited by this inter-NN volatility. Researchers Cunningham, Carney & Jacob (2000) carried out their research to provide the constancy in NNs. They have suggested the use k-fold cross-validation and ensemble neural network medical domain was used for the purpose of classification. Total 53 features and 1355 observations were considered, which relates less then to 10 observations per predictor variable. Very limited effective strategies are found in the literature for applying deep learning small biomedical datasets, and for validation of the same. Hence demands the methodology for application of NNs to medical domain with a small data set.

A subject-specific model for prediction of target class by applying regression Neural Network on small datasets can be validated using surrogate data and multiple runs of the NN. Multiple runs can break the effect of inter-NN volatility. Reliable evaluation on diverse NN designs can be achieved by engendering a large set of NNs- generally more than thousand. Small datasets generate random effects on NN, to account and remove the random effects in NN, surrogate data may be one of prominent solution. Surrogate data has successfully used by many researchers in the field of time series, neural coding and nonlinear physics. In present chapter Neural Network and surrogate data set are used to validate the results generated through NN designed for small data set. Dataset with electrical impedance measurements in samples of freshly excised tissue from the breast has been used for the experiments (Dua & Graff, 2019).

STEPS FOR TRAINING A NEURAL NETWORK

A neural network for deep learning may be designed and trained using the steps shown in figure 1.

VALIDATING THE PREDICTION

Since the aim of the study is to validate the result achieved on small dataset problem, we have used the method of multiple runs in which training is simultaneously done on large number of NNs having same design.

In each run the input to the NN and the scenario of testing of NN has been varied on three factors.

- First, starting values of Weights and biases were randomized.
- Second, test dataset was not changed, whereas training and validation datasets were varied.
- Third, the input order was varied for training and validation

Thousands of NNs were generated and trained with varied preliminary settings. A series of positive and negative NN were produced in the conceptualized environment. For the model, the NN which resulted in maximum throughput was selected.

Figure 1. Steps for Designing a Neural Network

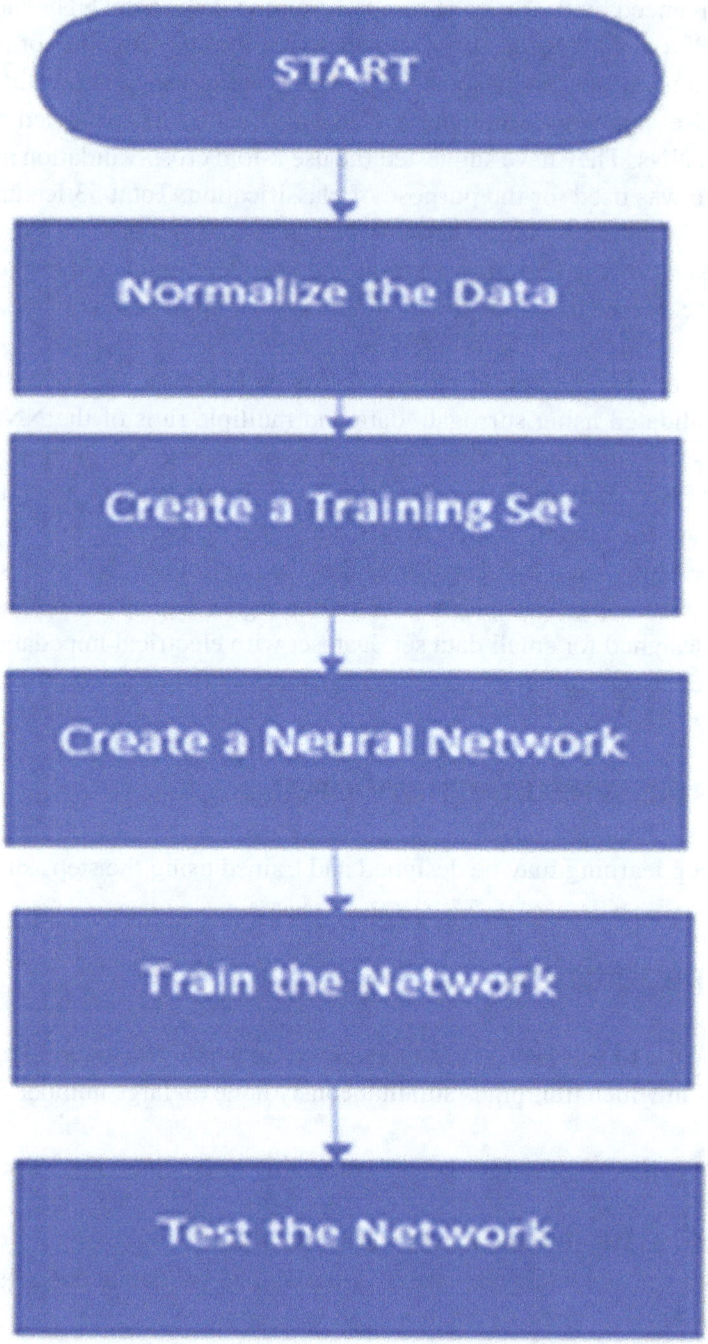

DATA SET

Dataset with electrical impedance measurements in samples of freshly excised tissue from the breast has been used for the experiments (Dua, & Graff, 2019). 106 instances were used. Total 10 attributes are used for class determination out of which 9 were used for features and 1 was used as class attribute.

Frequencies used for Impedance measurements: 15.625, 31.25, 62.5, 125, 250, 500, 1000 KHz.

Frequencies used for Impedance measurements of freshly excised breast tissue: 15.625, 31.25, 62.5, 125, 250, 500, 1000 KHz. Plotted in the (real, -imaginary) plane the weights represent the impedance spectrum from where the breast tissue features are computed.

In present research work the dataset has been used for predicting the classification of 4 classes by joining the fibro-adenoma, mastopathy and glandular classes whose discrimination is neither important nor can be accurately discriminated anyway.

Total nine features: Impedivity (ohm) at zero frequency, phase angle at 500 KHz, high-frequency slope of phase angle, impedance distance between spectral ends, area under spectrum, area normalized by DA, maximum of the spectrum, distance between I0 and real part of the maximum frequency point, length of the spectral curve have been utilized to classify the dataset. Data has been classified into six different classes viz: Carcinoma (Car), Fibro-adenoma (Fad), Mastopathy (Mas), Glandular (Gla), Connective (Con), Adipose (Adi) (Dua & Graff, 2019).

Electrical properties exhibited by biological tissues have been an area of curiosity. It was in late 1800s that the interest of scientist in this field compelled them to do more of experimentation to explore the electrical properties of living tissues. The curiosity in living tissues evolved a novel branch of physiology and the research focused on this branch has provided various insights in several mechanisms. Tissues comprise of cells and extracellular medium. The extracellular medium is primarily composed of ionic solutions. The tissue cells constitute of the cellular membrane and the intra-cellular fluid. The cellular membrane comprises of lipid bilayer and proteins. Composition of cellular membrane makes it capacitive. Since the membrane is selectively permeable, this acts as an exception which defies membrane conductivity. Selectively permeable is a physiological process of the living tissue cells. Intracellular fluid of the cell is an ionic solution of microscopic size and proteins also get charged in response to applied fields; these proteins also contribute to the tissue cell's electrical feature. Tissue cells demonstrate frequency dependent response. Hence when exposed to varied frequency, cellular constituents (intracellular fluid, cell membrane and extracellular medium) demonstrate impedance in varied amounts, unlike electrical components.

Usage of electrical impedance for analyzing biological tissues is increasing considerably as is comparatively low- cost diagnosis, is comfortable to the patients, and studies conducted until now suggest it to be effective in detecting disease in breasts tissues.

Analysis of electrical impedance of breast tissue is a quick and comfortable method which is more predictable in detecting cancers which have earlier gone undetected. Electrical impedance measurement has grown as an interest area for the scientists and medical fraternity too. Challenge is deployment and meaningful interpretation of this data for the benefit of clinical application.

Clinical application of electrical impedance shows its utility in breast cancer detection. Malignant breast tissues have shown higher electrical conductivity as compared to the normal breast tissue. Higher electrical conductivity shown by malignant breast tissue is still being researched upon, but researchers attributed this increased electrical conductivity to increased retention of cellular fluid, increased ionic nature and change in cellular membrane permeability. Impedance measurement in the tissue is utilized to map the electrical nature of breast tissue at various frequencies.

Tissue samples are normally classifieds into six groups. Normal breast tissues are glandular (Gla), connective tissue (Con), and adipose tissue (Adi). The other three are pathological tissue: mastopathy (Mas), fibroadenoma (Fad), and carcinoma (Car).

Standard deviation of all the tissues varied slightly from each other with frequency. Frequency dependent Standard deviation of the phase angle differed for tissue. Connective tissue and adipose tissue displayed highest value of standard deviation as their resistivity is more as compared to rest of the tissues of the group. There is a major difference in the impedivity of normal breast tissue as compared to the cancerous tissue cells.

IMPLEMENTATION

Neural Network was implanted in MATLAB 2019a using neural network tool. Number of neurons in the hidden layers are one of the most important features of a perceptual network. Network will not be able to model the complex data and fit will be poor if insufficient number of neurons are used. Training time will be worst in which network can fit the data if, too many neurons are used. Another drawback of overfitting is that random noise is generated by the network model. Though such type of models fits the training data successfully but fails to generalize new, poor and unseen data. Hence validity test becomes must for such type of models. At the initial stage one hidden layer and 10 neuron-based model was implanted. Figure 2 shows graphical representation of the neural network model implemented for the deep learning.

To achieve better result the no of neurons were increased in varied implementation. For final implementation of neural network with 20 neurons was designed. The network was run many times parallelly to record the best three result. Figure 3 represents the pictorial representation of designed network.

Figure 2. Neural Network Model With 10 Neurons

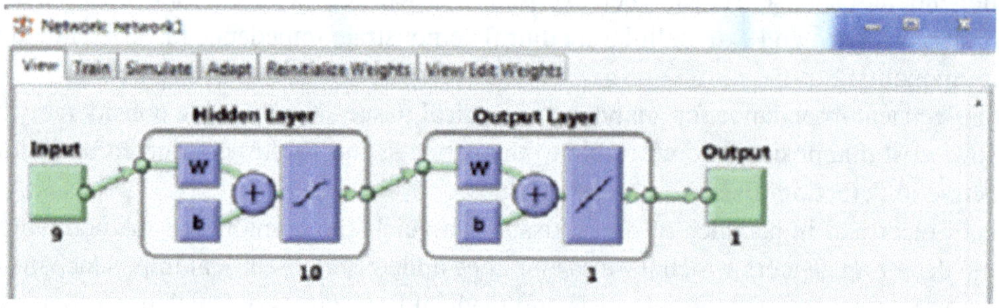

Figure 3. Neural Network Model With 20 Neurons

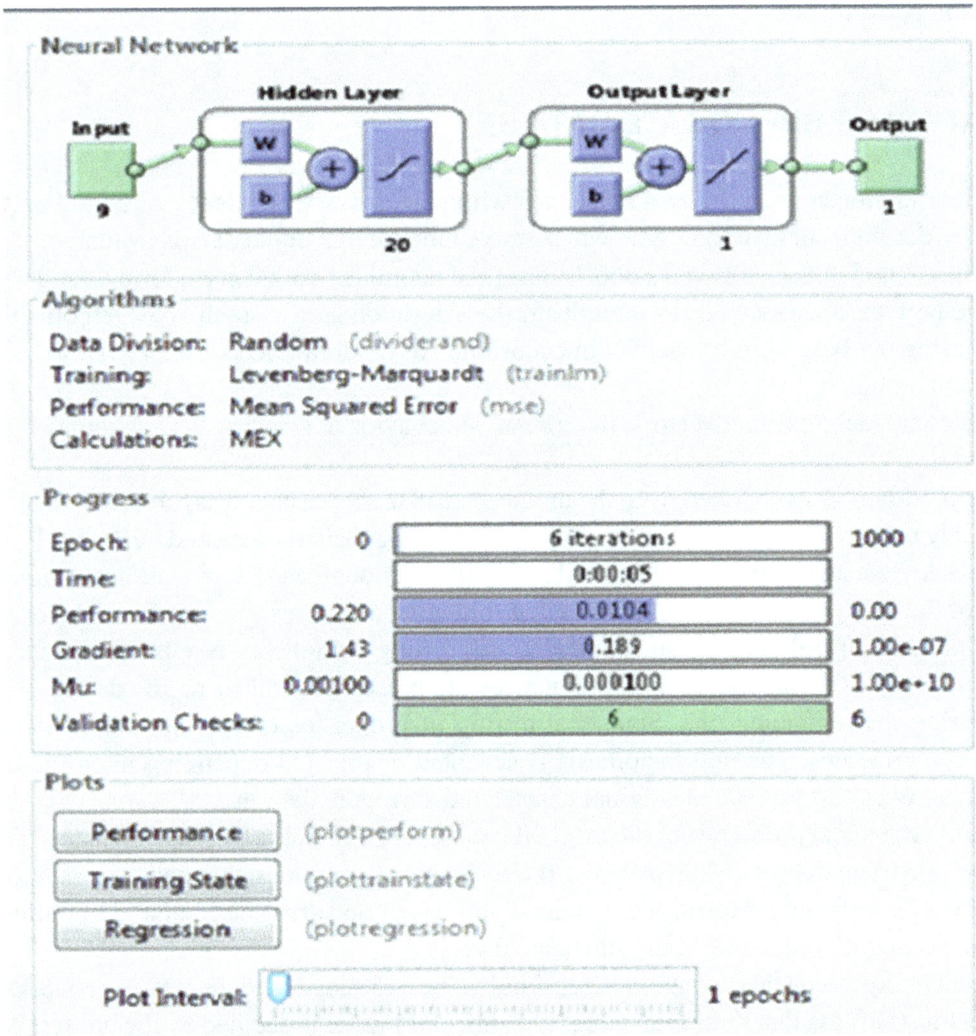

Backpropagation with momentum has been chosen as learning rule. Backpropagation is the most accepted training algorithm for neural network by the researchers. Calculation of gradient vector of the error surface is the policy of backpropagation. From the current point the line of steepest descent is pointed by the vector and the error will be decreased if we move along it from the present position. Subsequently systematic move will find a minimum distance for the convergence. The decision of size of step is a challenging task. Network may converge in lesser time if the large steps are chosen but it may result in going in wrong decision or may surpass the solution. By selecting very small steps, the algorithm may move to correct direction but will lead towards larger number of repetitions. In literature it has been stated that step size is proportionate to the slope and the learning rate. The precise setting for the learning rate basically decided by experiments as it is totally dependent on application. Learning rate could be decreased as the algorithm progresses i.e. it could be based on time. To ensure the movement in a fixed direction inclusion of momentum term is done by modifying the algorithm. Momentum is a well adopted technique. Use of momentum speed up the convergence as numerous steps are taken in the same direction. With the use of momentum, algorithm can escape local minimum and may maintain generalization performance.

GENERATION OF SURROGATE DATA SET

Since the interrelationships in the data correlates with performance efficiency of neural network deep learning provides high standard outcome when ample amount of sample data is available.

This scenario is changed and even a poorly designed neural network can perform extremely well and may achieve high performance on test samples if the size of dataset is small. To overcome this limitation and to bring out best learning via NN in occurrence of random effects use of surrogate data test is proposed in literature.

For each component of input vectors, the statistical behavior of real data set is simulated by the surrogate data set.

The alternate data sets generated from the unique true data set are called as Surrogate data. Surrogate data are widely used by many researchers for hypothesis testing (Scheinkman and LeBaron, 1989; Theiler et al., 1992; Schreiber and Schmitz, 1996; Small et al., 2001). Though these surrogate data maintain certain properties of the original true data set, at the same time they differ in some way from the original data.

For the purpose of utilizing the surrogate data for testing hypothesis, a null hypothesis is framed. Few characteristics of the action potential sequences are preserved, and surrogate dataset is generated by randomizing the remaining one. Statistical testing of properties of original dataset is performed through these surrogates. The null hypothesis is accepted or rejected depending upon the confidence factor obtained from test statistic of original dataset and surrogate dataset.

Though the statistical properties of the original data set are simulated by the surrogates, the complex dependencies between the several elements of the real dataset are not established. The neural networks may observe poor learning performance if trained and tested on surrogates as the correlation between the real data set is not established in the surrogate data.

Now again to overcome this constrain a threshold value is defined, and the neural networks designed for real data must surpass that threshold value. The threshold value is decided by the highest performing neural network based on surrogate data. Surrogate NN's maximum regression coefficient is set as the threshold the lowest performance of real data NN's regression coefficient.

Plenty of methodologies have been suggested by the researchers for generating surrogate samples. (Schreiber & Schmitz, 1996; Theiler et al., 1992; Li et al., 2007). Johnson (2011) has discussed Kolmogorov-Smirnov statistical test, using this test case surrogate

In order to achieve reduced normal distributions surrogates were produced via arbitrary numbers.

This arbitrary numbers were generated by estimating mean and standard deviation from the actual dataset. Range and size of the tissue samples were also estimated and approximated.

RESULTS AND DISCUSSION

Levenberg Marquardt backpropagation algorithm was used to train the dataset of breast tissue. Cost function expressed by MSE and was used to record the performance of the NN on training, validation and test samples during each iteration(epoch).

The iteration at which the validation performance reached a minimum is represented by the label Epoch. After training of first round over the 10-neuron network the best Validation performance was recorded at 0.058961 at epoch 3 (Figure 4). Figure 5 shows that training was stopped after continuing for 3 more iterations. This figure 4 indicates a very normal scenario of training. The problem in training is considered when the validation and test curves don't show similarity.

Performance of regression is shown in Figure 6. The percentage of validation achieved was 0.97%.

While running multiple NN parallelly, with changing order of input of test data and scenario at few cases overfitting was also recorder. Figure 7 depicts Overfitting as the test curve has increased significantly as compared to validation curve.

Figure 4. Validation of Performance on 10 Neuron Network

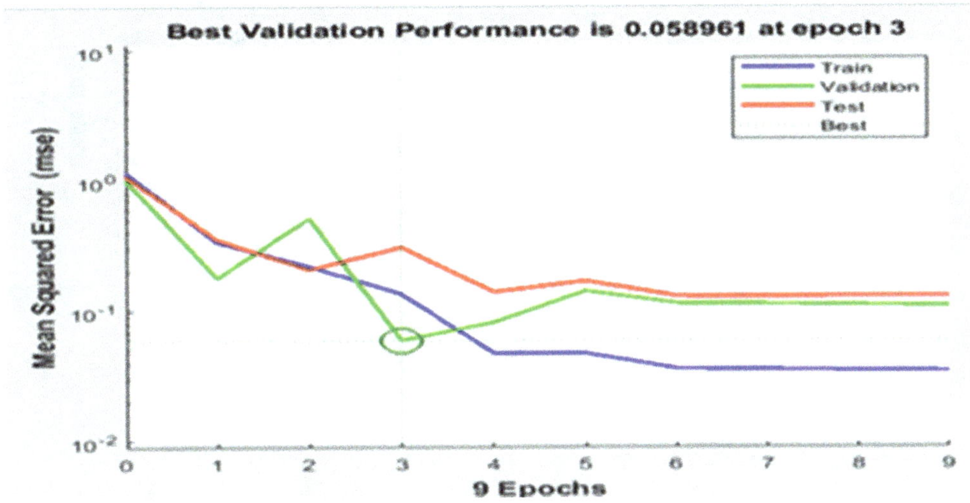

Figure 5. Algorithm for NN Designed on 10 Neurons

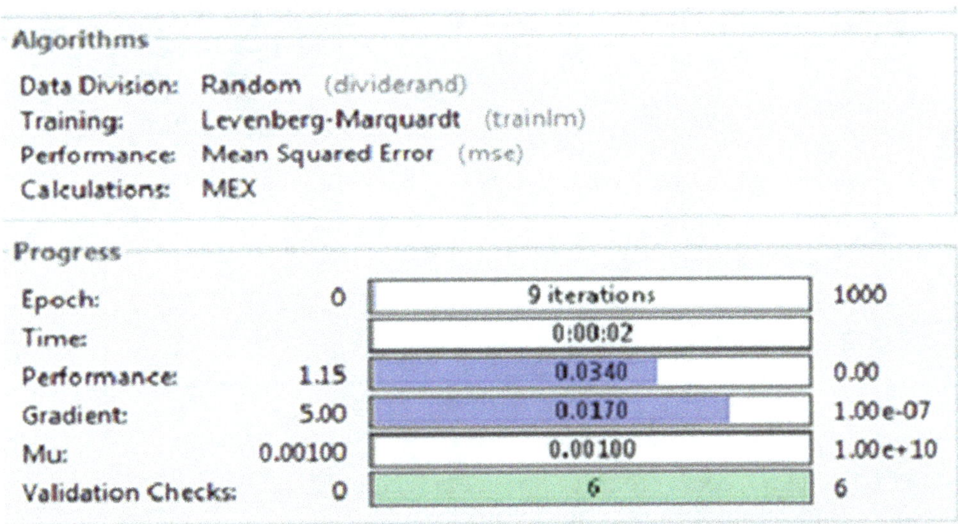

Figure 6. Regression Performance (First Test Run)

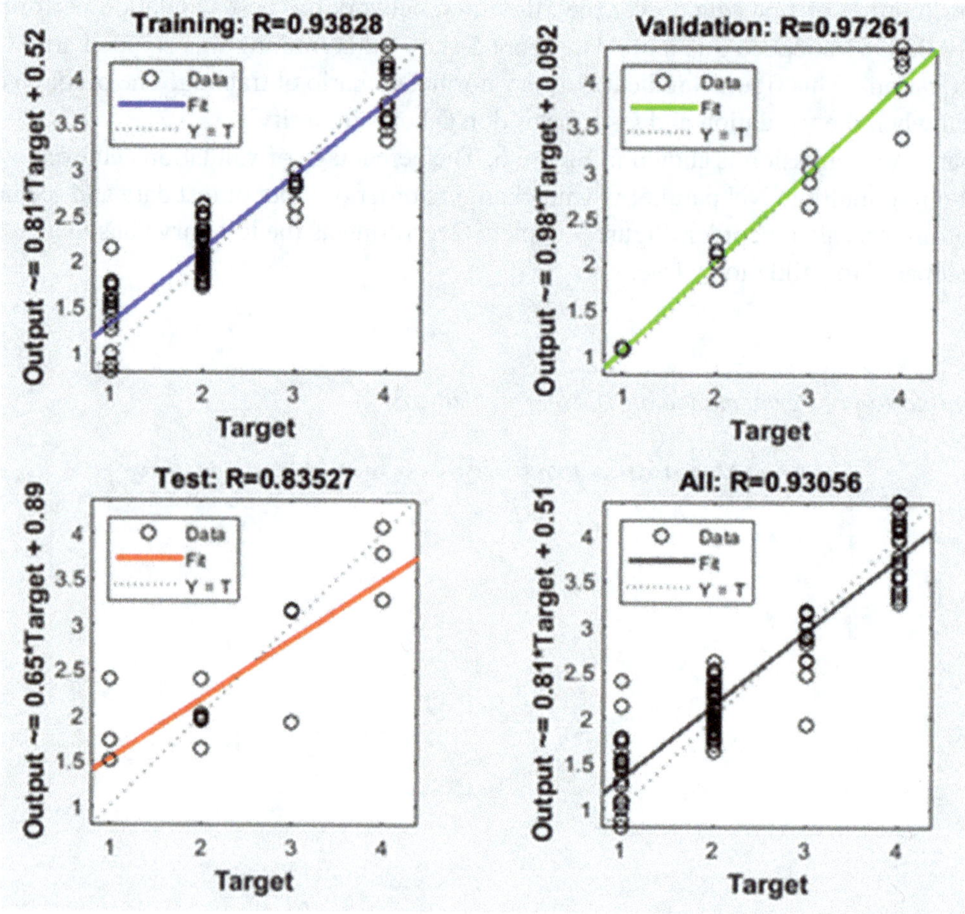

Figure 7. Validation of Performance for NN Designed on 20 Neurons (Varied Test Data)

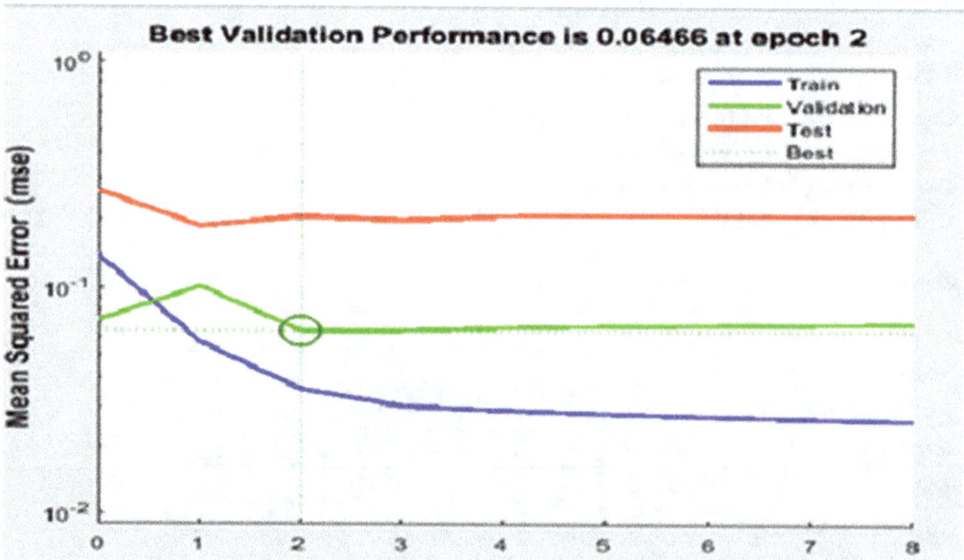

Regression coefficients R between the actual output (target) and predicted output were considered to monitor the criteria in order to major the performance of different NNs. The best performing NN was selected. For the entire dataset regression coefficients were calculated as (R_{all}). Regression coefficient was independently recorded for the training dataset as (R_{train}). Similarly, for validation dataset (R_{val}) and for testing dataset (R_{test}) were monitored. As it evident from various research in the field of regression analysis value of R may vary between 0 and 1. Highest model predictive performance i.e. 100% accuracy is represented by 1 with equal target and prediction values. Khovanova, Mallick and Shaikhina (2015) have conducted a statistical test over the bone dataset. As per the regression statistic R greater than 0.6 defines statistically substantial performance, i.e. $R_{all} \geq 0.6$, $R_{train} \geq 0.6$, $_{Rval} \geq 0.6$, and $R_{test} \geq 0.6$.

Across the run the mean regression coefficients for entire dataset was recorded as $\mu(R_{all}) = 0.91$ and the regression coefficient for test dataset was recorded at decreased values of $\mu\ (R_{test}) = 0.64$ (Figure 8).

When considering only statistically significant NNs (R > 0.7), the mean performance of all samples was recorded as 0.869 and individually for tests it was recorded as 0.766. Despite higher volatility, an undesirable distribution spread and lower mean performance, the maximal R values for the small dataset NNs were comparable with those for the large dataset NNs.

Figure 8. Varied Values Recorded for Mean Regression Coefficient

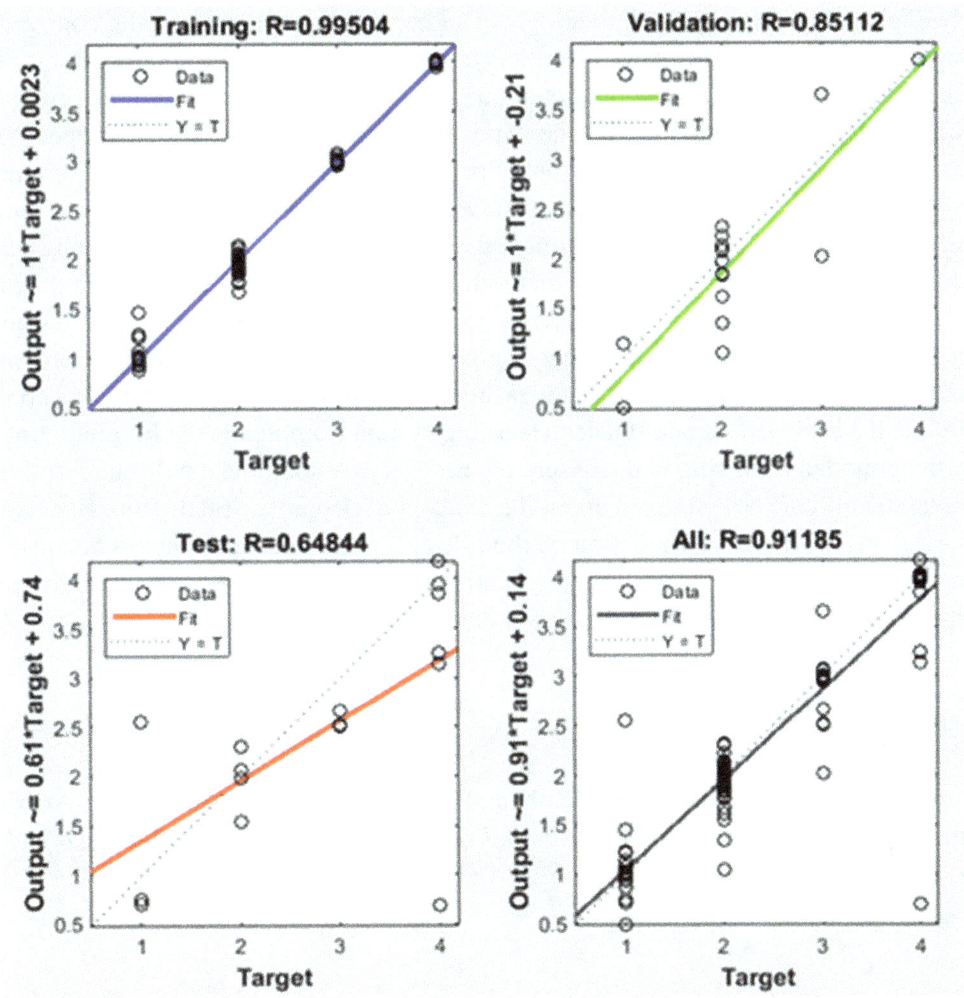

The overall performance of the NNs during a multiple run was valuated based on the threshold value. Those NNs were selected where the value for R was recorded more than 0.7. During multiple run statistically substantial performer networks having values of $R_{all} \geq 0.7$, $R_{train} \geq 0.7$, $_{Rval} \geq 0.7$, and $R_{test} \geq 0.7$ were used for validation.

CONCLUSION

The chapter has discussed in detail about the use of deep learning algorithm in health informatics. It is well acclaimed that deep learning-based system unlocks the full potential of healthcare intelligence if abundant dataset is available to train the deep learning model implemented via neural network. But the model does not guarantee the performance if the availability of training data is limited. Thus, designing and validating a deep learning based neural network becomes a matter of consent for the researchers. The solution for validating a deep learning model based on smaller dataset could be, running multiple runs of neural networks parallelly and use of surrogate data set. A cased study for validating a neural network based on a small dataset of breast tissue has been discussed in the chapter. Use of surrogate data ensures that proposed neural network can perform successfully on bigger set of data belonging to the domain. The introduction part highlights the major limitation of neural networks. The presented case study clearly depicts that discussed methodologies can be utilized to overcome the constrain of validity if smaller sample data set is available. Parallel running of multiple neural network on randomized data set with varied input validates the predicted output of proposed model. By applying multiple run of NN parallelly with varied inputs solves one major limitation of NN i.e. different speed of learning which was caused by change in sequence of input of trained data. Moreover, strategy of running multiple neural network with the use of Surrogate data resolves the second major constrain i.e. requirement of high volume of data set to train the mode. Author suggests that whenever a deep learning-based model is being designed over small data set, proper methodology must be adopted to validate the prediction.

Though the model based deep learning can be utilized for designing automation system in medical research, one major limitation of deep learning-based system is 'No reasoning is provided for the predicted output'. Research in the area of deep learning needs to focus on providing a deep insight and reasoning behind the achieved output. If a deep learning system is implemented for predicting treatment of a patient, the provided reasoning will reassure the accuracy. A doctor can only suggest the change in someone's treatment if he/ she is assured about the concept of diagnosis/ prediction. Hence, it could be concluded that along with proper validation methodology a neural network should be enriched with a justification about the prediction made. The justification will strengthen the trust of patients and doctors and will provide a learning behind the mistakes in diagnosis.

REFERENCES

Amato, F., López, A., Pena-Méndez, E. M., Vanhara, P., Hampl, A., & Havel, J. (2013). Artificial neural networks in medical diagnosis. *Journal of Applied Biomedicine*, *11*(2), 47–58. doi:10.2478/v10136-012-0031-x

Bazi, Y., & Melgani, F. (2006). Towards an optimal SVM classification system for hyperspectral remote sensing images. *IEEE Transactions on Geoscience and Remote Sensing*, *44*(11), 3374–3385. doi:10.1109/TGRS.2006.880628

Bowden, G. J. (2002). Optimal division of data for neural network models in water resources applications. *Water Recourses*, *38*, 1–11.

Cunningham, P., Carney, J., & Jacob, S. (2000). Stability problems with artificial neural networks and the ensemble solution. *Artificial Intelligence in Medicine*, *20*(3), 217–225. doi:10.1016/S0933-3657(00)00065-8 PMID:10998588

Dua, D., & Graff, C. (2019). *UCI Machine Learning Repository*. Irvine, CA: University of California, School of Information and Computer Science.

Foody, G. M., Mathur, A., Hernandez, C. H., & Boyd, D. S. (2006). Training set size requirements for the classification of a specific class. *Remote Sensing of Environment*, *104*(1), 1–14. doi:10.1016/j.rse.2006.03.004

Forman, G., & Cohen, I. (2004). Learning from little: comparison of classifiers given little training. In *Proceedings of the European Conference on Principles of Data Mining and Knowledge Discovery* (pp. 161–172). Academic Press. 10.1007/978-3-540-30116-5_17

Grossi, E., & Suzuki, K. (2011). Artificial neural networks and predictive emedicine: a revolutionary paradigm shift. In Artificial Neural Networks-Methodological Advances and Biomedical Applications (pp. 139-150). Academic Press.

Han, J., & Kamber, M. (2005). Data mining: Concepts and techniques. San Francisco, CA: Kaufmann.

Haykin, S. S. (1999). *Neural networks: A comprehensive foundation*. Upper Saddle River, NJ: Prentice Hall.

Hornik, K., Stinchcombe, M., & White, H. (1989). Multilayer feedforward networks are universal approximators. *Neural Networks*, *2*(5), 359–366. doi:10.1016/0893-6080(89)90020-8

Hsu, C. W., & Lin, C. J. (2002). A comparison of methods for multiclass support vector machines. *IEEE Transactions on Neural Networks*, *13*(2), 415–425. doi:10.1109/72.991427 PMID:18244442

Hudson, D. L., & Cohen, M. E. (2000). *Neural networks and artificial intelligence for biomedical engineering*. New York: IEEE.

Johnson, J. L. (2011). *Probability and Statistics for Computer Science*. New York: Wiley.

Jossinet, J. (1998). The impedivity of freshly excised human breast tissue. *Physiological Measurement*, *19*(1), 61–75. doi:10.1088/0967-3334/19/1/006 PMID:9522388

Khovanova, N. A., Mallick, K. K., & Shaikhina, T. (2015). Neural networks for analysis of trabecular bone in osteoarthritis. *Bioinspir Biomim Nanobiomater*, *4*(1), 90–100. doi:10.1680/bbn.14.00006

LeBaron, B., & Weigend, A. S. (1998). A bootstrap evaluation of the effect of data splitting on financial time series. *IEEE Transactions on Neural Networks*, *9*(1), 213–220. doi:10.1109/72.655043 PMID:18252443

Li, D. C., Wu, C. S., Tsai, T. I., & Lina, Y. S. (2007). Using mega-trend-diffusion and artificial samples in small data set learning for early flexible manufacturing system scheduling knowledge. *Computers & Operations Research, 34*(4), 966–982. doi:10.1016/j.cor.2005.05.019

Olutayo, O. & Singhal, G. (2009). Piecewise Multi-Classification Support Vector Machines, In *Proceedings of International Joint Conference on Neural Networks*. Academic Press.

Rong, H. J., Huang, G. B., Sundararajan, N., & Saratchandran, P. (2009). Online Sequential Fuzzy Extreme Learning Machine for Function Approximation and Classification Problems, IEEE Transactions on Systems, Man, and Cybernetics. *Part B, 39*, 1067–1072. PMID:19336333

Scheinkman, J. A., & LeBaron, B. (1989). Nonlinear dynamics and stock returns. *The Journal of Business, 62*(3), 311–337. doi:10.1086/296465

Schreiber, T., & Schmitz, A. (1996). Improved surrogate data for nonlinearity tests. *Physical Review Letters, 77*(4), 635–638. doi:10.1103/PhysRevLett.77.635 PMID:10062864

Shaikhina, T., Khovanova, N., & Mallick, K. (2014). Artificial neural networks in hard tissue engineering: another look at age-dependence of trabecular bone properties in osteoarthritis. In *Proceedings of the IEEE EMBS Int. Conf. Biomed. Heal. Informatics* (pp. 622-625). IEEE Press. 10.1109/BHI.2014.6864441

Small, M., Yu, D., & Harrison, R. G. (2001). Surrogate test for pseudo periodic time series. *Physical Review Letters, 87*(18), 188101. doi:10.1103/PhysRevLett.87.188101

Theiler, J., Eubank, S., Longtin, A., Galdrikian, B., & Doyne, F. J. (1992). (. Testing for nonlinearity in time series: The method of surrogate data. *Physica, 58*(1–4), 77–94.

Timmer, J. (1998). Power of surrogate data testing with respect to nonstationary. *Phys. Rev. E., 58*(4), 5153-5156.

Wasserman, P. D. (1998). *Neural computing: theory and practice*. New York: Van Nostrand-Reinhold.

Chapter 10
Managing the Scarcity of Monitoring Data Through Machine Learning for Human Behavior in Mental Health Care

Nitesh Kumar Dixit
https://orcid.org/0000-0003-0636-8642
Bhartiya Institute of Engineering and Technology, Sikar, India

Dileep Kumar Agarwal
Bhartiya Institute of Engineering and Technology, Sikar, India

Mahendra Kumar
Bhartiya Institute of Engineering and Technology, Sikar, India

ABSTRACT

Nowadays, in many fields, including medicine and public health, developments in information and communication technology have introduced a revolution. Due to the absence of effective machinery algorithms and many possibilities to enhance patient understanding of chronic diseases, information gathered from the distinct sources were ignored. Therefore, researchers are investigating information shortages of computer training methods. This work recommends a fresh strategy to produce stronger predictive models specifically intended for the problems. In order to address the scarcity of data, works propose to make use of a semi-managed learning environment while using all unlabeled data sets. The techniques suggested were implemented in the mental health care field of bipolar disorder. The methods suggested enhancing the efficiency of ranking to the accuracy of ≈ 73% to ≈ 90%. The results have been achieved by overcoming previous methods that use traditional monitored methods of learning.

INTRODUCTION

Health care is an important element of human existence and regular tracking of vital parameters such as therapy is a fundamental feature of health care. These procedures are even more essential in the therapy

DOI: 10.4018/978-1-7998-2101-4.ch010

of mental illnesses, for which qualified medical staff is required to track patient condition. Current practice for tracking these health fundamental parameters is only measured in discrete intervals from doctors or medical staff. In order to evaluate the efficacy of treatment (i.e. mental health), self-declared subjective health measures are also important, but these methods often lead to a loss of important data of the patient throughout the day or night.

Healthcare doctors have been using fresh sophisticated technology in the previous two decades to enhance healthcare facilities while increasing the quality of care and health results. In order to encourage health and health training and provide more cost-efficient care, this research focused particularly on the use of computers, smartphones, and other wearable devices.

BACKGROUND

A number of study projects have shown how potential the use of mobile technology to monitor human behaviour. Smartphones have been proposed as a promising candidate in order to infer human relationships and behavioural modifications in real-life operations (Mika et al., 2005, pp. 51-59). Researchers (Uwe et al., 2006, pp. 4-7; Mika et al., 2005, pp. 51-59) numerous benefits of smartphone signalling were recorded in continuously accumulating many kinds of qualitative information such as places, physical exercise, physical postures, expression-emotion etc.

The most dominating ideas in the field of health care include general computing, all-inclusive computing, and the creation and implementation of general health applications (Gaetano et al., 2007, pp 17-19). Patients and clinicians were mainly supported with mobile, comprehensive and all-encompassing computing technology. One of the researchers suggested that smartphones would help to control diseases by providing continuous feedback (Gabriela et al., 2011, pp. 1-8). The researchers emphasize the need for smartphones to handle mental illnesses through Variations of personal behaviour, daily routines and conscience-reported conduct. These systems evaluating information would help medical professionals react instantly and avoid patients migrating into severe illnesses. Furthermore, smartphones can also monitor physiological reactions that can stem from speech (e.g. expressing different feelings during telephone discussions) (Klaus R & Scherer, 1986, pp. 143-165). Various quantitative studies have shown the significance of nonverbal communication such as speech or body postures to evaluating the emotional state.

METHODS AND TECHNIQUES

In the following parts that will briefly define information gathered from the smartphone sensors and analysis behavioural for a mental health condition. These techniques can be defined as a processing chain that begins from raw sensory information and results in the user wellbeing forecast. Figure 1 shows the easiest instance of a left-to-right information stream which presents a mechanism for human behaviour.

As shown in Figure 1, information collection is the first step in this operation. The aim of pre-processing is to enhance signal noise by using filtering techniques, normalizing techniques and another removal of artifacts. Filtering methods are technologies that decrease noise from gathered information in order to improve the representation of behavioural patterns. The filtered information is often classified according to their significance and that will be done by the segmentation process. Some identification schemes

Figure 1. Supervised Learning Technique

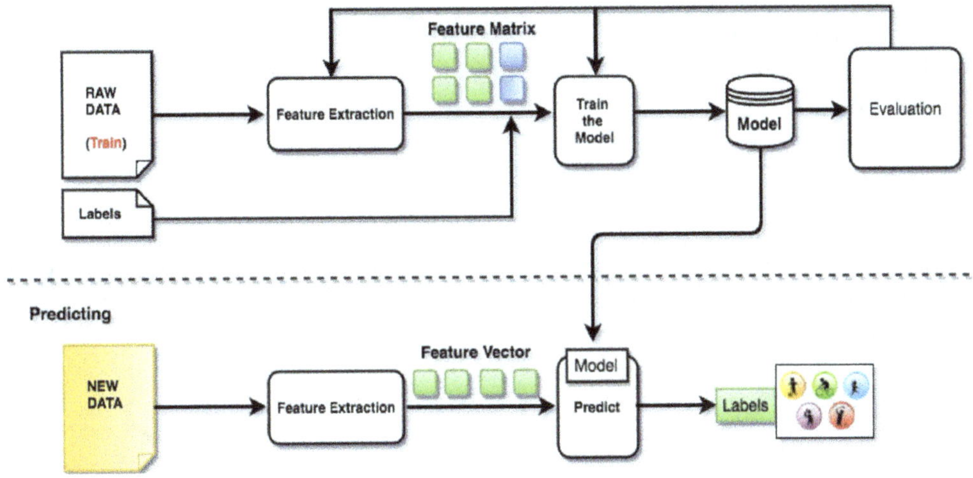

involve segmentation of each pattern in order to generate significant entities for extracting functions and for classifying them in the final stage.

It is the most significant problem to select the best set of characteristics that assist to decrease the size of data sets. Function extraction aims to reduce the number of functions extracted from the dataset and selects features according to their defined classes. Therefore, many specialists in the sector (Richard et al., 1997) stressed that the correct characteristics must be used to correctly recognize the behaviour.

The labelling method is that of the outputs for the next processing stage using the selected features from the entire database. The results of the classification are usually a confidential pick of one given category. The task of classifying the degree will instantly focus on characteristics common to each category. The performance exactness of the feature extraction phase is therefore substantially impacted. The learning methodology is used for extracting information from gathered information. The main objective of semi-supervised learning is to incorporate the benefit of regulated and unmonitored processes, by collecting facts identified and un-identified. The semi-supervised learning algorithms are one of the important subjects for studies in machine learning by using and exploiting the costless unlabelled information during the training phase. One of the researcher explained the technique used in semi-supervised learning studies (Rayid & Nigam, 2000, pp. 86-93).

Only one classification is needed, so only one function set is needed with the self-learning algorithm. The classification is based on current marked information and is applied to a series of unlabelled information. The classifier labels the unlabelled information for several iterations. Algorithm 1 displays the typical auto training algorithm as the pseudo code. Self-workout starts with marked information (L) and constructs a classification (C) that then applies to the unlabelled U information set. T is the set of cases most confidently anticipated. The marked set is introduced and the classifier is then retrained for fresh cases with several iterations.

Algorithm 1: Self-Training Algorithm
Input: $L = (x_i, y_i)$; Identified Information sets.
$U = (x_i, ?)$; Unidentified Information sets

T; the threshold
while U $\neq\varnothing$ or U'$\neq$ $\varnothing$ do
Prepare classifier (C) with learning information (L)
Classification information done through Classifier (C)
If (confidence > T) then
L = L + U'
U = U - U'

This fresh enhanced information is used to induce a fresh model for producing fresh projections of the decreased information (see Algorithm 1). It is constantly repeated until or exceed the threshold or empty the unmarked data.

Transfer Learning

Throughout this session analysis took the approach of addressing the shortage of dataset: first, to use the data available to develop a Ti template for a new subject. And equate the design to the remaining T models for the other subjects. In Algorithm 2, which used assessment algorithm trees to induct the subject model. Transfer learning could not be implemented in proposed model data set gathered by patients with bipolar disorder because of the small number of respondents and the differing status and would lead to adverse transmission.

Algorithm 2 Transfer Learning Algorithm.
Let D_T ; dataset from target user
Let $\{D_1, \ldots, D_n\}$; datasets from other users
Let $M_{all} = \{M_1, \ldots, M_n\}$;
Let Th = threshold value
for each $M_i \in M_{all}$ do
Find similarity value with M_T ($sim(M_T,M_i)$)
end for
Sort M_{all} using $sim(M_T, M_i) | M_i \in M_{all}$
If Naıve then
Select model M_i
identify D_i and generate new model M_T with condition $\{D_T \cup D_i\}$
else if (for threshold condition)
$M_{sim} = \{U_i M_i | sim(M_T,M_i) > Th\})$
Let D = $\{U_i$ Di | Di was used to induce $M_i \in M_{sim}\})$
Induce new model MT with $\{D_T \cup D\}$
else if (for Sampling condition)
Let M_K = initial K elements in dataset
Let D = $\{U_i D_i | D_i$ was used to induce $M_i \in M_K\})$
Let $D_0 = \{ U_i$ sample $D_i \in D \propto sim(M_T, M_i)\}$
Induce new model M_T with $D_T \cup D'$
else if (for Ensemble Condition)
Let M_L = first L elements in dataset

M_T S_L i=1 $w_i M_i | w_i$ = sim(M_T, M_i)∧ M_i∈ M_T (for weighted model)
end if

For Learning follow these steps:

- To predict mood variables associated with surveys, use initial raw data captured from smartphone evaluation.
- A classifier has been instructed to anticipate weighted (on the grounds of exactness) values for each of the survey factors.
- Triggering a model which predicts a patient's episodic status in a bipolar disorder using the collected information.

Testing steps are

- Implement smartphone data to calculate a weighted array of mood factors with intermediate models (depending on the precision).
- To preview the final model, use smartphone data and expected mood variables.

The data from the questionnaires are characterized by three factors for bipolar disease. Thus, in Bipolar and Stress apps, algorithm induce three and six classifiers.

INTERMEDIATE MODELS

The latent variables are used by certain methods to produce better prediction models. These hidden variables were developed artificially and are used to create better models as intermediate data. So intermediate model algorithm 3 will use for this purpose.

Algorithm 3
Let D_1; Dataset from smartphones
LetD_2; Dataset from variables questionnaires
Let Y; set associated classes
For x_i∈ D_2 do
Train a classifier C_i with training data (D_1, x_i)
end for
for every value of C_i do
for e_j∈ D_1 do
Use e_j as input to C_i
end for
end for
instruct a C_{final} with labelled information data ((D_1∪ $\dot{D}_2$),Y)

TRAINING

Semi-monitored methods for Training to target scarce information have been suggested and researched extensively. A broader study is submitted in semi-supervised learning literature survey with the most significant algorithms in this region (Xiaojin, 2006). Semi-supervised learning's primary goal is to connecting the strengths of monitored and unmonitored training through the experience of marked and unmarked facts.

Co-Training

Co-training utilizes two classifiers for predicting unlabelled information. Learning comparable to self-training. Similarly, co-training is a wrapping technique using two C1 and C2 classificatory which can allocate a reliability score to their projections (as shown in Algorithm 4). Nothing from one training set (i.e. V1 to L2 and V2 i.e. L1) the two categorizers trained on two' views' information (v1 and v2) offer their trustworthy unlabelled forecast (Johnson & Zhang, 2007, pp. 1489-1517).

To create a healthy classification, adequate labelled information will be provided in each perspective (v1, v2). Based on the class label, both opinions are dependent. The clearest presumption is that there are two distinct v= [v1, v2] opinions. If both assumptions exist, co-trainers can learn from labelled and unlabelled information effectively. The above assumptions were examined for the processing of natural languages (Rayid & Nigam, 2000, pp. 86-93) and study (Johnson & Zhang, 2007, pp. 1489-1517). This technique can be used for datasets without distinct opinions or various classification kinds.

Algorithm 4. Co-Training
Input: $L = (x_i, y_i)$; Marked labelled
$U = (x_i, ?)$; Unmarked labelled and instruct C_1, c_2 classifier
T; As a threshold
for $U \neq \varnothing$ or $U \neq \varnothing$ then
Train C_1, c_2 classifier and
Explore C_1' and C_2' as most-confident prediction
$L_1 = L_2 + U'$
$U = U - U'$

Semi-Supervised SVM (S3VM)

In the classifier's teaching phase, half-supervised methods are very important. Taking into account that the use of unmarked information to learn can contribute to the improvement of classifiers performance (i.e. Through the forecasts contain useful new predictions).

Semi-controlled SVM (S3VM) training was initiated by optimizing the initial SVM (see Equation 1) (Thorsten, 1999, pp. 200-209) first.

$$\min\left[\frac{1}{2}\cdot\|w\|^2 + C.\sum_{i}^{i=1}\varsigma\frac{d}{i} + C^*.\sum_{j}^{u}\varsigma^*\frac{d}{i}\right] \tag{1}$$

Where u shows the number of unlabelled information and unlabelled instance parameters included in the stage of learning. The margin shall be evaluated by 1 and by minimizing the norm that corresponds to the maximization of the limit and the fulfilment of the limit for each information stage (Thorsten, 1999, pp. 200-209). The performance gap between monitored SVM and semi-monitored S3VM was proved (Thorsten, 1999, pp. 200-209). The objective of the S3VM is to identify unlabelled instances so that the maximum margin of the decisions is provided for labelled instances and new labelled instances.

EXPERIMENT SETUP

In this section the survey schemes are presented, the configuration of the research and the original data analysis are also presented. The new generation of embedded-sensor mobile systems has developed possibilities to explore fresh contextual facilities, and such information can be helpful.

The primary issues of self-monitoring technologies can be described as follows in real-world situations:

- Most current devices are constructed under supervised conditions, where marked information are important for model construction.
- It takes more energy and time to have adequate marked cases.
- These schemes depend on the accuracy of the information marked by the user.
- The effective participation and encouragement of user (i.e. reminders, feedback) which is sometimes lacking in self-monitoring.
- Although most structures do not use unlabelled cases, these cases can also contain significant data.

Monitoring systems

This scheme included five parts: a smartphone, an exercise screen, a new Galvanic Skin Response (GSR) detector, a gateway, and a permanent EEG unit for regular readings. 10 participants (9 women and 1 man) were included in the research unit. As inclusion parameters, the ability and readiness of all patients to use modern smartphones were identified as bipolar disorder (with frequent episode modifications) and patient's age were between 18 and 65. A personalized smartphone was provided to each of the patients in any manner. The device has mounted an ongoing monitoring implementation (DFKI) 4 that stored information on the record of the device and periodically transferred the information to an independent server. All detecting modalities including smartphone, accelerometer, GPS, Wi-Fi, Bluetooth, SMS, mobile calls and their duration have been examined. Figure 2 shows the mobile application software for monitoring patient health that continued to run in the backdrop. The software was created to collect appropriate disease elements in near co-operation with the psychiatrists. The inner affective status of the patient was measured by means of questionnaires and behaviour was measured through phone-sensor sampling.

Patient Psychiatric Evaluation

The psychiatrists have put the patient-interviews to reduce the memory effect, which preventing partial assessment results. During the patient assessment, the clinicians used the following standard scales.

Figure 2. Patient monitoring application for Bipolar Disorder.

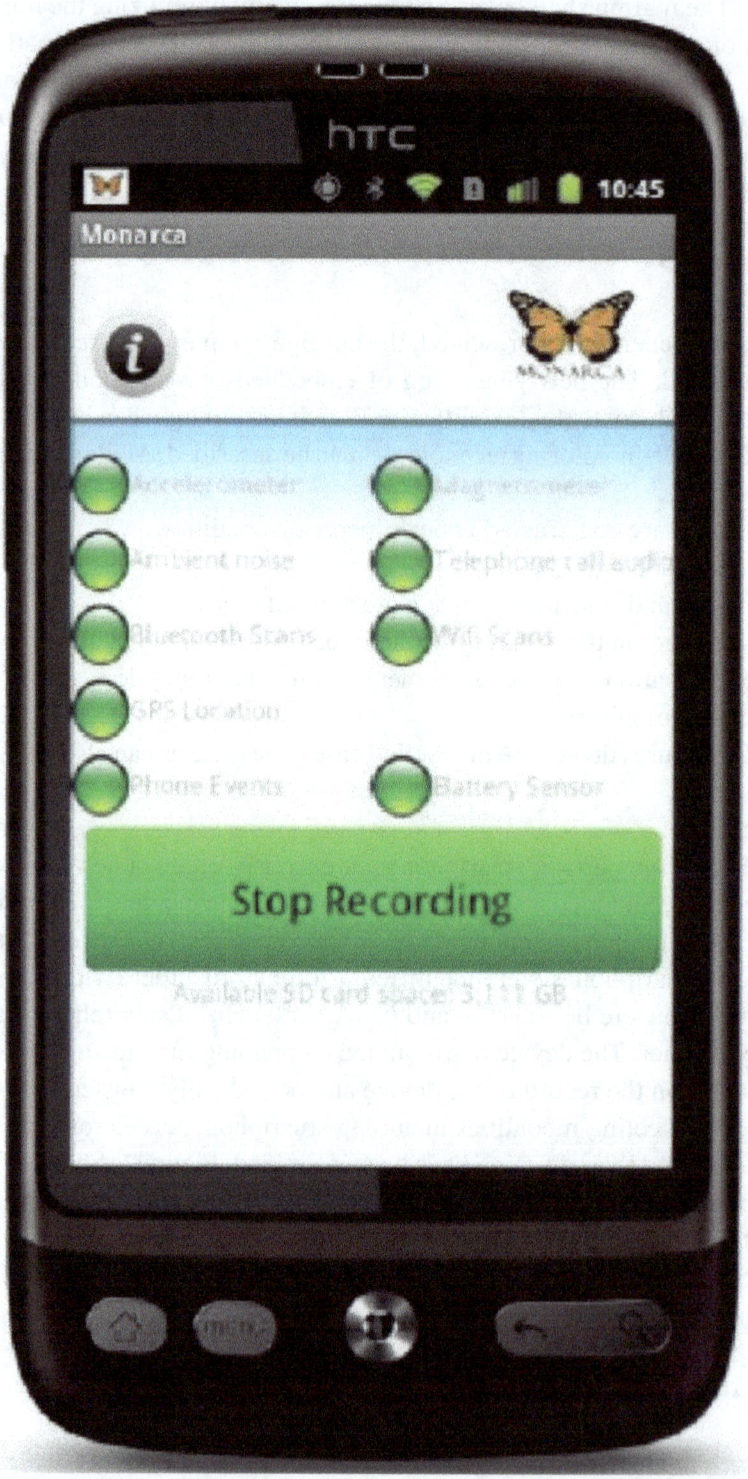

Table 1. Psychiatric Evaluation of Patients

P.ID.	1st Observation	2nd Observation	3rd Observation	4th Observation	5th Observation
P601	+1	+0.5	+0.5	+0.25	0
P602	-0.5	0	0	0	-1.5
P603	-1.5	-1	0	0	0
P604	-1.5	-	-1.5	-	-1.5
P605	0	-	-1.5	-1	0
P606	-0.25	-0.5	0	NA	-
P607	-1.25	-1	-0.25	-1	-1
P608	-1.5	-0.5	0	-	0
P609	0	0	-1	-0.5	-1
P610	+0.5	-0.5	-1	-1.25	-

- Hamilton Depression Scale: This extent has been implemented to evaluate the seriousness of depression in a patient by assessing a variety of symptoms. The greater the symptom size, the greater the disease intensity scale.
- Young Mania Rating Scale: This is the most commonly used rating extent for overexcited signs assessment. The basis results may vary in particular based on the clinical characteristics of the patient such as sadness and obsession.

For 10 patients with bipolar illness, there were five measurement points as shown in table 1. During the full test, a person (P606) showed no episodic change. Furthermore, the person (P0606) dropped out of a clinical trial owing to the situation experienced at that time. In this work, purposed model also analyzed the telephone-conversation and classified the information. In addition, there were not enough phone calls to be employed in the evaluation model in patient P605. Only five participants have given enough information for and classes owing to re-recurrence (i.e., more than two modifications occurred) to enable us to categorize this research into their state (P602, P603, P606, P609, P610).

Given that the test was performed under uncontrolled circumstances, it could not be ensured that the patients always brought the mobile with them during their normal regular lives. Furthermore, there have been many practical difficulties. In certain cases, some patients switched off their detecting application during the night resulting in information breaks. For the whole sampling period, this has considerably improved an amount of lacking information. The real quantity of accessible sensor information ranged from 19 to 71 datasets per person per detector mode. Fortunately, on the smartphone, a day-to-day self-rated mood has been evaluated so that model can draw on the patient's behaviour and self-reporting mood at real time.

State Calculation

At 4 Hz to 10Hz system have continually recorded 3-axial linear speed, which varies due to working circumstances of Android system like scheme charges and battery standards. At 5 Hz set frequency (25.6 seconds), the accelerometer pulses have been re-sampled. An average of 2 GB of pure accelerometer

Table 2. List of appeals and classes based on medical reviews.

Patient	Depression			Ordinary	Soft Manic	Total	Additional Data
	Strict	Sensible	Soft				
P602	18	-	56	74	-	149	217
P603	67	-	-	49	-	117	99
P607	-	56	19	-	-	75	58
P609	-	71	-	80	-	151	89
P610	-	-	17	-	81	98	14
All	85	127	92	203	81	590	531

information was available for each patient. The square roots of the sum of the components of each acceleration axis are determined shown in equation 2.The size variation (as shown in Equation 3) for each n = 128 sample given an event rating range within a three-state threshold, namely 'none,' 'moderate,' and 'strong,' as described in the FUNF structure (Aharony, Pan, Ip et al., 2011, pp. 643-659).

$$SVM = \frac{1}{n}\sum_{i=1}^{n}\sqrt{x_i^2 + y_i^2 + z_i^2} \tag{2}$$

$$\text{var}\, Sum(n) = ((SVM(n) - avgSVM(n))^2 - \left(\frac{n}{n-1}\right) - 2SVM(n)$$

The purposed system have therefore mixed the two effective states (' moderate ' and ' high ')(3) to create a final rating for this study, which was concerned in changing overall exercise rates. The analysis of accelerometer and audio voice characteristics was done during a telephone discussion. We analyzed and chosen patients with sufficient data during their telephone discussion who constitute a range of disease severities in their mental assessment. In this study, the auto-assessment questions for motor exercise, such as emotional self-reportedness, physical state and degree of exercise, have also been included. Table 2 also demonstrates additional information (last column) showing the number of mobile calls that are not connected with any event.

Feature Extraction

The app created for research captures microphone voice transmissions only during telephone conversations through a sample rate of 22 Hz and amplitude of 16 points. In order to prevent its first reconstruction while maintaining the characteristics needed for analysis of the speech, algorithms were created to shrink the real message. The acoustic characteristics included in this study are shown in Table 3. The characteristics have been split into two different kinds: the presidium and the vocal tract.

A summary of mobile discussions during the trial can also be seen in Table 4. This chart demonstrates daily the total amount of telephone conversations of psychological assessments. The model explores the relation between the lengthy expression breaks throughout depressive moods of depressed patients, as

Table 3. Choose speech characteristics relevant to bipolar conditions.

Group	Features Type
Prosodic: Energy, Times P_0V, F_0	"LOG energy", "Zero crossing rate", "Probability of Voicing"
Spectral: "MFCC" "MEL" "SEB" "SROP" "SFlux" "SC" "SpecMaxMin"	"MFCC" "MEL Spectrum" "Spectral Energy in bands" "Spectral roll of the point" "Spectral flux" "Spectral Centroid" "Spectral max and min with DFT."

Table 4. Total number and time of telephone calls (entrance, exit) in psychiatric evaluations (Mean ± SD)

Patient ID	1st-2nd	2nd-3rd	3rd -4th	4th -5th
P602	200(4.395±2.69)	102(2.55±3.7)	76.5(2.02±1.605)	96.5(2.68±1.895)
P603	84.5(3.38±1.7)	59.5(2.83±4.73)	79(3.53±2.26)	42.5(2.655±1.665)
P607	60.5(3.05±2.165)	25(2.5±1.505)	62.5(3.73±2.735)	59.5(3.2±2.46)
P609	86(5.03±3.545)	54(4.355 ±2.88)	92.5(2.44±2.425)	-
P610	65(6.58±4.005)	108(5.68±6.3)	-	-

Table 5. Interaction between duration and number of lengthy calls and clinical test outcomes

P.ID.	Dur. Avg. / Long Pauses Avg.	Dur. Avg. / Long Pauses Avg.	Diff. (%)	Dur. Avg. / Long Pauses Avg.	Diff. (%)
P602	28.78/0.26 (MiD)	19.9/0.14 (N)	-15.45/-26.07	37/0.027 (SeD)	48.49/51.25
P603	65.43/0.575 (SeD)	43.97/43.5 (N)	-16.40/-12.17	n/a	n/a
P607	27.075/0.265(MoD)	35.915/0.33 (N)	82.05/78.02	59.08/0.045 (MoD)	-8.02/-12.05
P609	47.32/0.375 (N)	65.43/0.55 (N)	13.45/14.28	n/a	n/a
P610	42.98/0.31 (MiM)	111.48/0.751 (N)	37.16/72.26	n/a	n/a

(N) = Normal; (MiD) = Mild Depression; (MoD) = Moderate Depression; (SeD) = Severe Depression; (MiM) = Mild Manic.

shown in Table 5. It shows that average delays in depressive condition and response delays have been generally more frequently introduced than during non-depressive condition. This reduction can be seen in P602, P603, and P609 patients. In P602 and P603, when the average call duration /average lengthy pause amount between the phrases was from 115(sec.)/0.84 in a depressed condition, 79.54(sec.)/0.56 in a regular state (P602) and in P603 in patients with an average mobile call length and amount of lengthy periods from 260(sec.)/2.30, in a depressed state, it is more apparent in P602 and P603. The number of intervals between changes from an occurrence of psychosis through to a breakdown (P610) is given by Figure 3 and Figures 4. The patient's personality event ate allocated of general voice sections in conversation shown in Figure 5 and Figure 6.

Figure 3. Overall mean values of a number of long pauses (p610).

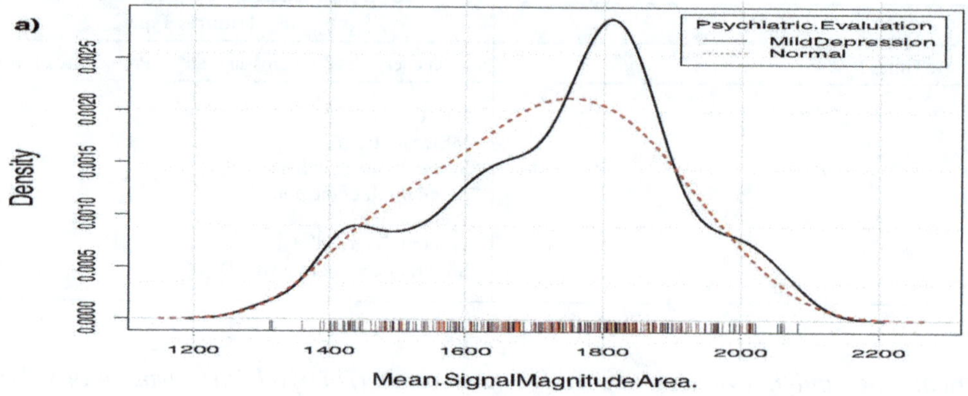

Figure 4. Mean total length values of long breaks (p610).

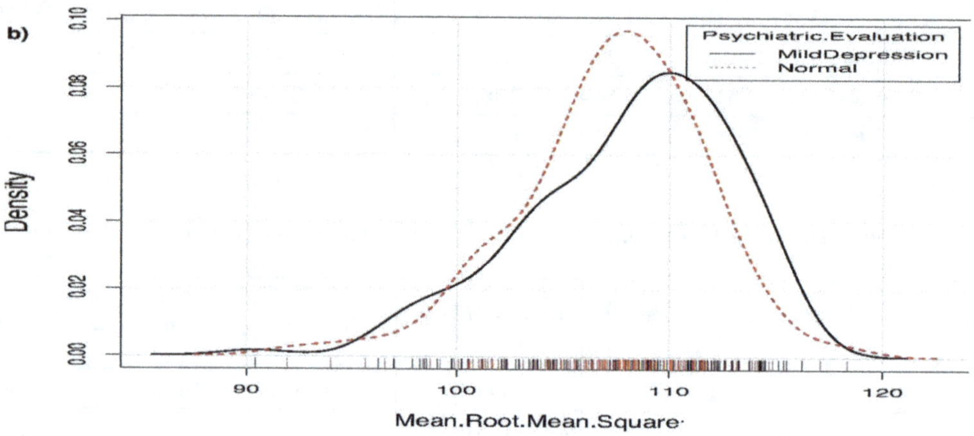

Figure 5. Maximum mean values for the number of segments (p607).

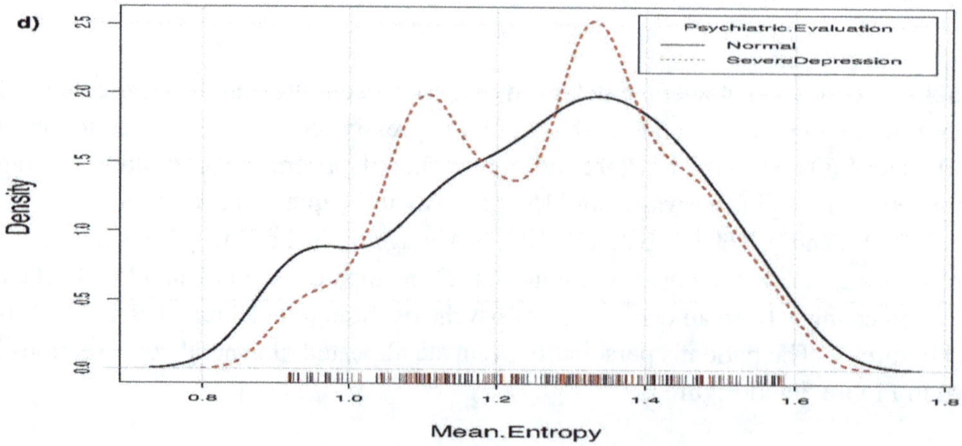

Figure 6. Maximum average values for maximum speech length (p602).

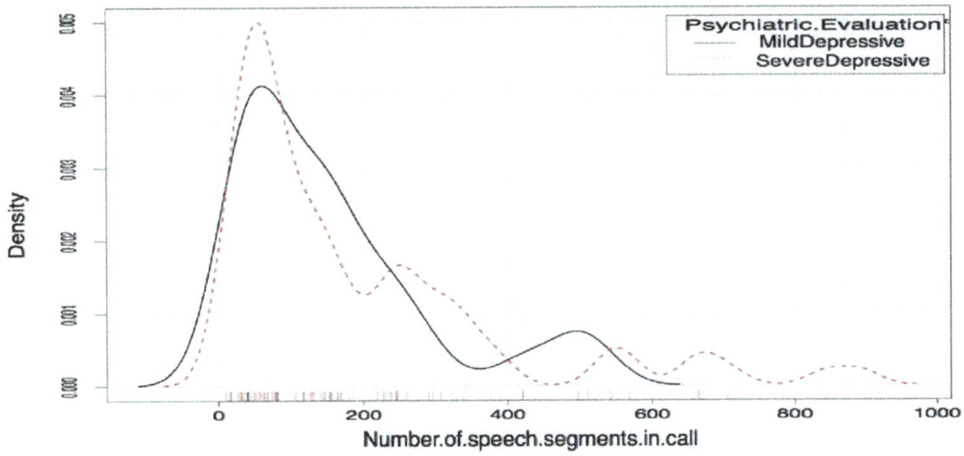

Figure 7. Average overall values of simultaneous speech length (p603) – left side.

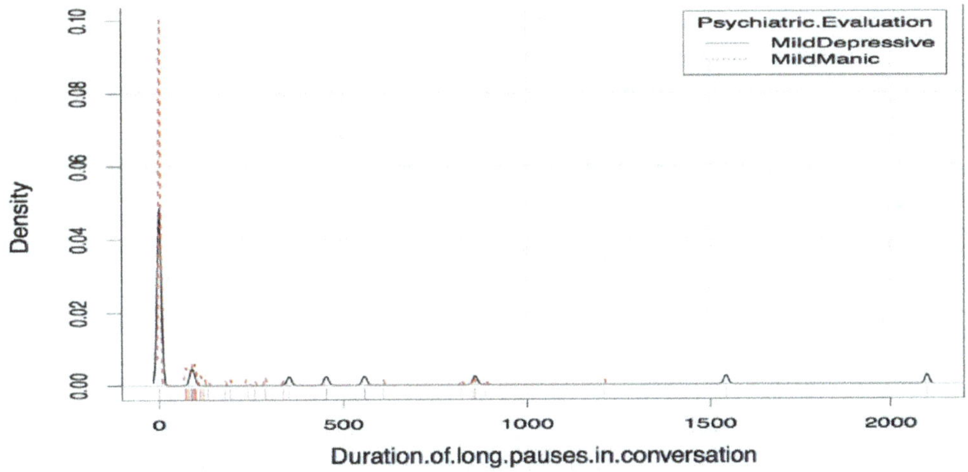

Figure 8. Total mean length values not superposed to psychiatric assessment (P610)-on the right-hand side.

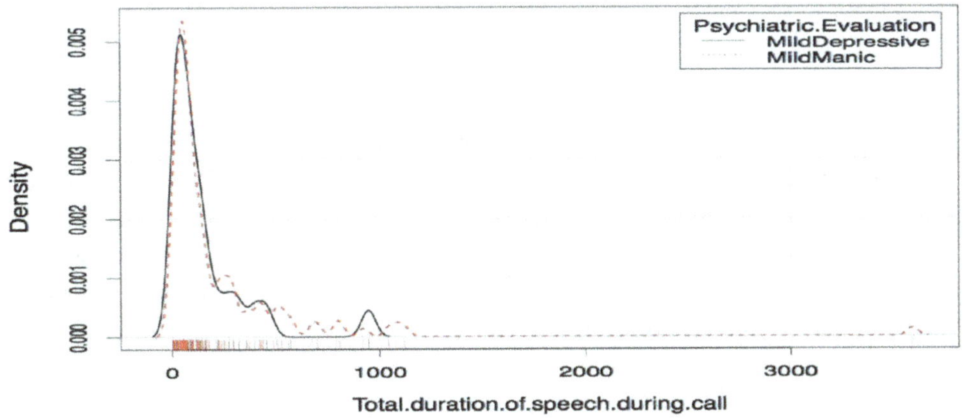

Figure 9. Distribution of satisfaction rate (p610).

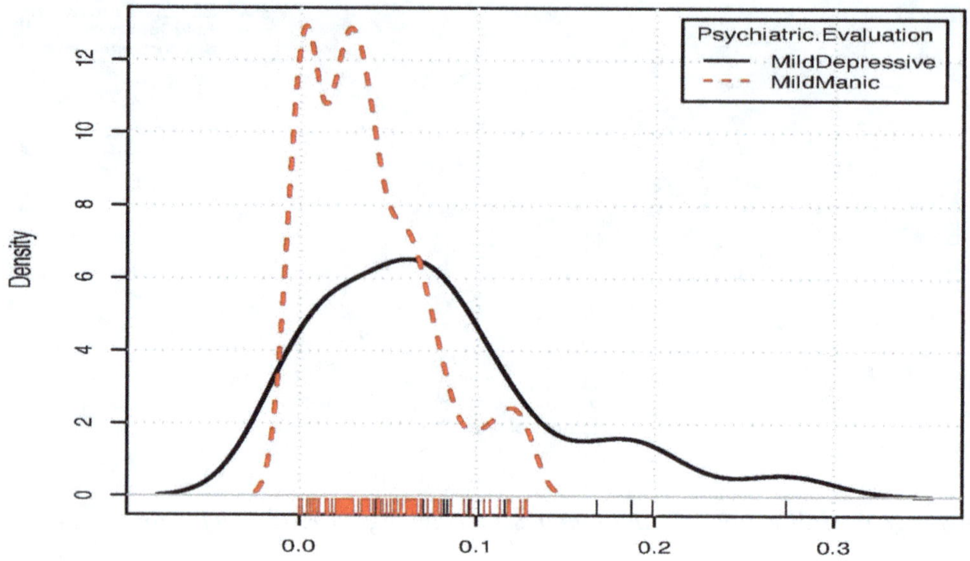

P1002 can be seen for the person who had a manic episode, as shown in the research (Nicola et al. 2012, pp 2104-2107) as a reverse pattern, where a person had lowered its average long pauses. During the depressive episode, the average length and number of lengthy intervals has risen to 73.27%/143.54% during the depressive episode. During telephone conversations, the system also examined speech overlap, speech performance, and mental characteristics. Voice performance tests effective voice frames determined by an energy-based voice exercise. During a mobile conversation, we studied the regularity and reactions of both effective participants. The regularity of the conversation was observed by speaking overlapping. A relation of overlapped depression (P0302) to overlapped manic episode patients ' voice (P1002) is presented in Figures 7 and 8.

Similarly, the system discovered a distinct proportion of happiness from the manic episode in conversation in Figure 9. Also, in low depression, the equanimity characteristic showed a lower percentage, while model discovered less equanimity during the telephone conversation in the ordinary state (as shown in figure 10). Table 6 provides a description of all the qualities used in the experimentation. The machine evaluated various sets of these attributes in the experiments.

RESULTS

The suggested method in classifying the levels of movement in various bipolar disorder states is summarized in this section. The process start with the significance of real-life operations of monitoring physical activity in bipolar disorders. The model also uses a semi-monitored learning technique to solve the scarcity of information. The model addresses the difficulties of developing exact designs to predict the development of the disease. The section contains the proposals on methods to enhance understanding about their state (e.g., self-training, intermediate models).

Figure 10. Distribution through psychiatric assessment of the level of equanimity (p602).

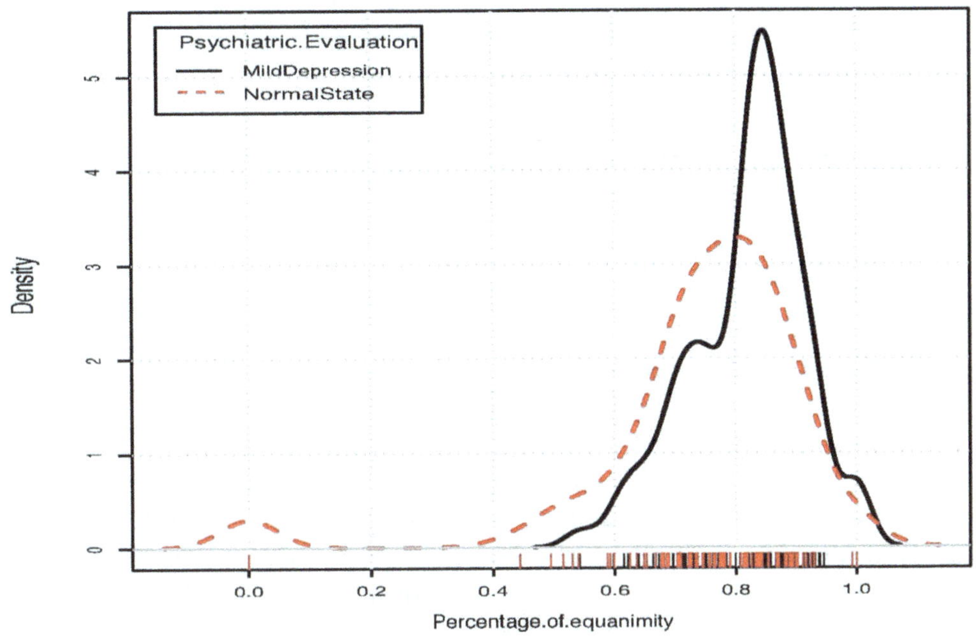

Monitoring Bipolar Disorder Patients

In fact, mortality in those with bipolar disorder is high and estimated to be 2 to 3 times higher compared with overall population mortality (Belmaker, 2004, pp. 476-486). The recurrence of bipolar patients rises with the period of time and the recurrence can differ between a few months. Thus, lifelong retention treatment is needed in patients with bipolar illness (Richard, 2004, pp. 18-26).

The classification of bipolar disease is focused on a clinical evaluation of results obtained by comparative psycho-pathological scales established in the mid-1960s (e.g., BRAMS, YMRS) and further new variants (e.g. BSDS). Such assessments and questionnaires are well described and elaborated in a detailed manual (Maria et al., 2012, pp. 457-463). However, other methods include regular reports, because often they depend on the present attitude episode (Sims et al., 1999, pp. 152-157). Treatment is the primary cure of bipolar disorder at the present time, but depends heavily on the dose timing and has

Table 6. A selection of innovative features.

Feature	Number
Accelerometers	
1) Time Domain 2) Frequency Domain	30 15
Audio:	
1) Emotional 2) Spectral	2 5
Questionnaire	4

Table 7. Correlation of the patient state to overall levels of physical activity. ($p < 0.05$, $N = 5$).

Patient ID	r
P601	0.336
P602	0.1885
P603	0.148
P604	-0.074
P607	0.142

to be adjusted differently according to the patient's state of mind. Treatment can be very efficient if given at the start of the patient shift to another state, but in serious cases where diseases occur and persist to a considerable degree, treatment can be less efficient. The following variables can have a considerable effect on the surveillance of patients suffering from mental disorders: Mental disorders symptoms are mainly manifested by patient behaviour changes. Depression, by example, occurs through motor delays in which behaviour changes can be captured by analysing mobile information from motion sensors. Typically, a psychiatric evaluation of mental disorders is done using a questionnaire. The questionnaire focuses on patients who recall previous events such as the quantity of physical activity recorded by the patient but a number of problems affecting self-reporting, including:

- Recall bias: Where it is difficult for subjects to recall occurrences in the past;
- Subjectivity: The current emotional condition of the subject may affect self-reporting
- High effort: Self-reporting needs a great deal of commitment to collect high-quality information, specifically in epidemiological studies where data is stored through self-reports or by observatory from third parties.

Physical Activity Observation

An essential experiment component is the accurate physical activity assessment to track the well-being of individuals and calculate the correlation between physical activity and the outcome of chronic diseases. The state of the physician is connected to the complete physical involvement, as shown in Table 7. The association is highest for P601 (r = 0.336), but for P603 (r = -0.148), which shows a decrease of the overall rate of physical activity (as evaluated by phones) as patient's condition improved (Patient P603 passed from the significant depressive event(-3) to normal (0)).

Taking these outcomes into account, the model chose to further explore to know how the regular rates of behaviour relate to incidents of manic disorder. In this regard, we split the day into four periods, namely Morning (06:00 to 12:00), Afternoon (12:00 to 06:00), Evening (06:00 to 12:00) and Night (12:00 to 06:00). There will clearly be distinct behaviour patterns for distinct patients so that a split of the day has been set examining at a certain interval every six hours the relation among physical activity and patient status.

Once the days were split into periods, compared to the psychiatric assessment of the patients, the model explored patterns of physical activity concentrations. The model deliberate the amount of all the percentages in hours of every one day to normalize work rates. This gives the hour and day an overall amount of operation. Dividing the operations into hours enabled us to match standard average rates of

Table 8. The association between total physical activity (PA) and mental evaluation in the depressive / manic episode.

P.ID.	No. Evaluations	Average of PA (Score)				Decrease of PA
		Depression State	Improved State	Factor of Improvement	Depression State	
P601	4	2.85% (+1.5)	0.54% (+0.5)	40%	n/a	n/a
P602	4	6.24% (-1.5)	7.21% (0)	07.05%	3.26% (-3)	22.10%
P603	4	8.85% (-1)	22.05% (0)	89.07%	17.8% (-3)	07.03%
P604	4	2.21% (-1.5)	6.08% (0)	89.06%	n/a	n/a
P607	4	7.26 (-1.5)	10.45% (-0.5)	22.11%	6.68% (-2)	18.15%

exercise in distinct hours of the day. With reference to scientific research in the treatment of bipolar patients, model examined associations between morning physical exercise concentrations and mental results in depressed patients (Maria et al., 2012, pp. 457-463), as shown in Table 8. In the morning, a significant distinction occurred in mean PA concentrations when patients moved from depression to normal condition. This rise is most noticeable in the case of P0201 patient, where average physical movement increased from 8.85% in depressed conditions to 22.03% for regular conditions and P603 patient with an increase of average PA.

The two other patients P601 and P607, which increased from normal to depressive, showed a significant reduction in physical activity. As a result, physical activity rates decreased by 55.20% for patient P601 from ordinary to serious anxiety (rating of -3), with physical activity decreasing by 36.25% in patient P607 due to an a-2 depressive episode. The inverse pattern have seen, comparable to the studies recorded in the P0101 manic incident for the individual (Agnes et al., 2014, pp. 1-8). In a manic episode, average PA reduced from 5.70% to 1.14% in a moderate manic episode. Because of the low level of exercise reported by the manic person, Telephone use for the patient was very low, one sign of mania incidentally. The recording of the mobile user records (supplied by the software) also verified this, leading in the availability of small accelerometer information for evaluation.

The previous chapter dealt with the morning exercise rate and its interaction with the psychiatric assessment. In this session, the program measured the coefficient of association between the daily exercise level and the assessment psychological level for all patients. The purposed model also wanted to investigate whether the physical activity level is correlated over other daily intervals. Table 9 shows the outcomes of the correlation.

Table 9. Correlation in day cycles among patient status and exercise levels ($p < 0.05$, $N = 5$, $N^{**} = 3$)

Patient ID	Morning	Afternoon	Evening	Night
P601	n/s*	0.107	-0.025	n/d*
P602	0.290	-0.271	0.318	n/d*
P603	0.132	0.275	0.125	n/d*
P604	0.445	-0.421	-0.357	0.302
P607**	-0.416	0.106	0.225	0.003

One of the important results from the analysis of patient's activities is that the connections between the person daily intervals are much greater than those for the overall exercise concentrations (see Table 9). These findings can be shown in patient P601 with an overall rate of activity r = 0.377 and the greatest daily range connection r = 0.318 (Evening). The same pattern also emerges in other patients, such as P602, when values are R = 0.156 compared to R = 0.276 for daily interval; P603, with r = -0.071 (average) compared with r = 0.428 (average); and in P607, where the person had a powerful adverse correlation between concentrations of physical activity and psychiatric ratings, for r = 0.140, (overall) vs. r = -0.37 (interval).

Except in the case of P601, patient correlations with overall concentrations of exercise are significantly greater (r = 0.358) than the regular interval correlations (r = 0.107). The model can only speculate on the factors for these outcomes without further studies. The patient had a manic incident at the start of the test with the condition of seriousness declining by the finish of the test. One possible interpretation may be that the overall level of exercise of the patient may well have linked with its state; however, it is difficult to see whether these periods influenced the total correlation rating owing to the lack of information for the day and night periods.

CLASSIFICATION OF BIPOLAR DISORDER EPISODES

The most coherent indicator of bipolar disorder is progressively proof of motor activities. The motor function includes many fields such as body movement, motor reaction time, psychomotor activity and speech-related motor activity. Motor activity data may be used in bipolar patients to identify event type, which is extremely significant since serious disease and manic conditions can lead to death.

This section presents a scheme that can classify patients with bipolar disorder by means of sensible smartphone data. The method also demonstrates evaluation outcomes from different classification systems, different types of characteristics and the role of questionnaires in classifying cases of bipolar disorder. Finally, the purposed model presents a new strategy for monitoring daily mobile conversations in order to identify people with bipolar disorders with impaired lives. Motor exercise is often used to define a set of diseases that vary from moderate to extremely serious and are prevalent characteristics of bipolar disturbance. An important aspect of psychiatric assessments has always been assessing the motor exercise of patients. The patients had elevated active concentrations through pressurized to speak incoherently.

Movement agitation was also shown for pursuing ideas and decreased sleep requirements. In blended and depressed periods, the motor side delays and irritable times can also occur in patients (Maria et al., 2012, pp 457-463). Therefore, motor exercise surveillance is essential to the classification of the critical condition of the disease. For this intent, the smartphone provides technological feature. Sensor information obtained on smartphones that provides an enormous ability of the behaviour of bipolar patients in their real lives using computer learning methods. In comparison to other research, the model demonstrate that bipolar mood episodes are only possible in mobile calls to predict patients using data acquired. Two types of traits acquired, i.e. voice characteristics (prosodic, spectral) and the intensity of telephone discussion (time and frequency features) are illustrated in Figure 11.

Figure 11. The method suggested in bipolar disorder patients in attempt to identify motor behaviour.

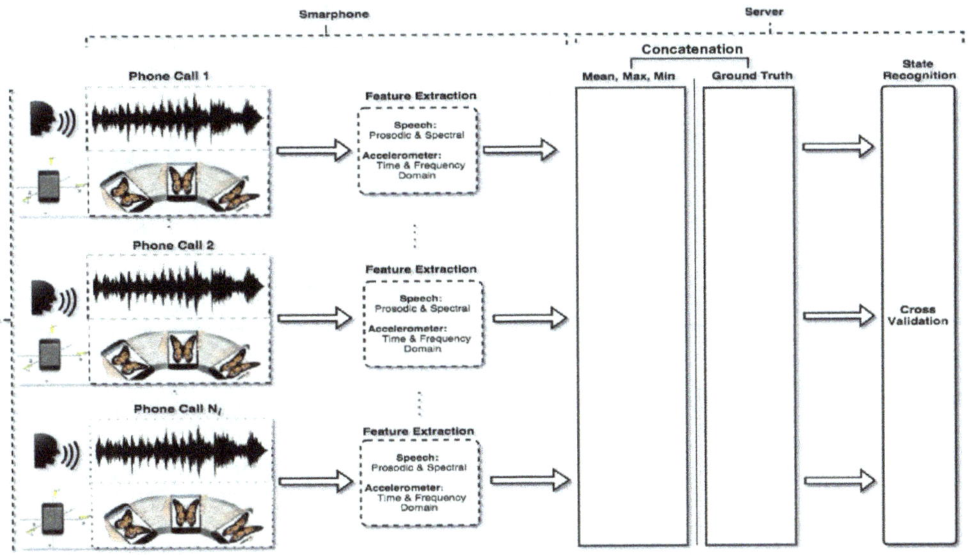

EXPERIMENTAL RESULTS

This section demonstrates the four laboratory outcomes to validate our model for classifying sequences of bipolar disorder as accessible:

- Comparing the efficiency of distinct data classifiers.
- Choosing a number of characteristics that correspond to the task.
- Assessing the impact of the questionnaires on depression understanding of patients.
- Use a training approach to solve the problem of how information from phone calls can be used unlisted to increase the accuracy and the relation between data from the complete data collection and marked data from bipolar disturbances.

The process discovered a model for each participant as well as a separate model for combining all the data from all the patients. For all the studies, conducted 10-fold cross-validation and record overall accuracy, precision and recall scores for each episode.

The outcomes of mental and sensory audio functions with accelerometer frequency-specific domain features and the survey data can be seen in Table 10 and Table 11 other pairs of characteristics produced similar outcomes. The tables indicate the precision outcomes, their mean and outcomes for distinct patient classifications with data from all patients (the last column is "All P."). As shown in the table 10, all data sets have no leading classification, even if the choice treaties are on median stronger than most other classification. With data from all the patients, it was also conducted remarkably well.

The process evaluated various feature sets. The table 12 shown the characteristics of the accelerometer (time domain versus frequency domain), audio characteristics (mental and spatial), and mixing characteristics of the accelerometer with distinct audio characteristics. Collected data from the questionnaires was also included in all of these outcomes.

Table 10. Accuracy results from Frequency-domain features and all Audio features.

Classifier	P602	P603	P607	P609	P610	Avg. (SD)	All P.
C4.5	44.96	42.73	39.40	43.89	42.89	42.26(± 4.17)	38.25
Random Forest (RF)	43.62	42.31	35.43	44.72	41.88	41.09(± 7.24)	35.30
SVM	46.14	37.60	30.79	41.75	43.91	41.43(± 7.52)	38.52
Naïve Bayes	35.90	31.19	30.30	31.35	78.17	32.17(± 7.35)	58.29
k-NN (1)	43.95	31.84	25.30	39.77	39.08	37.20(± 12.14)	38.03
AdaBoost. M1	42.28	43.59	37.08	44.88	43.04	42.25(± 6.06)	25.10
Bagging	44.63	43.16	36.02	44.72	43.14	43.14(±7.45)	58.01

Table 11. Precision results from the frequency and spectrum characteristics of the field.

Classifier	P602	P603	P607	P609	P610	Avg. (SD)	All P.
C4.5	45.15	42.28	34.42	43.40	55.40	43.14 (±2.17)	36.25
Random Forest	45.03	29.45	35.43	45.25	42.35	43.58 (±3.45)	36.42
SVM	46.05	52.05	38.08	43.44	43.40	41.49(±3.22)	33.15
Naïve Bayes	36.24	30.18	32.45	31.25	34.18	34.35(±3.38)	23.83
k-NN	42.08	32.18	32.25	36.45	42.36	37.21(±5.23)	28.29
AdaBoost. M1	42.28	42.09	36.08	45.06	48.42	42.06(±3.08)	26.10
Bagging	44.13	43.16	36.58	43.08	43.15	42.45(±3.53)	39.56

The tests reveal that the findings of the frequency domain characteristics with only the characteristics from accelerometers are somewhat greater than 80 times on average. It is also important to note that the output of the sound characteristics is comparable when both types (mental and spectral) are regarded in isolation. The highest outcomes are acquired by combining audio with frequency domain characteristics from the accelerometers in both the spectral and emotional characteristics.

To produce a fully independent implementation, it is essential to assess the effect on the outcomes of the questionnaires. This is important because the self-assessment for depressed patients can be counterproductive since they are daily reminded of their depression condition with the questionnaires. The model tested the frequency domain characteristics with and without questionnaire data. The findings are given in Table 13.

However, the findings achieved from the surveys, have decreased slightly, but the average findings are still more than 82%. This makes the creation of an automated surveillance instrument sensible. The table 13 shows the only way to produce highly profitable outcomes is to use data from questionnaires.

Motor Movement Categorization

Table 2 shows more than 900 phone calls without a related event. We agreed that the model should use a semi-supervised algorithm to see whether all accessible information can enhance the efficiency of past outcomes. The model followed a straightforward strategy, by splitting the information into ten layers, by using the training data for the classification of unlabelled information.

The weight of this classification was related to the classified value. All classified data with the initial training set has then been used to develop an extended training set. With this collection, the process

Table 12. Precision comes from various sets of features

Description		P602	P603	P607	P609	P610	Avg. (SD)
Accelerometer	Time Domain	44.76	36.54	36.09	41.91	42.64	40.39(±3.33)
	Frequency Domain	44.76	41.88	37.75	43.85	42.89	42.27(±2.15)
Audio	Emotional + Spectral	45.35	31.40	37.08	43.23	46.23	41.12(±4.15)
	Spectral	45.30	36.45	37.08	46.06	43.12	42.42(±3.15)
	Emotional	45.30	36.11	37.08	44.08	41.36	40.25(±4.09)
TD + Spectral		43.41	35.47	36.24	43.25	43.14	39.25(±4.45)
TD + Emotional		89.52	74.36	70.20	43.10	42.13	40.15(±3.55)
TD + (Emotional +Spectral)		89.53	70.09	69.54	42.10	42.14	42.16(±5.06)
TD + (Emotional +Spectral) Without Questionnaire		50.0	59.40	70.86	25.08	41.11	31.12(±6.07)
FD + Spectral		45.13	43.95	25.41	42.39	42.26	43.19(±42.22)
FD + Emotional		45.15	42.26	36.43	42.39	43.29	42.25(±2.52)
FD + (Emotional +Spectral)		45.42	42.26	36.19	41.39	42.58	43.281(±2.08)
FD + (Emotional +Spectral) Without Questionnaire		48.29	42.08	36.13	44.25	42.15	41.28(±2.20)

Table 13. Precision outcomes using questionnaire data.

Patient	With Questionnaires	Without Questionnaires	Only Questionnaires
P602	44.96	39.76	45.3
P603	42.73	42.06	38.46
P607	39.40	37.41	37.08
P609	44.28	44.69	44.77
P610	42.89	42.89	41.37
Avg.	42.77	41.27	41.42
All P.	38.25	30.58	29.88

Table 14. Accuracy is a semi-monitored approach to training.

Patient	Supervised	Semi-Monitored
P602	42.25	45.38
P603	43.47	42.25
P607	62.42	31.25
P609	43.25	44.69
P610	42.38	41.62
Avg.	41.31	40.43
All Patients:	32.25	36.24

produced a model and tested it on the experiment panel and then achieved 10 times the result. Table 14 provides the outcomes.

As the outcomes demonstrate, the addition of information from other calls doesn't greatly change the initial results. A wide variety of semi-monitored algorithms are available to improve results.

While the overall performance outcomes may sound good, the individual readings of accuracy and recall are essential to analyze in order to see how efficient positive designs are for each episode. Table 15 shows the results for each patient for Mild Depression (MiD), Moderate Depression (MoD), Severe Depression (SeD), Mild Manic (MiM), and Normal (N) state. It is important to remember that the pur-posed have more than 80% of outcomes in most instances. These results show the effective diagnostics for depressive episodes can be used by Smartphone technology.

Predictive Classes vs. Expert Evaluation

The last set of studies was intended to demonstrate how inductive designs are to identify the future occurrence of patient events for all phone calls accessible. We only demonstrate outcomes for patients P0201 (Figure 12) and for patients P0702 (Figure 13) for the worst outcomes. Both figures show the psychiatrist's assessments at the top and the classified states in the middle, the model's weight or con-fidence at the bottom of the model.

Induced models closely follow the assessment of the clinicians and establish acceptable types for psychological evaluations in the middle states, as the statistics show. The statistics also indicate the mistakes generated by the model classification in red. In specific, it can be seen that the designs do not have a lot of mistakes that can be further reduced when a weight range of less than 0.8 is withdrawn.

VOICE FEATURES EXTRACTION

In the above section, the process show the significance of analysing the behaviour in relation to motor activity to determine the patient condition. This model contrasted the conventional techniques supervised with semi-supervised techniques of learning. In periodic surveys, we used a psychiatric assessment as-sessed by the psychiatrist and semi-supervised learning methods. This study based on data collected on a daily basis from self-reported wellness questionnaires. The main benefit of this strategy is to enhance the efficiency of monitored classification and we suggest using new intermediate patterns. In order to create a template for evaluation of the episodic state in bipolar disorders, the model create three auxiliary designs using the captured objects i.e. physical, activity and psychological conditions.

Is it feasible to enhance identification precision by integrating intermediate hidden variables relating to the well-being of the patients before creating the ultimate model? The current work attempts to respond to the study issue by comparing surveys and motor activity-related behaviour in a phone conversation.

An experimental assessment was conducted using actual information. There are two elements to the studies:

- To finish the designs for subjects with lacking information, using semi-supervised learning.
- Prediction of attitudinal variables that are incorporated into the primary model to boost prediction accuracy by using intermediate models.

Table 15. Evidence of reliability and recall for some medical states.

Patient	State	Precision		Recall	
		+Questionnaire	-Questionnaire	+Questionnaire	-Questionnaire
P0201	Mild Depression	1.065	0.425	0.567	0.517
	Normal	0.455	0.406	0.452	0.445
	Severe Depression	0.368	0.252	0.368	0.365
P0302	Severe Depression	0.463	0.425	0.445	0.458
	Normal	0.421	0.415	0.404	0.358
P0702	Moderate Depression	0.425	0.436	0.433	0.415
	Mild Depression	0.421	0.365	0.265	0.284
P0902	Normal	0.448	0.458	0.458	0.442
	Moderate Depression	0.436	0.425	0.440	0.441
P1002	Mild Manic	0.442	0.540	0.268	0.524
	Moderate Depression	0.315	0.502	0.265	0.364
All Patients					
Severe Depression		0.269	0.365	0.226	0.208
Moderate Depression		0.450	0.369	0.306	0.341
Mild Depression		0.390	0.350	0.320	0.280
Normal		0.425	0.436	0.362	0.362
Mild Manic		0.412	0.405	0.451	0.325
Average		0.348	0.396	0.303	0.308

Figure 12. Evidence from the clinical model P602 and the psychiatrist's evaluations.

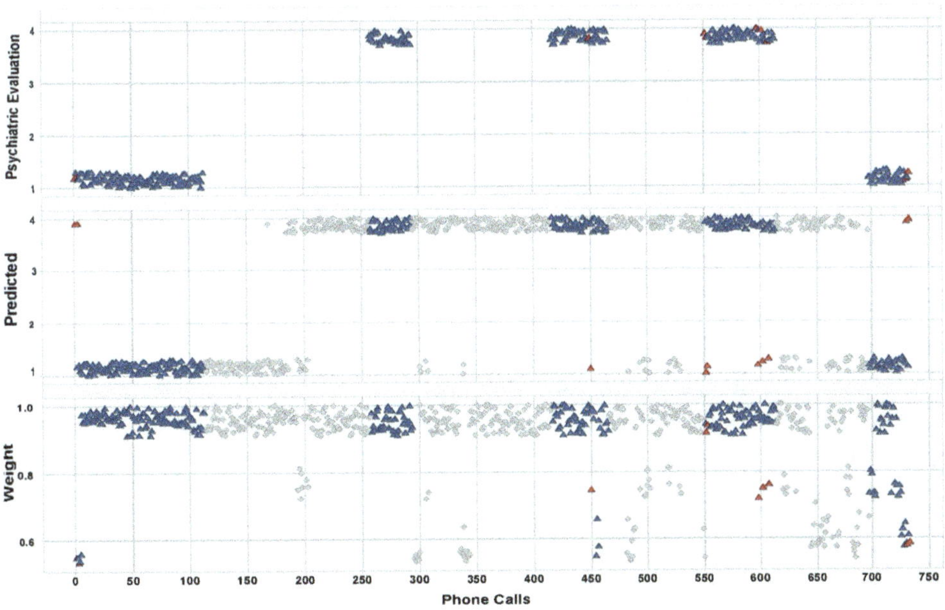

Figure 13. Patient model mediated outcomes P607 and doctor evaluations.

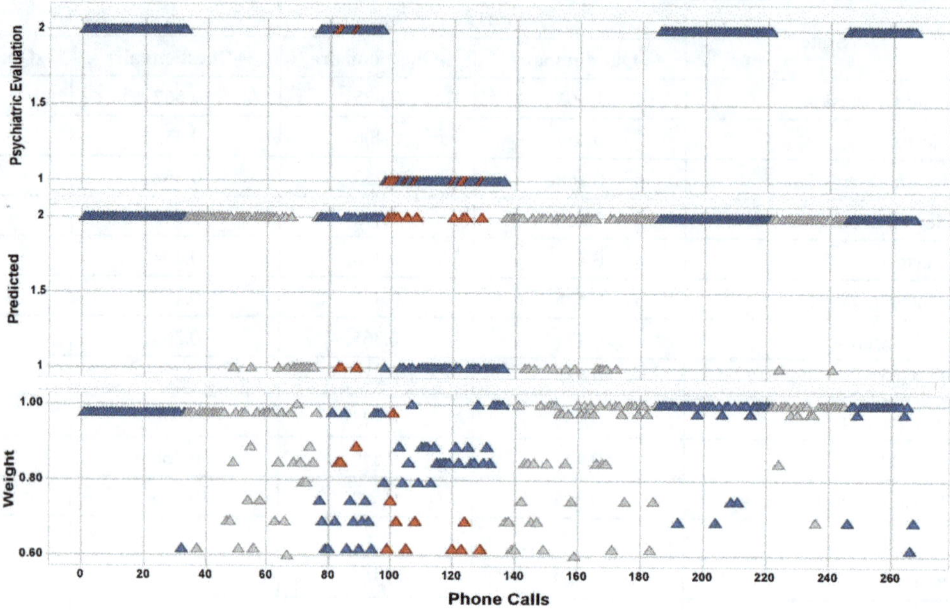

Figure 14. Intermediate model.

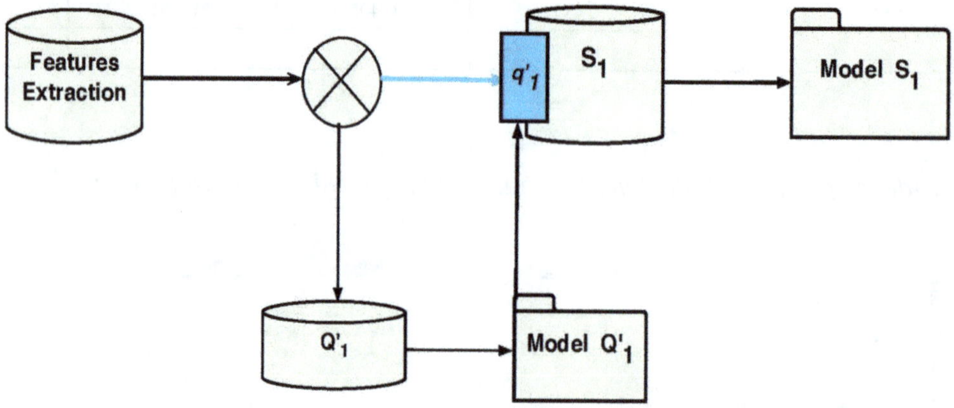

Experiments

Similar to prior studies, during the phone conversation, the model analyze information with accelerometers where the model know that patients have their smartphones. In order to classify the path of episodic state modifications, process assumed that analysing statistics from accelerometer measurements during the mobile conversation is appropriate. The second sort of data analyzed for this study involves personal information on the physical, active and psychological well-being of patients.

Intermediate models based on the smartphone accelerometer information, 30 frequency domain characteristics are obtained. These are used in the construction of the optimal mood models, Q1; and the stress model, S1. Both designs are combined via a weighted linear mixture to estimate the pressure amount in the forecast phase. Patient data via questionnaires is very helpful, but it is a tedious job for patients. In this study, the model suggests predicting the well-being factors connected with questionnaires using mobile information to reduce the strain on patients. The anticipated mood factors with all the other smartphone information are then used to identify the patients ' episode status. The model call these designs the factors of the intermediate systems questionnaire psychological and well-being circumstances as they are used for the ultimate predictive model. While additional variables such as latent parameters have been used previously in literature (Li et al., 2009, pp. 2036-2043). The method for constructing medium designs is illustrated in Figure 14.

Three factors obtained from physical, activity and psychological conditions have been used in these studies to construct 3 optimal designs. The self-reported questionnaires obtained from the regular self-evaluation are used to train each classifier individually. The intermedia designs got the data from smartphones during the prediction phase to forecast a weighted range of welfare conditions. The smartphone information and the mood factors were then used to provide the introduction of the ultimate episodic model state.

EXPERIMENTAL RESULTS

The experiments were aimed at the following:

- Compare the information efficiency of various classifiers.
- To increase knowledge of self-reported mental state, measure the impact of intermediate models in a person who has bipolar disease.
- Use SSL to deal with the problem of how unlabelled information can be used to expand the precision of accuracy.

The purposed have used Weka classifiers with their standard parameters for all tests (Mark et al., 2009, pp. 10-18). This work has developed a system for the object and 10 times all experiments have been cross-validated. Overall reliability and correct results are reported. In the earlier session, the model have proved that the data derived from the accelerometers is higher identification accuracy in all audio characteristics. Various characteristics were evaluated using the intermediate models. A different result of characteristics are obtained like mental and spatial and a combination of mental or discrete characteristics of the frequency domain as shown in table 16 and table 17 that shows data outcomes. The outcomes are over 81% on average only with accelerometer characteristics in the frequency domain. However, with audio only, the output is less than with accelerometer characteristics. The highest outcomes are achieved

Table 16. IM: Precision comes from the use of various sets of functions.

Features		P602	P603	P607	P609	P610	Avg. (±SD)
Accelerometer	Time Domain (TD)	29.56	31.05	37.12	28.16	40.25	32.55(±5.25)
	Frequency Domain (FD)	41.17	42.36	33.12	43.09	43.56	41.02(±3.40)
Audio	Emotional + Spectral	28.60	27.63	35.19	26.58	39.82	32.06(±5.17)
	Spectral	29.55	36.82	35.29	26.50	39.25	32.05(±5.05)
	Emotional	36.55	32.58	32.13	28.19	38.05	31.06(±5.15)
TD + Spectral		29.40	37.26	35.40	30.12	38.18	32.06(±5.53)
TD+ Emotional		32.17	27.96	35.52	38.14	39.78	35.62(±5.30)
TD+ Emotional + Spectral		30.09	29.32	35.25	30.24	38.14	35.06(±4.21)
FD + Spectral		43.08	42.36	35.43	48.24	41.08	42.06(±5.08)
FD+ Emotional		41.59	42.25	35.46	48.42	41.52	41.25(±4.02)
FD+ Emotional + Spectral		43.65	42.96	35.76	49.25	42.26	41.36(±3.25)

Table 17. Intermediate models and semi-supervised learning - Accuracy results from using different sets of features

Features		P602	P603	P607	P609	P610	Avg. (±SD)
Accelerometer	Time Domain (TD)	36.06	38.46	58.07	28.08	44.50	38.4(±5.23)
	Frequency Domain (FD)	45.13	42.95	37.59	43.44	43.16	42.36(±2.32)
Audio	Emotional + Spectral	43.17	36.38	48.30	46.24	40.25	39.21(±3.14)
	Spectral	36.42	42.24	42.35	36.70	41.59	39.05(±2.09)
	Emotional	32.04	38.25	42.05	28.35	41.17	36.78(±6.06)
TD + Spectral		39.39	33.87	42.52	30.63	38.22	39.01(±5.95)
TD+ Emotional		46.25	35.41	46.13	38.03	39.90	39.38(±3.42)
TD+ Emotional + Spectral		42.52	34.35	40.45	30.21	38.60	36.30(±4.62)
FD + Spectral		45.44	45.58	42.78	48.72	43.15	45.45(±2.95)
FD+ Emotional		49.42	45.58	42.57	42.62	46.19	46.29(±2.37)
FD+ Emotional + Spectral		45.44	45.52	40.58	53.36	42.51	44.22(±2.39)

in combination with the spectral and emotional characteristics of the sound with the accelerometer's frequency domain. In this research there was a new approach to identifying people with bipolar disorders from the accelerometer and speech features from smartphones, namely the intermediate process. The well-being of the intermediate designs has shown that the precision for the classification of bipolar episodic disease is improved. The use of data derived from the accelerometer frequency characteristics leads to greater identification precision than the data extracted from audio recordings. When the spectral was incorporated, it improved by combining the information from audio characteristics with the accelerometer functions. Although the use of the self-reports questionnaires on the mobile phone suggests that personalized designs with low data sets could be appropriate to automatically change behaviour recognition and that would assist the psychiatrist in the nearest future.

CONCLUSION

The purposed methods have regarded how to deal with the problems of mental health and human behaviour with unlabelled and scarce information. In compliance with semi-monitored training, by introducing new frameworks and transferring alternative learning techniques to concerns. The research has examined ways of addressing the issue of the classification of patient behaviour from smartphone information. This work starts to address several open issues in machine learning. As mentioned previously, it is complicated to collect information labelled as a patient annotation must make an attempt to labelled information. In previous sections mentioned that unlabelled information is often abundant, for example, mobile captures, internet queries, metadata, sensors, places, and other records.

Introducing a new intermediate model to improve ultimate model precision and the environment of semi-supervised learning, the research suggests a solution to problems in the field of machine learning. This study shows that SSL and TL are extremely beneficial to be incorporated into monitoring schemes which can be benefited by new unlisted information. The outcomes demonstrate that with few labelled learning cases present, the training designs have been guided and the output of the ST algorithm evaluated. The model described the distinction in results precision between monitored and semi-supervised learning techniques. The techniques monitored were mildly stronger (by 0.75%) for semi-monitored teaching. The findings from additional data from intermediate models have shown that the overall accuracy is improved (from 73 to 90%).

The primary contributors to this work are described below: The following are:

- The initial work was to handle scarce information, using smartphone information gathered to monitor individual mental health and behaviour.
- The purposed model suggested using Self-learning techniques for a conventional semi-supervised training technique aiming at increasing the accuracy and precision of any existing monitored.
- In order to enhance the predictive precision of the destination model, model suggested a methodology that obtains data on a different source model.
- Finally, the new Intermediate Models have been provided as an input to the predictive final model. The model also contributed to human behaviour comprehension.
- In healthcare, scientists in the sector frequently drop scarce data resulting in the lack of information in current monitoring technologies. The model has suggested machine learning designs that use this limited information to enhance the understanding and precision of monitored subjects.

Lastly, purposed model suggested new techniques for collecting background information from the raw smartphone information and for understanding the resemblance or de-similarity of subject behaviour in the surveillance days, also techniques were suggested in order to create accurate designs. The work shows the significance of using machine-learning methods to process limited information from mobile sensors for mental health monitoring. However, the use of suggested methods and a restricted number of respondents are concerned with several problems. The model has a restricted number of subjects involved in the studies in this study. It is clear that increasing the number of objects and the collection of ongoing data on long-term evaluation of topics would increase statistical significance and precision.

REFERENCES

Agnes, G., Venet, O., Gernot, B., Jose, C., Stefan, O., Oscar, M., ... Paul, L. (2014). Using smart phone mobility traces for the diagnosis of depressive and manic episodes in bipolar patients. In *Proceedings of the 5th Augmented Human International Conference*. ACM. doi:10.1145/2582051.2582089

Aharony, N., Pan, W., Ip, C., Khayal, I., & Pentland, A. (2011). Social fMRI: Investigating and shaping social mechanisms in the real world. *Pervasive and Mobile Computing*, *7*(6), 643–659. doi:10.1016/j.pmcj.2011.09.004

Belmaker, R. H. (2004). Bipolar disorder. *The New England Journal of Medicine*, *351*(5), 476–486. doi:10.1056/NEJMra035354 PMID:15282355

Christophe, A., D'Alché-Buc, F., & Grandvalet, Y. (2001). Semi-supervised margin boost. In Advances in neural information processing systems (pp. 553–560). Academic Press.

Gabriela, J.E.B. & Silvia, G. (2011). A framework for overcoming challenges in designing persuasive monitoring and feedback systems for mental illness. In *Proceedings of the 5th International Conference on Pervasive Computing Technologies for Healthcare (PervasiveHealth)*. IEEE. doi:10.4108/icst.pervasivehealth.2011.246097

Gaetano, S. V., Narayanaswami, C., & Menning, W. (2007). Guest Editors' Introduction Pervasive Computing in Healthcare. *IEEE Pervasive Computing*, *6*(1), 17–19. doi:10.1109/MPRV.2007.11

Johnson, R., & Zhang, T. (2007). On the effectiveness of Laplacian normalization for graph semi-supervised learning. *Journal of Machine Learning Research*, *8*(July), 1489–1517.

Klaus, R. (1986). Vocal affect expression: A review and a model for future research. *Psychological Bulletin*, *99*(2), 143–165. doi:10.1037/0033-2909.99.2.143 PMID:3515381

Li, L. J., Socher, R., & Fei-Fei, L. (2009, June). Towards total scene understanding: Classification, annotation and segmentation in an automatic framework. In *Proceedings of the 2009 IEEE Conference on Computer Vision and Pattern Recognition* (pp. 2036-2043). IEEE. doi:10.1109/CVPR.2009.5206718

Maria, F. J., Brage, S., Vinberg, M., Christensen, E. M., Knorr, U., Jensen, H. M., & Kessing, L. V. (2012). Differences in psychomotor activity in patients suffering from a unipolar and bipolar affective disorder in the remitted or mild/moderate depressive state. *Journal of Affective Disorders*, *141*(2), 457–463. doi:10.1016/j.jad.2012.02.020 PMID:22391514

Mark, A. H., Eibe, F., Holmes, G., Bernhard, P., & Reutemann, P., & Ian, H.W. (2009). The WEKA data mining software: an update. ACM SIGKDD explorations newsletter, 11(1), 10–18. doi:10.1145/1656274.1656278

Maurer, U., Smailagic, A., Siewiorek, D. P., & Deisher, M. (2006, April). Activity recognition and monitoring using multiple sensors on different body positions. In *Proceedings of the International Workshop on Wearable and Implantable Body Sensor Networks (BSN'06)* (pp. 4-pp). IEEE. doi:10.1109/BSN.2006.6

Nicola, V., Guidi, A., Gentili, C., Werner, S., Bertschy, G., Valenza, G., . . . Scilingo, E. P. (2012). Speech analysis for mood state characterization in bipolar patients. In *Proceedings of the 2012 Annual International Conference of the IEEE Engineering in Medicine and Biology Society (EMBC)* (pp. 2104–2107). IEEE. doi:10.1109/EMBC.2012.6346375

Raento, M., Oulasvirta, A., Petit, R., & Toivonen, H. (2005). ContextPhone: A prototyping platform for context-aware mobile applications. *IEEE Pervasive Computing*, *4*(2), 51–59. doi:10.1109/MPRV.2005.29

Rayid, G., & Nigam, K. P. (2000). Analyzing the effectiveness and applicability of training. In *Proceedings of the ninth international conference on Information and knowledge management* (pp. 86–93). ACM. doi:10.1145/354756.354805

Richard, M. (2004). The early warning symptom intervention for patients with the bipolar affective disorder. *Advances in Psychiatric Treatment*, *10*(1), 18–26. doi:10.1192/apt.10.1.18

Richard, O.D., Peter, E.H., & Stork, D.G. (1997). Pattern Classification. John Wiley & Sons.

Sims, J., Smith, F., Duffy, A., & Hilton, S. (1999). The vagaries of self-reports of physical activity: a problem revisited and addressed in a study of exercise promotion in the over 65s in general practice. Family Practice, 16(2), 152–157. doi:10.1093/fampra/16.2.152

Thorsten, J. (1999). Transductive inference for text classification using support vector machines. In *Proceedings of the Sixteenth International Conference on Machine Learning (ICML)* (pp. 200–209). Academic Press.

Xiaojin, Z. (2006). *Semi-Supervised Learning Literature Survey*. University of Wisconsin-Madison.

Chapter 11
Machine Learning Is the Future for Lung Cancer Prognosis and Prediction

Ayshwarya Balakumar
Kristu Jayanti College, India

Senthil S.
REVA University, India

ABSTRACT

Lung cancer is one of the major reasons for the death if it is not diagnosed in the early stages of cancer. It is the one among the most dreadful disease which affects in the lungs function. It can be identified only after the disease spread into the deeper parts of the lungs and then only it will make a life threading problem. Lung cancer prognosis which was done based on the various parameters such as age, sex, condition of smoking, duration of smoking and count of smoking per day. The proceedings were done using the algorithm for the time to first cigarette after awakening which is represented as TTFC. The expert doctor says that the back-propagation network is a great deal in the recognition of the lung cancer without any involvement by them. This research is based on the classification of lung cancer and its stages using the establishment of the BPN and predicts the recurrence. Similarly, with this BPN, an algorithm that is inspired from its habitat known as ant lion optimization algorithm is also used in the optimization of weights and parameters of the BPN. The use of the ALO algorithm provides an improved convergence mechanism by improving the proposed technique's accuracy. The use of this proposed method with the BPN optimizes the network and the ALO optimizer provides an accurate prediction of the lung cancer by the earlier stage and even predicts the changes for reoccurrence after diagnosis. The prognosis analysis was made by the various comparative study between the characteristic features of HIV and the unaffected person using the algorithm such as the Wilcoxon rank-sum test. This algorithm will continuously classify the viral load and CD4 count which is based on factors such as age, sex, and smoking activities. It will be useful for early diagnosis and future prediction. Lung cancer rates can be analyzed based on the incident rates of affected and unaffected persons to HIV infections.

DOI: 10.4018/978-1-7998-2101-4.ch011

INTRODUCTION

The unrestricted development of cells in the lung tissues causes the lung cancer which is termed as lung carcinoma. Lung carcinoma is a malicious lung cancer. The growth would spread outside the lung which process is termed as metastasis to the adjacent tissues and the other parts of the body. The classification of lung cancer is as follows: Non-small cell lung cancer (NSCLC) and small cell lung cancer (SCLC). The performance is segregated depending on the observation of the equipment of tumor cells using the microscope. These divisions of cancer are handled, developed, and dispersed by various methods. The major reason for lung cancer is cigarette smoking which would include various diseases such as peripheral arterial disease and coronary artery disease. Cigarette smoking may lead to atherosclerosis which would decrease the blood flow by thickening the arteries.

The lung cancer mostly belongs to the SCLC category for about 10%-15%. The lung cancer will be highly damaging and the rapidly developing one is the SCLC which poses 10%-15% in proportion of lung cancer. Smoking of cigarette that has nicotine content and the deposition of toxins is the main cause of the lung cancer. The SCLC's are identified only after it is rapidly spread over several parts of the body till a significant level. Among the range of lung cancer category, the NSCLC is the most affected and 85% of the portion is this case in the entire lung cancer cases.

Stages of NSCLC:

Stage I: Identification of cancer only in the lung zones. Stage II: Identification of cancer spread over the adjacent lymph nodes of the lung. Stage III: Identification of cancer developed towards the chest from the lungs and lymph nodes which is said to be the advanced stage. Stage IV: The entirely advanced stage. This state exists when the disease covers both the lungs and in the collection of other fluids inside the lungs or the development in other organs.

However, undergoing with the remedial treatment, around 30% - 55% of the patients who have NSCLC have a chance of reoccurrence and perish. Likewise, after surgery several lung cancer patients preferably sooner or later pass away cause of reoccurrence. Also, undergoing this treatment itself poses a high possibility of danger. Yet, the mortality associated treatment is a rare occurrence, still the persistence of hazards in death and the patients maximally will also meet with a reduced act after the surgical treatment. So, although with all the developed surgical treatments, the remedy for the cancer with the surgical removal of affected portions does not plays a vital role, the complete elimination of the affected portion is reasonable.

The proposed work is inspired to build the system with the performance of the computer to provide the support of spontaneous identification to make the medical decisions in an automated technique as its routine. And it should conclude with the procedures like detecting the disease at earlier stage with the radiologist's portion which could effectively diagnose the patient's scenario. Besides the prior detection of lung cancer presence, this work also subjects the significance of the reoccurrence of disease prediction before and after the surgical treatment undergone by the medical specialists either the radiation therapy way or the medical surgery.

The rest of the part are followed by various sections like, Section II: Introduction to automatic prediction of lung cancer of several research survey proposed by different scholars using classification section. Section III: Illustration of the proposed strategy. Section IV: Description of the evaluated results of the proposed technique. Section V: Conclusion of the work.

RELATED WORKS

According to the study of Cruz and Wishart, proposed and legalized revisions that the machine learning scheme significantly improves the cancer prediction exactness for about 15%-25% of its vulnerability, mortality and repetition than in ANN process. It also states that machine learning improves the elementary knowledge of the cancer progress and development.

The examinations of Yao et al., the cellular heterogeneity from varied cell types was been quantifiably illustrated by the progress of a computational approach in H&E marked compulsive images. They implied a deep learning approach for the classification of the cell subtype and then presented a reckonable feature to describe cellular information. They resulted on two lung cancer data sets survival models built from the clinical imaging biomarkers have better prediction power.

Studies said approximately 84% to 91% are of non-small cell lung cancers (NSCLC) and it was diagnosed by using the Artificial Neural network (ANN) model to achieve the accuracy level. The prediction of Lung cancer improved medication with timely diagnosis using the ANN model and the accuracy was 100%. Just Neural Network (JNN) was used for the training and valuation and testing, according to the research done by Kashf et al. (2018).

The study of the successful research by the Ministry of Health and Welfare, Taiwan (2016) for the prediction of the non-small cell lung cancer survival patients rate by the diagnosis completed by Lee et al, was achieved by the Artificial Neural Network (ANN) and Logistic Regression (LR), with a precision rate of LR model: Peculiarity = 73.8, Sensitivity = 77.3 and with AUROC (Area Under ROC curve) of 81%, In ANN model: Peculiarity = 76.8, Sensitivity = 77.6 and with AUROC of 83% which obviously states that the precision rate of the ANN is greater than that of the LR model.

The two most predominant lung cancer subtype is that the Adenocarcinoma and squamous cell carcinoma. Thus, the researchers Coudray et al., (2018), designed the deep convolution neural network (DCNN) model on the histopathology images. The Cancer Genome Atlas (TCGA) provides the images of histopathology which exactly describes the images of whole-slide pathology obsessed by squamous cell carcinoma, adenocarcinoma or the normal lung tissue. trained a deep learning convolutional neural network (CNN) model (inception v3) on histopathology images obtained from The Cancer Genome Atlas (TCGA) to accurately classify whole-slide pathology images into adenocarcinoma, squamous cell carcinoma or normal lung tissue. They performed multiple mutations and obtained the cross entropy for every individual and finally achieved the test by the tiles present in LUAD classifier.

Jiang and Xu., claimed the most mutual NSCLC subtype is that the LUAD, which in turn accounts around 40% of the histological types and likely to its reappearance. Utilizing the study on the TCGA datasets and by applying the ANN technique in the medication and the testing and prediction sequence they primarily examined the LUAD's survival diagnosis in which the factors gets affected (Daoud and Mayo, 2019).

The gene expression dimension and their noise are reduced by means of neural network filtering methods. The amount of network's hidden nodes and the hidden layers are classified and determined by the trial and error method whereas the binary class and the multi class taxonomy uses the convolution neural network and the MLP classification methods. By achieving great clustering exactness, they make the neural networks to decide the accuracy and the network architecture.

PROBLEM STATEMENT

The framework with any such conditions is stated to be considered to poses the objective of twofold. At first the discrepancy in the conclusion by the varied physicians in observing and evaluating danger of the lung cancer minimization. Indisputably the reliability between varied physicians was enhanced by computer-supported strategies in several medical background, indulging the identification of the cancer affected node and CT used screening and in classifying the node it might predict and wait for so called resolution by supporting challenges could bring the identical benefit. Secondly, within the classification that aids the non-skilled physicist or least knowledgeable physicist in the valuation of the risk of a particular malignant node it could provide an improved functionality.

The classification of lung cancer in this examination practices the ANN (i.e., artificial neural network). Besides the artificial network, a meta-heuristic habitat inspired methodology labelled such as ant lion optimization (ALO) technique is used for the parameters of the ANN to optimize. The prediction of the existence of lung cancer till a considerable level is enhanced by the classification of the accuracy of ANN which is used besides the technique of the ant lion optimization.

PROPOSED METHODOLOGY

Lung cancer arises in various health diseases such as chronic obstructive pulmonary disease (COPD) which is found familiar in most of the lung cancer affected community people. The prognosis may occur by taking the account of various factors such as age, sex and the smoking records which will be useful in lung cancer prevalence. The death reason out of all the existing cancer's the most important least chance for the continued existence of the patients as per the various cancer communities providing the online lung database from the internet sources and is describing the process by the proposed system is that the Lung cancer. The following phases are from the proposed system methodologies, Phase 1 is about the pre-processing, and the phase 2 is about the feature extraction phase, the phase 3 is about feature selection and the phase 4 is the final phase for the organization and development of the taxonomy process. The figure 1. explains about the entire process clearly.

Datasets

The datasets are quite sufficient for us to analyze even though it is a least amount, they are supposed to be there in the real-world conditions and so they are enthralling and appropriate. The machine learning and Intelligent Systems at the University of California, Irvine accommodated and conserved the datasets in the Center. The employment of the designed technique uses the lung cancer data set [1] from UCI Machine learning repository.

Pre-Processed Data

The data Processing is the primary phase of the suggested techniques in which the data set is given for training and testing for further analyzation by converting the raw data into an appropriate format.

Table 1.

Input: $x = (x_1, x_2 \dots . x_M)$

M – Maximum number of features

1. Find mean $\bar{x} = \frac{1}{M}\sum_{i=1}^{M} x_i$
2. Calculate deviation ← mean $\Phi_i = (x_1 - \bar{x})$
3. Find Covariance matrix (A) // A is (N × M) matrix→ Φ_i $(i = 1 \dots M)$ // through $C = \frac{1}{M}\sum_{N=1}^{M} \Phi_N \Phi_N \equiv AA^T$
4. Compute eigenvalue (C) as $C: \lambda_1 > \lambda_2 \dots . \lambda_N$
5. Compute eigenvector (C) as $C: \mu_1 > \mu_2 \dots . \mu_N$ // C will form symmetric basis, (i.e. any vector x or $x_1 - \bar{x}$,originally essential as a proportional combination of the eigenvectors): $x_1 - \bar{x} = b_1\mu_1 + b_2\mu_2 \dots . + b_N\mu_N = \sum_{i=1}^{N} b_i\mu_i$ //
6. Arrange (λ_i, μ_N) //descending order//

$$pc_1 > pc_2 \dots \dots > pc_l$$

// l is the transformed number of features//

Reduction of Dimension Using the Principal Component Analysis

The PCA utilization in diminishing the measurement of the statistics safely protects the original data's modifications that existed in it. The reason behind the usage of PCA for converting the input vectors to the fresh examination area changes the input vectors in the fresh exploration area. There are 7 features chose by the usage of the PCA algorithm. The PCA algorithm be a sign of the tryouts.

PCA Algorithm

Table 1 gives an example of the PCA algorithm.

Training and Testing Trials

The back-propagation network is used for purpose of employing the input samples of data for training and examination. Formerly the input data are allowed to arbitrarily select the weights of the neural network. For the purpose of learning the neural networks, it is acknowledged to use the sample set of the data for performing the exercise and testing the set of data. They perform the taxonomy methodology and the result of the arrangement for the analyzed set of facts is given with the weights to inspect the percentage at which the bugs occur or the bugs in the frequency error whilst operating the practice of taxonomy method and by changing the weights the error is modified.

The Neural Networks in medicinal Taxonomy

For the purpose of inspecting problematical concerns where the connections amongst the input and the output data are vaguely described, the ANNs work as an effective technique. In things like the detection of the disease imaging report, choosing for the specific disease its specific drug, the role of the Artificial Neural Networks is been capably used on such type of health care.

The BPN

In Learning the multilayer neural networks through the least rate of learning the back-propagation technique recognized about the proposed work, specifically in using the large size learning of the group. The proposed technique which uses the back-propagation technique through the best period (the seen time), it could be imposed with the vast means of the network with a considerable size.

Steps of the BPN Algorithm

1. Utilizing the pseudorandom sequence generator rearrange the whole connection weights W with the least random value.
2. Repetition until conjunction (As far as the gradient vE(t)/vW is smaller in contrast amid the predefined value or whilst the predefined value is greater than the error E)
   (1) Estimate the enhancement factor exploiting,

$$\Delta W(t) = -\eta \frac{dE(t)}{dW} \tag{1}$$

   (2) Improve the weights with

$$W(t+1) = W(t) + \Delta W(t) \tag{2}$$

   (3) Estimate the error E(t+1).

Here t denotes amount of repetition, W denotes weight to the connection weight and h means to the rate of exercise taking place. The variation between the prime y_j and the expected result d_j is computed by the limitation, Mean Square Error (MSE) and by picking the error value E.

$$\mathrm{E} = E = \frac{1}{2}\sum_{i=1}^{n_j}\left(d_j - y_j\right)^2 \tag{3}$$

Using the word known as momentum will be the modest approach to evade fluctuation difficulties while testing the surface of error as of the least benefit:

$$\Delta W(t) = -\eta \frac{dE(t)}{dW} + \alpha \Delta W(t-1) \quad (4)$$

In the proposed method, for the purpose of stimulating the convergence methodology the flexible value of training would be implemented. The training rate might be varied as trails for the group learning technique.

$$\eta(t) = \begin{cases} \beta\eta(t-1) & \text{if } E(t) < E(t-1) \\ \theta\eta(t-1) & \text{if } E(t) > kE(t-1) \\ \eta(t-1) & \text{Otherwise} \end{cases}$$

Where through the iteration the rate of the process of training will be known as h(t), and β, θ and k would be chosen to $\beta > 1, 0 < \theta \langle 1 \, and \, k \rangle 1$ although the training rate might be improvised operating, the learning approach also might be advanced.

$$\eta(t) = \eta_0 + \lambda E(t-1) \quad (5)$$

With the aid of ignoring practice, the teaching method will be the methodology that could miss the unemployment associates. It is common for the weights associated with the overlooking procedure to be strengthened with the assistance of

$$\Delta W'(t) = \Delta W(t) - \varepsilon sgn(W(t)) \quad (6)$$

Where sign(x) denotes the sign function and the ε is the amount at which the takes place. According to the second term on RHS, the appropriate rate of the weight would be present with the reduction aided for y. Meanwhile this one least spending during the processing reveals a better outcome, the examination of the conjugate gradient's technique is utilized (Polak, 1971). Therefore, the reporting of the related weights are done with the aid of,

$$W(t+1) = W(t) + \eta(t)d(t) \quad (7)$$

$$d(t) = -\nabla E[W(t) + \beta(t)d(t-1) \quad (8)$$

$$d(0) = -\nabla E[W(0) \quad (9)$$

Where d(t) signifies conjugate gradient, E denotes the gradient, h(t) would mean step wide, and with the aid of Polak-Ribiere function the b(t) is intended.

Ant Lion Optimizer

The back-propagation network uses the ant lions in the optimization of the parameter enhancement. This approach improves the prediction and speeds up the convergence process and eliminates the problem of being trapped within the local minima clutches.

i) The development and design of the ALO algorithm utilizing optimization math concepts.

When enhancing, the following setups are imposed:

¬ Using the varied arbitrary walks, the ants move around the examination area.
¬ For the detailed calculation of bees, arbitrary navigation will be implemented, using tricks created by antlions, arbitrary navigations will be affected.
¬ Antlions with bigger holes are more likely to get hold of ants.
¬ Each antlion is going to get antlions to grasp every move, so they attempt to turn out to be the most right antlion.
¬ During the fall of ants in the way of the stated animals, the diversity of the arbitrary steering would be reduced.
¬ Whilst the ant improves the endurance relative to the antlion, it refers to the use of holding and dragging the antlions.
¬ When the antlions capture any new prey it automatically relocates itself and starts to build another new snare in there by improving the chance of hitting a greater number of prey for each upcoming hunt by the enhancement of handling altered model.

ii) Ant's Arbitrary walks:

The communication that occurs within the antlions and the ants in the snare is utilized in the ALO technique. In this case the ants must forcibly travelling through the examination area to test the communication, and by utilizing the fitness of traps the antlions will be given permit for them to perform the hunting process. A random walk has to be picked up for making the prototype of the ants navigation as trials as the ants naturally move in a randomly determined manner for finding its own prey.

$$X(t)=\left[0, cumsum\left(2r(t_1)-1\right), cumsum\left(2r(t_2)-1\right) \dots cumsum\left(2r(t_n)-1\right)\right] \tag{10}$$

Where n denotes the chief quantity of steps, t states the phase wherein the arbitrary move it belongs to, sum calculates the cumulative sum, and the stochastic function that follows the following format is explained with r(t)

$$r(t)=\begin{Bmatrix} 1 & if\ rand > 0.5 \\ 0 & if\ rand \leq 0.5 \end{Bmatrix} \tag{11}$$

Whereas t indicates the step whither the random navigation and for reading there would be any random value formed in accordance with the uniform distribution between [0,1] Expression 10 may not be explicitly to improve the position of ants. We will be structured using the corresponding expression to maintain the random walks inside the examination area.

$$X_i^t = \frac{(X_i^t - a_i)*(d_i - c_i^t)}{(d_i^t - c_i)} \tag{12}$$

Where a_i would denote the arbitrary navigation of ith variable, b_i denotes the greatest rate at which the random walk belongs, c^t_i would denote smallest value in i^{th} variable for t^{th} iteration of the ith variable and d^t_i indicates the greatest value for the ith variable through the tth step. Thus, in the being of every random moves with the examination area the expression has to be applied in each step.

iii) Acquiring the prey in Antlion's pits

In place of mentioning in the above definition the snares of the antlions can affect arbitrary walks of the ants.

$$c_i^t = Antlion_i^t + c^t \tag{13}$$

$$d_i^t = Antlion_i^t + d^t \tag{14}$$

Where d^t signifies the vector calculating the greatest of whole variables through the tth step, and the c^t is the smallest of the whole variables at i^{th} iteration. The variables for $Antlion^t_j$ and i^{th} ant describes the location of the selected j^{th} antlion in the tth repetition.

iv) Building trap

A roulette wheel will be familiarized to establish the hunting ability of the antlion. Ants are expected to have confined with a solitary antlion selected. When making the optimization task using the roulette wheel operator on picking up the antlions based on the suitability, they use the ALO algorithm.

v) Sliding ants towards antlion

Using the predicted techniques or tactics, antlions will be able to build the snares relative to suitability and the ants will be forced to maneuver subjectively. None less after realizing that the ant is in the snare, the antlions blocks the sand away towards the middle of the trap. The subsequent expression of the above-mentioned definition will be predicted.

$$c^t = \frac{c^t}{I} \tag{15}$$

$$d^t = \frac{d^t}{I} \tag{16}$$

Where I denote ratio, c^t -smallest of the whole variables through t^{th} step, and d^t subjects to the vector comprising, greatest value of the whole variable during t^{th} step.

vi) Catching prey and re-building the pit

The Final hunting process will be when the ant arrives at the bottom of the hole and is trapped inside the antlion's head. The antlion drags the antlion after the above process and takes the sand that is inside and eats the ant's body.

$$Antlion_j^t = Ant_i^t if\ f\left(Ant_i^t\right) > f(Antlion_j^t \tag{17}$$

Where t portrays the current step, $Antlion_j^t$ shows the location where the particular j^{th} antlion must be present in, and for the Ant_i^t postulates the location where the ith ant must be in through the tth step.

Detection of Parameter and ALO Optimization

Commonly, an unspecified parameter that recognizes the problem in the recognized structure and selected procedure could be changed to an optimization question. A defined objective purpose must be stated together with the authentic results of the process that would be established as the system results after activating the actual mechanism. Unidentified parameters that subsequently consider the vector as the particle and the objective function in the optimization procedure must be minimized. While the input from the actual system and known structure will fit together more healthily, parameters expected might be closer to the original rate.

Target of Function

The unbiased purpose of the expected methodology is to achieve amidst the training and testing samples the optimal classification efficiency. The new objective function is projected together with weights that characterize the value of the weights and each parameter are determined in the corresponding unconventionality. Among the outcome of vectors original and predicted, the weighted least square is the smallest motivation. The following description of the function:

$$C_{IOF}(\theta) = \sum_{k=1}^{L}\sum_{j=1}^{n}\left(w_j(z_j(k) - \widehat{z_j(k)}\right)^2 \tag{17}$$

Figure 1. Flowchart for Proposed BPNALO

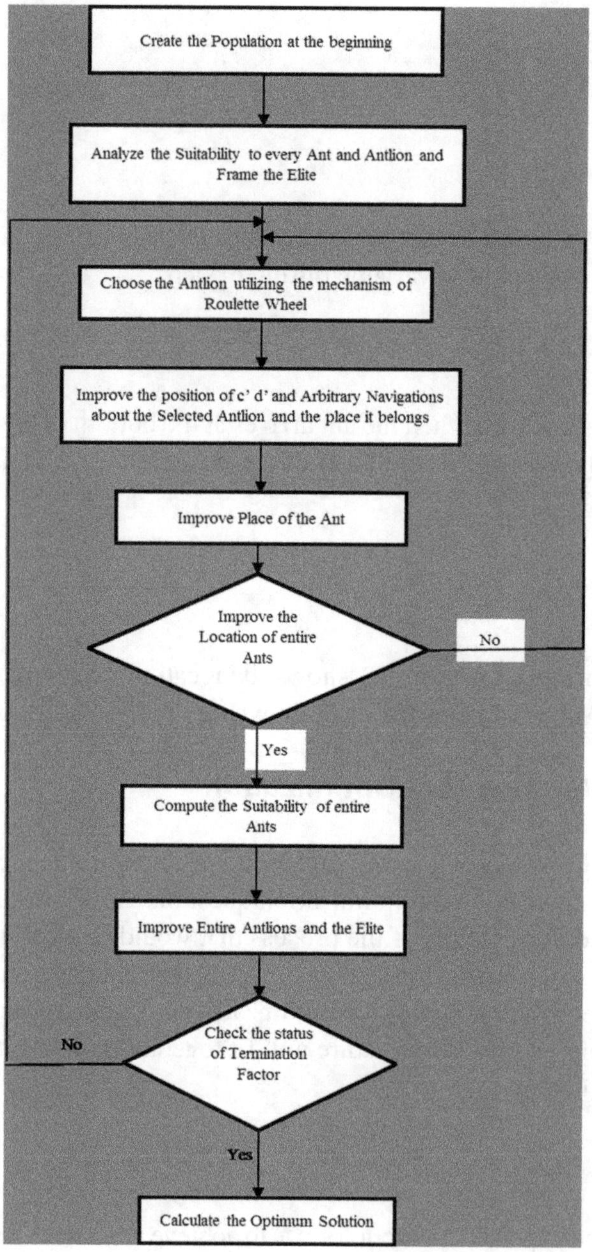

Where z = [x y m_t] subjects to the result of vector of the original structure, zÆ= $\left[x\text{Æ}\widehat{y},\ \widehat{mt} \right]$ mentions about the vector of expected prototype, L denote sample quantity, n means to the magnitude of the result vector for the construction along the value n = 3. While calculating the weights in inspiration the result of vector will be figured for several varied times. The Calculation of the weight of vector w = [w1 w2 w3] would be done in the act of consequent phases:

(1) Mount every vector parameter with a value each as $\theta_i, i = 1, 2 \ldots m$ i, (m denote the parameter size of vector θ, m = 5), and attain the system result of vector z = [z_1(k), …, z_n(k)], k = 1, …, L.
(2) Loop: i = 1:m

Adjust the ith parameter's value, $\theta_{new} = \theta_i * (1 + \Delta\%)$ and get the system result of vector^zi = [^zi1(k), …, ^zin(k)].
End Loop.

(3) Figure out,

$$g_j = \sum_{i=1}^{m} \sum_{k=1}^{L} \left(z_j(k) - \hat{z}_{ij}(k) \right)^2$$

(4) Compute the jth weight

$$w_j = \frac{g_j}{\sum_{j=1}^{n} g_j}$$

The Strategy of Detecting Parameter

The Fig. 2 depicts the illustration of that incorporates the process of the BPN parameter dependent on ALO realization. Formerly, a appropriate input signal would be picked up for activating the definite system and the system estimated. To calculate the suitability, the obtained administered result and the exhibited result is utilized as the inputs in the suitability evaluator. Later, the anonymous parameter vector $\hat{\theta}$ would get established by lowering the sufficient function $s\ of(\hat{\theta})$ is done by grasping the

Figure 2. ALO's Parameter Identification Block Diagram

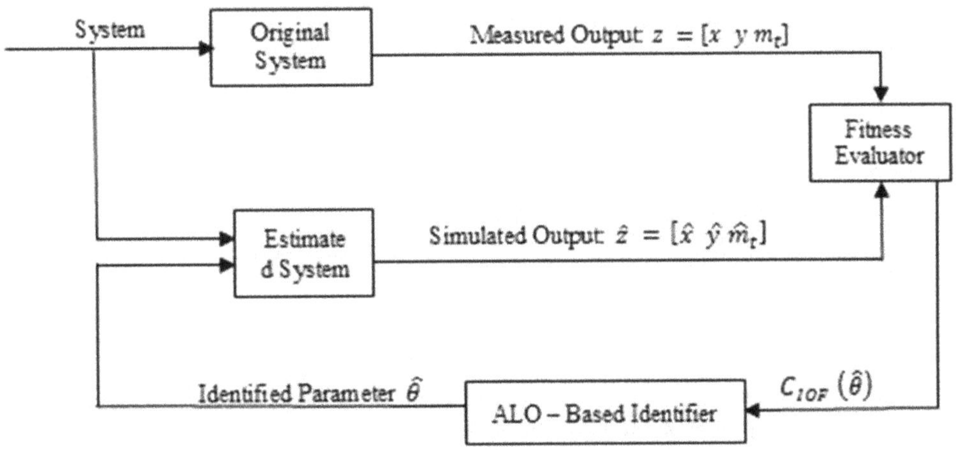

ALO-reliant. Thus, the procedure is repeated, and the documented parameters assessed to flow in the direction of closer to definite values gradually. The fig.3 displays the parameter identification strategy.

The Parameter Acknowledgement accuracy is evaluated through the aid of the following Parameter Error (PE) expression:

$$PE = \left| \frac{\theta_i - \widehat{\theta}_i}{\theta_i} \right| * 100\% \tag{18}$$

and average parameter error (APE):

$$APE = \frac{1}{m} \sum_{i=1}^{m} \left| \frac{\theta_i - \widehat{\theta}_i}{\theta_i} \right| * 100\%$$

where θ_i is the original system's parameter, $\widehat{\theta}_i$ denote the estimated system's parameter, m subjects to the size of θ.

EXPERIMENTAL ANALYSIS

The entire dataset split into two parts one for training and other for testing. The major part of the data 70% is used for training and other 30% is taken for testing the functionality of the proposed classification model. The proposed classification model is evaluated and the obtained results compared with BPNGA, BPNWO on the evaluation metrics which is given in Table 1. In the classification model BPN uses the structural neurons of 7-14-1 (i.e.) 7 input neurons and 14 hidden neurons and one in output layer.

Prevalence Concerning Smoking, HIV and Nicotine

Lung cancer is independent of factors such as HIV, nicotine, age, sex and smoking history. The prevalence was done by the weight and when considering the lung cancer cases it has been rated with high prevalence in control (p, 0.001) and lesser amidst the control (p, 0.001) in the existing smoking. The proposed algorithm consists of features which is independent of HIV, nicotine, age, sex and smoking history.

The findings of the prognosis results in the analysis of the lung cancer diagnosed patients who were also affected by HIV were grownup and most of them were to be expected of being current smokers and nevertheless been a nonsmoker in comparison with the HIV affected patients without evolving the lung cancer. The HIV affected and Uninfected persons will differ based on the race were $p < 0.001$. p indicates the race factors which tend to evaluate affected and unaffected persons of lung cancer. The prevalence was done by considering the TTFC in the lung cancer patient that the hazard of possessing lung cancer whose TTFC > 60 min had been drastically inferior about the range of OR = 0.24 (95% CI 0.08, 0.69). Lung cancer does not have any association with diabetes and heart attack as they have contact with aortic atherosclerosis. There exists the statistically important risk for those associated with hypertension (OR = 2.34). The BMI and risk consisting (OR = 0.93) as an significant factor inverse

Table 2. Confusion Matrix

		Predicted Class: **Positive**	**Predicted Class**: **Negative**	
Actual Class	**Positive**	True Positive (TP)	False Negative (FN) Type II Error	**Sensitivity** $\frac{TP}{(TP+FN)}$
Actual Class	**Negative**	False Positive (FP) Type I Error	True Negative (TN)	**Specificity** $\frac{TN}{(TN+FP)}$
		Precision $\frac{TP}{(TP+FP)}$	**Negative Predictive Value** $\frac{TN}{(TN+FN)}$	**Accuracy** $\frac{TP+TN}{(TP+TN+FP+FN)}$

association. Limiting the analysis to ICD 440 only, the associations were very similar. For example, the odds ratio for TTFC > 60 min was 0.30 (95% CI 0.08, 1.06).

The functionality of the proposed classifier is evaluated in with the help of the confusion matrix. It is a matrix of plotted against the ground truth of the provided information. The Ground truth is the actual class of the data used for the training or testing.

Evaluation Metrics Used

The overall predication results will be evaluated in terms of quality of the classified results. The predicted results which will be original class of the actual data is termed as accuracy. Generally, it will be expressed in percentage. The formula for accuracy calculation is,

$$\text{Accuracy}(\text{A}) = \frac{(\text{TP}+\text{TN})}{(\text{TP}+\text{TN}+\text{FP}+\text{FN})}$$

Sensitivity

The sensitivity clearly signifies the prediction system confirms the existence of the cancer precisely.

$$\text{Recall}(R)\,\text{or Sensitivity} = \frac{\text{TP}}{(\text{TP}+\text{FN})}$$

Table 3. Performance Analysis Prediction of Lung Cancer at Third stage using BPN- ALO technique

PREDICTION MODEL	Accuracy (%)	Specificity (%)	Sensitivity (%)
BPN-GENETIC ALGORITHM	95.40	91.70	93.50
BPN-WO	98.10	95.20	90.30
PROPOSED BPN – ALO	99.10	96.80	88.60

Specificity

The sensitivity clearly signifies the prediction system confirms the non-existence of the cancer precisely (i.e.) who does not suffer from lung cancer.

$$\text{Precision}\left(\text{P}\right)\text{or}\left(1-\text{Specificity}\right)=\frac{\text{TP}}{\left(\text{TP}+\text{FP}\right)}$$

Table 3, Table 4, and Table 5 describes the analysis of functionality for the projected technique neural network and ant lion optimization concerning functionality metrics like accuracy, specificity, and sensitivity for prediction of all stage's cancer.

Table 3, Table 4, and Table 5 summarizes the obtained results in terms of functionality metrics accuracy, specificity, and sensitivity for prediction of all stage's cancer. This clearly reveals that the proposed prediction model functioning well while analyzing the functionality metrics.

The comparison chart of various stages of cancer is plot in Figure 3. The obtained accuracy of various stage data is predicted using proposed BPNALO model and reveals the better performance. Out of the techniques available for the prediction of Lung Cancer, the proposed BPNALO performs better by having a considerable accuracy of nearly 100% for detecting the lung cancer at stage 3 and stage 2 it is having the prediction accuracy of 93% and even at stage 1, it is having the prediction accuracy of 87%. From the results, it is inferred that the proposed BPNALO technique outperforms well.

Table 4. Performance Analysis prediction of Lung Cancer at Second stage using BPN- ALO technique

PREDICTION MODEL	Accuracy (%)	Specificity (%)	Specificity (%)
BPN-GENETIC ALGORITHM	84.30	82.60	90.50
BPN-WO	87.60	86.40	86.70
PROPOSED BPN – ALO	93.20	89.60	84.30

Table 5. Performance Analysis prediction of Lung Cancer at First stage using BPN- ALO technique

PREDICTION MODEL	Accuracy (%)	Specificity (%)	Sensitivity (%)
BPN-GENETIC ALGORITHM	78.70	75.20	83.70
BPN-WO	85.20	80.70	78.60
PROPOSED BPN – ALO	87.10	85.30	74.70

Figure 3. Accuracy Comparison of Prediction of Lung Cancer at Various Stages

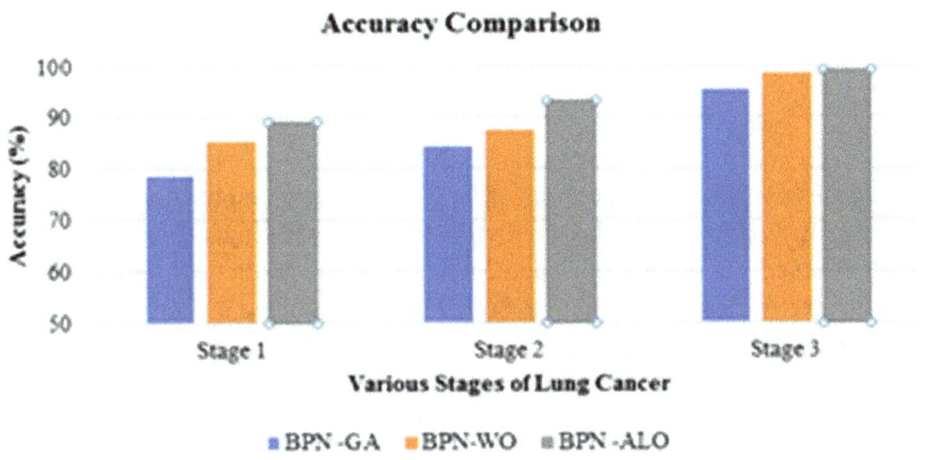

Figure 4. Specificity Comparison of Prediction of Lung Cancer at Various Stages

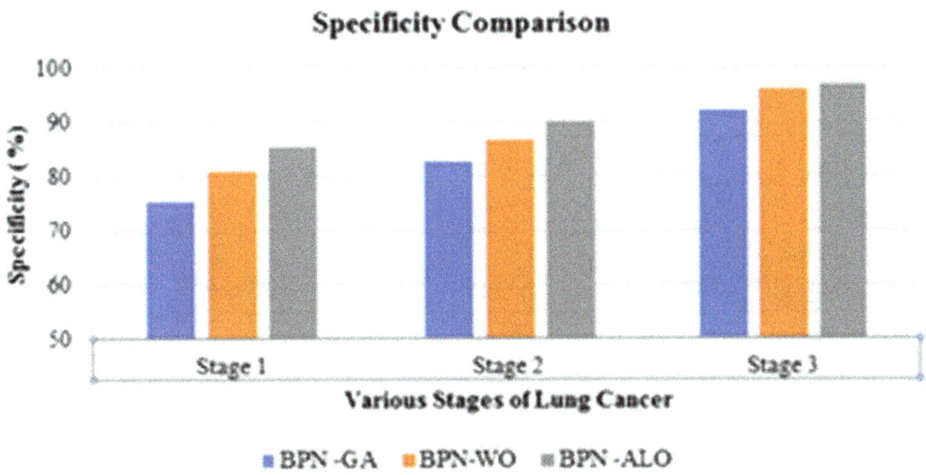

Figure 5. Sensitivity Comparison of Prediction of Lung Cancer at Various Stages

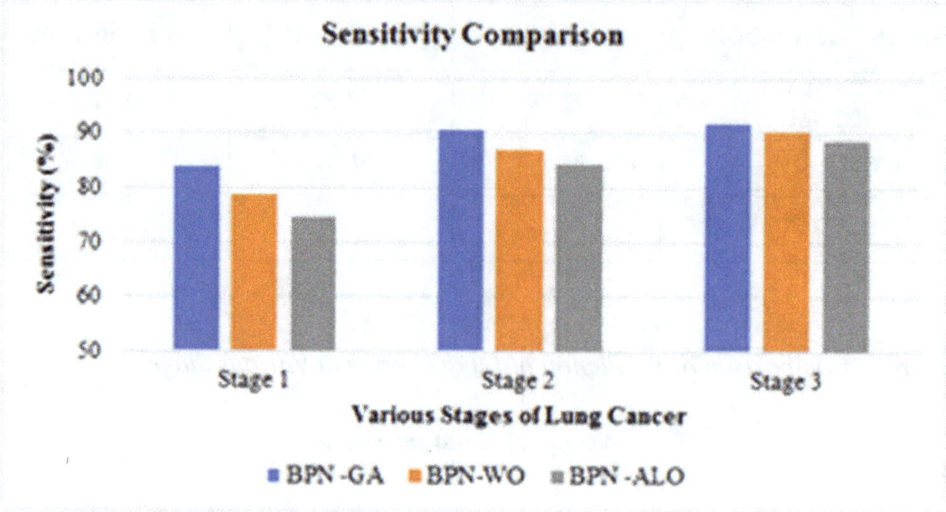

Figure 4 establishes the specificity analysis of lung cancer at three phases of lung cancer. The proposed BPNALO performs better than other prediction models by having a substantial precision of 97% for detecting the lung cancer at stage 3 and stage 2 it is having the prediction precision of 90% and even at stage 1 it is having the prediction accuracy of 86%. From the attained outcomes it is observed that the proposed BPNALO technique performance is the best in comparison with other techniques.

Figure 5 shows the sensitivity examination of lung cancer at all stages of lung cancer. The proposed BPNALO outperforms better than other prediction models discussed in the literatures by obtaining the sensitivity values of 89% for detecting the lung cancer at stage 3 and stage 2 it is having the prediction precision of 85% and even at stage 1, it is having the prediction accuracy of 75%.

Table 6 and Table 7 establish the Chance of Prediction of Recurrence affected by Lung Cancer during second at First Stage.

From Figures 6 and Figure 7 it is observed that comparison of various parameters for predicting the chance of recurrence for Stage 2 and Stage 1 respectively. The proposed BPNALO technique has

Table 6. Performance Analysis Prediction of Recurrent at Second stage using BPN- ALO technique

PREDICTION MODEL	Accuracy (%)	Specificity (%)	Sensitivity (%)
BPN-GENETIC ALGORITHM	66.7	64.1	71.6
BPN-WO	70.9	68.7	67.2
PROPOSED BPN – ALO	72.3	70.4	65.7

Table 7. Performance Analysis Prediction of Recurrent at First stage using BPN- ALO technique

PREDICTION MODEL	Accuracy (%)	Specificity (%)	Sensitivity (%)
BPN-GENETIC ALGORITHM	61.2	60.4	63.4
BPN-WO	63.2	62.6	61.7
PROPOSED BPN – ALO	67.8	64.5	59.3

Figure 6. Comparison of Various Parameters for Prediction of Recurrence Lung Cancer at Second Stage

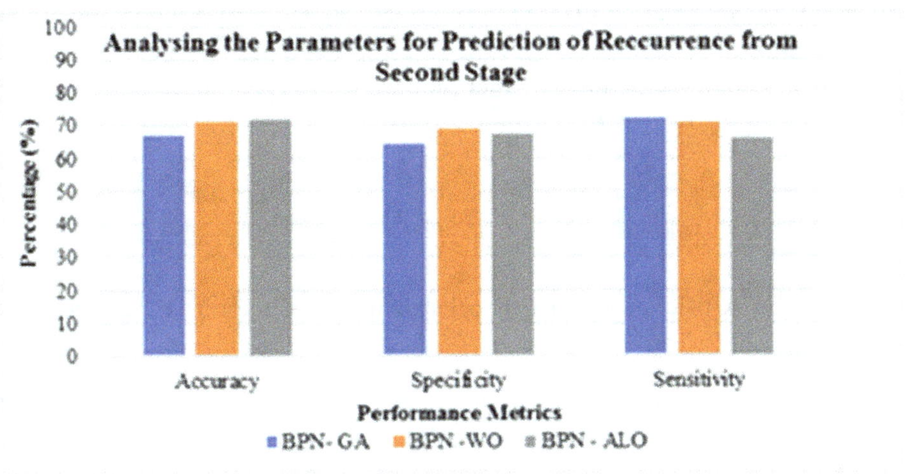

Figure 7. Comparison of Various Parameters for Prediction of Recurrence Lung Cancer at Various Stages

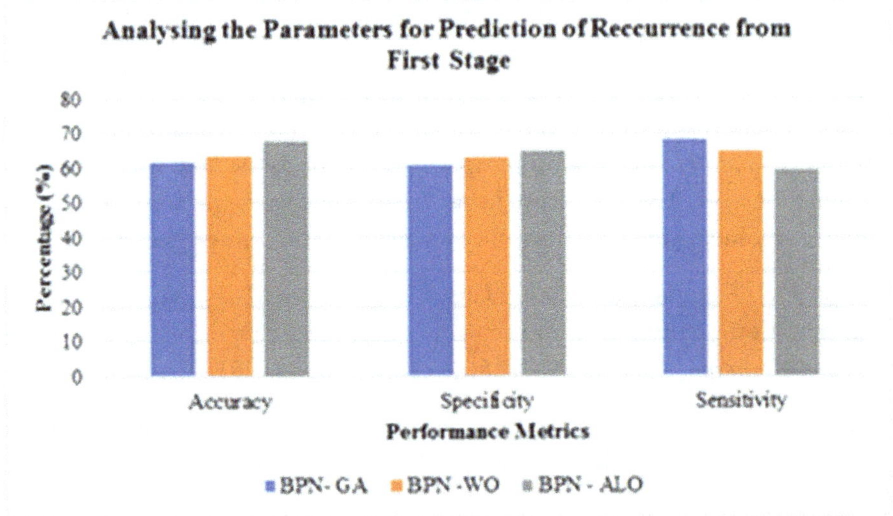

better prediction accuracy for the chance of recurrence for stage 2 patients of 73% and stage 1 patients prediction accuracy of 68%. Though the prediction of the chance of recurrence is having a good impact in recurrence lung cancer studies. This complete evaluation results of the proposed prediction model achieves improvement of appreciable performances and hence proved by the experiments performed.

CONCLUSION

The research paper focused explicitly on predicting the existence of lung cancer using the BPN by choosing the BPN optimization parameter using the Meta Heuristics techniques Enthused by Nature to improve the correctness and consistency for the prediction of lung cancer at the earlier phase itself. Besides, in forecasting the possibility of reappearance after undertaking the medication the proposed BPNALO technique is utilized. The output from the both would be very obliging in determining the nature and deepness of the medication offered to the lung cancers. From the results attained from the Surveys achieved the proposed BPNALO that it has an improved performance in forecasting the possibility of recurrence and attained extremely exact outcomes in expecting the presence of lung cancer at an earlier phase.

REFERENCES

Al-Shayea, Q. K. (2011). Artificial neural networks in medical diagnosis. *International Journal of Computer Science Issues*, *8*(2), 150–154.

Aljarah, I., Faris, H., & Mirjalili, S. (2018). Optimizing connection weights in neural networks using the whale optimization algorithm. *Soft Computing*, *22*(1), 1–15.

Amato, F., López, A., Peña-Méndez, E. M., Vaňhara, P., Hampl, A., & Havel, J. (2013). Artificial neural networks in medical diagnosis.

Bhuvaneswari, P., & Therese, A. B. (2015). Detection of cancer in lung with k-nn classification using genetic algorithm. *Procedia Materials Science*, *10*, 433–440. doi:10.1016/j.mspro.2015.06.077

Brause, R. W. (2001, October). Medical analysis and diagnosis by neural networks. In *Proceedings of the International Symposium on Medical Data Analysis* (pp. 1-13). Springer. 10.1007/3-540-45497-7_1

Brownlee, J. (2015). Practice Machine Learning with Datasets from the UCI Machine Learning Repository. Machine learning mastery. Retrieved from https://machinelearningmastery.com/practice-machine-learning-with-small-in-memory-datasets-from-the-uci-machine-learning-repository/

Coudray, N., Ocampo, P. S., Sakellaropoulos, T., Narula, N., Snuderl, M., Fenyö, D., ... Tsirigos, A. (2018). Classification and mutation prediction from non–small cell lung cancer histopathology images using deep learning. *Nature Medicine*, *24*(10), 1559–1567. doi:10.103841591-018-0177-5 PMID:30224757

Cruz, J. A., & Wishart, D. S. (2006). Applications of machine learning in cancer prediction and prognosis. *Cancer Informatics*, *2*. doi:10.1177/117693510600200030 PMID:19458758

Dandıl, E. (2018). A Computer-Aided Pipeline for Automatic Lung Cancer Classification on Computed Tomography Scans. *Journal of Healthcare Engineering*. PMID:30515286

Daoud, M., & Mayo, M. (2019). A Survey of Neural Network-based Cancer Prediction Models from Microarray Data. *Artificial Intelligence in Medicine*, *97*, 204–214. doi:10.1016/j.artmed.2019.01.006 PMID:30797633

Greco, F. A., & Oldham, R. K. (1979). Small-cell lung cancer. *The New England Journal of Medicine*, *301*(7), 355–358. doi:10.1056/NEJM197908163010704 PMID:223051

https://www.cancer.net/cancer-types/lung-cancer-non-small-cell/stages

Griffiths, D. (1986). Pit construction by ant-lion larvae: A cost-benefit analysis. *Journal of Animal Ecology*, *55*(1), 39–57. doi:10.2307/4691

Gupta, A., & Shrivastava, M. (2012). Performance of ANN using Back Propagation Algorithm for Medical Diagnosis System. *International Journal of Advanced Computer Research (IJACR)*, 2.

ICS. (n.d.). Datasets. Retrieved from https://archive.ics.uci.edu/ml/datasets.html

Jiang, N., & Xu, X. (2019). Exploring the survival prognosis of lung adenocarcinoma based on the cancer genome atlas database using artificial neural network. *Medicine*, *98*(20), e15642. doi:10.1097/MD.0000000000015642 PMID:31096483

Kashf, D. W. A., Okasha, A. N., Sahyoun, N. A., El-Rabi, R. E., & Abu-Naser, S. S. (2018). Predicting DNA Lung Cancer using Artificial Neural Network. *International Journal of Academic Pedagogical Research*, *2*(10), 6–13.

Kose, U. (2018). An Ant-Lion optimizer-trained artificial neural network system for chaotic electroencephalogram (EEG) Prediction. *Applied Sciences*, *8*(9), 1613. doi:10.3390/app8091613

Kuruvilla, J., & Gunavathi, K. (2014). Lung cancer classification using neural networks for CT images. *Computer Methods and Programs in Biomedicine*, *113*(1), 202–209. doi:10.1016/j.cmpb.2013.10.011 PMID:24199657

Lee, H. A., Chao, L. R., Rau, H. H., & Hsu, C. Y. (2018, July). Constructing Prediction Model of Lung Cancer Treatment Survival. In *Proceedings of the International Conference on Frontier Computing* (pp. 1925-1933). Springer Singapore.

Mirjalili, S. (2015). The ant lion optimizer. *Advances in Engineering Software*, *83*, 80–98. doi:10.1016/j.advengsoft.2015.01.010

Nall, R. (2018). What to know about lung cancer. Medical News Today. Retrieved from https://www.medicalnewstoday.com/articles/323701.php

Naresh, P., & Shettar, D. R. (2014). Early Detection of Lung Cancer Using Neural Network Techniques. *Prashant Naresh Int. Journal of Engineering Research and Applications*, 4.

Selvanambi, R., Natarajan, J., Karuppiah, M., Islam, S. H., Hassan, M. M., & Fortino, G. (2018). Lung cancer prediction using higher-order recurrent neural network based on glowworm swarm optimization. *Neural Computing & Applications*, 1–14.

Teramoto, A., Tsukamoto, T., Kiriyama, Y., & Fujita, H. (2017). Automated classification of lung cancer types from cytological images using deep convolutional neural networks. *BioMed Research International*. PMID:28884120

Tharwat, A., & Hassanien, A. E. (2018). Chaotic antlion algorithm for parameter optimization of support vector machine. *Applied Intelligence*, *48*(3), 670–686. doi:10.100710489-017-0994-0

Tian, T., Liu, C., Guo, Q., Yuan, Y., Li, W., & Yan, Q. (2018). An improved ant lion optimization algorithm and its application in hydraulic turbine governing system parameter identification. *Energies*, *11*(1), 95. doi:10.3390/en11010095

Tkacz, E. J., & Kostka, P. (2000). An application of a wavelet neural network for classification of patients with coronary artery disease based on HRV analysis. In *Proceedings of the 22nd Annual International Conference of the IEEE Engineering in Medicine and Biology Society* (Vol. 2, pp. 1391-1393). IEEE. 10.1109/IEMBS.2000.897999

Uramoto, H., & Tanaka, F. (2014). Recurrence after surgery in patients with NSCLC. *Translational Lung Cancer Research*, *3*(4), 242. PMID:25806307

Win, S. L., Htike, Z. Z., Yusof, F., & Noorbatcha, I. A. (2014). Cancer recurrence prediction using machine learning. *International Journal of Computational Science and Information Technology*, *6*(1).

Wu, Y. C., Wei, N. C., Hung, J. J., Yeh, Y. C., Su, L. J., Hsu, W. H., & Chou, T. Y. (2017). Generating a robust prediction model for stage I lung adenocarcinoma recurrence after surgical resection. *Oncotarget*, *8*(45), 79712. doi:10.18632/oncotarget.19161 PMID:29108351

Xie, Y., & Minna, J. D. (2008). Predicting the future for people with lung cancer. *Nature Medicine*, *14*(8), 812–813. doi:10.1038/nm0808-812 PMID:18685594

Yamany, W., Tharwat, A., Hassanin, M. F., Gaber, T., Hassanien, A. E., & Kim, T. H. (2015, September). A new multi-layer perceptrons trainer based on an ant lion optimization algorithm. In *Proceedings of the 2015 Fourth international conference on information science and industrial applications (ISI)* (pp. 40-45). IEEE. 10.1109/ISI.2015.9

Yao, J., Wang, S., Zhu, X., & Huang, J. (2016, October). Imaging biomarker discovery for lung cancer survival prediction. In *Proceedings of the International Conference on Medical Image Computing and Computer-Assisted Intervention* (pp. 649-657). Springer. 10.1007/978-3-319-46723-8_75

Chapter 12
Effective and Accurate Diagnosis Using Brain Image Fusion

Sivakumar Rajagopal
https://orcid.org/0000-0001-8486-7960
Vellore Institute of Technology, India

Babu Gopal
Velammal Institute of Technology, India

ABSTRACT

Medical imaging techniques are routinely employed to create images of the human system for clinical purposes. Multi-modality medical imaging is a widely used technology for diagnosis, detection, and prediction of various tissue abnormalities. This chapter is focused on the development of an improved brain image processing technique for the removal of noise from a magnetic resonance image (MRI) for accurate image restoration. Feature selection and extraction of MRI brain images are processed using image fusion. The medical images suffer from motion blur and noise for which image denoising is developed through non-local means (NLM) filtering for smoothing and shrinkage rule for sharpening. The peak signal to noise ratio (PSNR) of improved curvelet based self-similarity NLM method is better than discrete wavelet transform with an NLM filter.

INTRODUCTION

The imaging process in medicine is mainly used to provide visual information about the internal parts to provide better decision making for clinical purposes and further procedures (Anjali Wadhwa et al., 2019). An important advantage is the extraction of prior knowledge for the prevention of diseases. Nowadays the most frequent and severe syndrome created by Alzheimer's disease, which affects the human memory and thinking process to lead everyday life (Yujun Hou et al., 2019). Multimodal Image acquisition is generally affected by the faulty instrument noise, manual handling of medical instruments,

DOI: 10.4018/978-1-7998-2101-4.ch012

the imperfect process followed in the acquisition procedure and improper fusing methods used, and due to the error introduced by the transmission process and the type of compression techniques used for transmission (Mzoughi et al., 2019).

Magnetic Resonance Imaging (MRI) image acquisition depends on the various parameters. It depends on the strength of the magnet used to generate static field, the patient size, handling the of the machine, selection radio frequency (RF) coil, frequency of radiofrequency coil, pulse sequence used to transmit and receive RF pulse, positioning of gradient coils for slice selection, various parameters set for acquisitions process, the type reconstruction technique (Gudjartsson & Patz, 1995).

Image restoration often requires the decomposition of a degraded image as approximation and details. In this research work, smoothening by improved Non-Local Means Filter (NLM) (Buades et al., 2011) and sharpening by Soft thresholding shrinkage rule (Chang et al., 2000) play the role of decomposition. The decomposition of degraded image restores line discontinuities by employing Fast Discrete Curvelet Transform.

The three-dimensional imaging can be used to identify the depth information which can be realized by the vision system (Cootes et al., 1992). The anatomical variations in the different individual's images can be analyzed using brain image registration. It is useful to combine information from different sources, analyze the individual variations, localizing and detecting various diseases and fuse the images for better decision making (Babu & Sivakumar, 2017). The similarity-based brain image registration is initiated for minimizing geometric distortion.

Multimodal fusion techniques applied to brain image analysis is used to reduce the redundant information and increase the required details from different imaging techniques. A multimodal image fusion provides clear feature details to enable the clinician to make an efficient decision for disease analysis Data fusion in medical images is introduced to merge multimodal (anatomical and structural information) and multi-patient images for the identification of structures (Piao et al., 2019; Padmavathi et al., 2019). Image fusion is focused on data combination, identification of anatomical structure based on image geometrical features and statistical image features (Barillot et al., 1993). The main drawbacks are poor resolution and mis-registrations which are overcome by improved curvelet based self-similarity measured in MRI.

A fuzzy-based algorithm proposed by Stelios Krinidis and Vassilios Chatzis (2010) integrates both the gray level and spatial level details. The performance of the integrating process can be enhanced by fuzzy local information C Means (FLICM) (Zhang et al., 2019). The FLICM is mainly used to retain most of the image details and make image insensitive to noises. The image segmentation and clustering process can be made effective using the Fuzzy based. They utilize a fast, generalized, Fuzzy C Means (FGFCM) algorithm to integrate both the gray level and spatial level image information. In their research work, the improved curvelet based NLM method is applied in Fuzzy C Means (FCM) to classify aging syndrome from due to Alzheimer's disease.

The majority of older people are suffering from Alzheimer's disease. It is also affecting the people in the age group between the forties and fifties. The effect of the disease becomes more severe at the later stages. It is a degenerative disease, where symptoms gradually worsen over several years. The effect of disease on memory loss at the initial stage is less, but it becomes worse at a later stage, individuals finding it difficult to respond to any conversation. The progress of the disease can be classified into four different levels (Robert Katzman et al., 1988). The early level does not make any significant change in everyday routine and it is known as Mild Cognitive Impairment (MCI) (Peterson, 2004). The cognitive loss and decrease in independence are increased in the second and third levels of the disease and are called Mild and Moderate AD (Nygard, 2003). The overall reduction in personality and dependency on care takes are increased in the last level of disease and it is known as severe AD.

Yujun Hou et al. (2019) found that more than 18 million persons are affected by Alzheimer's disease globally. It may increase to 34 million in the year 2025. Most of the developing countries will contribute to this increase due to the increase in the older people population. It is found that more than 9 million developing countries people are affected by Alzheimer's disease and it may increase to 12 million by 2025. In India, there is a possibility of more urban areas people are prone to Alzheimer's disease than the rural people. Currently more regress action globally ongoing to identify the disease at an early stage to prevent severe stages. Early-stage detection and treatment will improve and stabilize behavioral and cognitive activities. Using the accurate early detection of disease levels, modern therapeutic methods can be used to correct the pathological changes.

Image registration and fusion are important for better image feature selection and extraction. The goal of the registrations process is to make different modality images to align each image modalities. Through the Image fusion process, more clear information and details can be obtained from medical images. Nowadays, due to the rapid advance of technologies in medical imaging, anatomy with functional details can be acquired with more information and good resolution (El-zhara et al., 2016; Fereshteh et al., 2019).

Image registration is mainly used for geometric correction and sharpening. Image fusion is employed for the enhancement of certain features not visible in single-shot images. The brain abnormal functional location can be identified by combing MRI and Positron Emission Tomography (PET) images (Goshtasby, 2005). In many medical image analysis applications, the image registration process is an essential fundamental analysis (Mzoughi et al., 2019). Many pathological details can be detected using medical image registration. Self-similarity-based image restoration is applied to the context of image registration which provides better geometric alignment (Babu & Sivakumar, 2017).

NLM similarity-based restoration is applied to the fusion of medical images by combining images of various modalities. The radiologists utilize the spectral information and spatial information for disease diagnosis, monitoring, and research. The fusion framework is used for classifying the different brain defects. The fused image has enhanced the visualization for medical images. Kirankumar and Shenbaga Devi (2007) has implemented wavelet and KL transforms for fusing CT and MRI. The existing method is used to extract required information by different fusion rules; it is limited to retain the important information about high-frequency details like edges of the multimodal fused image. Sivakumar (2007) exploited the curvelet transform in a more detailed way with multi-scale information. Curvelet transform is a special member of the multi-scale geometric transforms. Curvelet transform provides better results compare to the wavelet transform in image reconstruction of objects with more edges.

To preserve the long edges with small features an image fusion method has been proposed by applying wavelet transform and contourlet transform (Shutao Li et al., 2011). This method required a longer time of execution. Stationary wavelets transform (SWT) overcomes the problems related to translation-invariance in the Discrete Wavelet Transform (DWT) implementation. The features obtained by DWT may change remarkably due to the dithering of the brain MR image (Shift variant). The centers of the two images from one subject are located at slightly different positions by using DWT based classification.

Shutao Li et al. (2011) compared the image fusion performance of the various multi-resolution transforms with different decomposition levels. The experimental results implied better image fusion. A medical image fusion method based on the Neuro-fuzzy technique provided a good objective and subjective evaluation of performance and it is free from image degradation, loss of fine image detail information and contrast reduction (Sudeb Das & Malay Kumar Kundu, 2013). The main drawback was time complexity.

The fused image quality can be improved by using a slant transform-based technique with computation complexity (Arathi & Latha Parameswaran, 2013). It had limited selection capability for threshold and decomposition coefficients. Vivekangoth et al. proposed an image fusion-based algorithm using the wavelet transform to detect brain tumors; the paper utilized complementary and redundant details from two different imaging modalities (Dwith et al., 2013). It considers only PSNR and does not include statistical evaluation parameters namely, mean, entropy, standard deviation, correlation coefficient, and similarity measure.

A new medical image fusion using multimodal was proposed using a few coefficients for two different modal images (Zhaodong Liu et al., 2014). In this method, two different types of fusion rules are employed for both low frequency and high-frequency coefficients; pulse coupled neural network fusion rule is employed to fuse low-frequency coefficients; it does not reduce time complexity. Anbumozhi and Manoharan (2014) depicted brain tumor detection using multimodal image fusion (CT and MRI); the method reduced redundancy and uncertainty. A cascade of wavelet and NSCT method described two different types of medical imaging techniques (MRI&CT) and it is useful to provide better phase details, variance, and directional information. The main drawback is the temporal localization due to shift-invariance (Vikrant Bhateja et al., 2015).

A curvelet transform local energy-based image fusion for medical images employs anisotropic property to capture edge points in an image (Richa Srivastava et al., 2016). This method is good for line discontinuity and also provides better evaluation parameters namely, correlation coefficient, edge similarity measure, and average pixel intensity. Pritika and Sumit Budhiraja (2016) provided the guided image filter with edge preservation for the multimodal images; the guided image filter reduced the ringing artifacts in the image. Paul Hill et al. (2016) introduced multi-resolution transforms. This method is computationally complex and requires longer running time; the resulting image has low entropy.

The self-similarity measure is applied in the context of image segmentation. Yong Yang et al. (2017) proposed the different types of wavelet transform and contourlet transform which are employed for medical image fusion. These transforms have better results compare to the basic wavelet transform. These techniques demand larger memory and high computational complexity. Image fusion using the multimodal sensor adopted the analysis of multistate geometric of the NSCT and fuzzy logic-based fused rule of the high-frequency band. This method preserves information better and enhances the condition of the fused image. This work does not extract approximation in intermodal image fusion.

The clustering process can be used to classify objects and patterns. The different clusters are having samples with very close similar samples (Zhang et al., 2019). There are two different types of clustering techniques based on fuzzy and hard clustering. On many occasions, the efficiency of a hard clustering method is reduced by the noise, lessor contrast, and inconsistent intensity and overrun contrast issues. Fuzzy clustering, as a soft segmentation method is implemented in image clustering and segmentation successfully.

Maria Elena and Fernando Flores developed an automatic brain structure detection and segmentation algorithm to classify MRI images (Maria Elena Algorri & Fernando Flores Mangas, 2004). The NLM fuzzy clustering information is concentrated in a small subdivision of a larger image. The knowledge base algorithm exploits a small subset of semi-automatically classified images that are combined with a set of fuzzy indexes that captured the experience and expectation a human expert uses during recognition tasks. A semi-automatically identified image is used to identify the structure of the brain. Their techniques utilize algorithm uses minimal image processing techniques for segmentation, then justifies or appropriate the segmentations, and by utilizing the fuzzy indexes the criteria at a maximal level can be measured for the final classification decision.

MRI is used to find changes in brain tissue atrophy and more specific in a gray matter (Peter & Nick, 1998); white matter is not featured for AD. The higher fat content tissues are shown as bright and the Cerebrospinal fluid (CSF) content areas are shown as dark. MRI assesses breakdown of tissue characteristics which induce signal modifications on a few sequences such as white matter hyperintensities on T2-weighted MRI. MR sequences are diffused due to AD that has microstructural changes. Diffuse cerebral atrophy with widened sulci and dilation of the lateral ventricles can be observed. The early stage of Alzheimer's disease can be diagnosed using the dilation of the Parahippocampal fissure, with a very high level of accuracy (Ferris et al., 1980). The brain features are extracted using the structural MRI and the existing methods can be divided into voxel-wise tissue probability, cortical thickness and hippocampal volumes (Friston et al., 2007). The fusion of brain image is essential to extract vital details from multimodal information which is useful to clinically detect and predict various diseases. The improved curvelet based self-similarity method is proposed in this chapter which is applied in the context of brain image fusion which helps in diagnosing Alzheimer's disease accurately. This method utilizes lesser storage space required to store one multimodal image compare to storing each mode details separately.

The fusion methods are assorted into three different types using the representation of different levels such as pixel, feature, and decision-based level (Shivsubramani & Soman, 2010). Pixel-based fusion technique is applied to the acquired medical images; most of the original details are retained. In feature level based fusion technique, the important features are extracted from the segmented acquired medical images and each region features are used for fusion. In a decision based fused methods is a complex method and is mainly utilized for highly of fusion. In general, pixel-based image fusion methods are divided based on the domain; spatial based and transform-based. Spatial based methods are applied directly to medical images using local spatial features; MAX, MIN, MEAN and Principal Components. The spatial domain-based fusion method introduces distortions and any spectral related information cannot be fetched. However, the pixel-based fusion methods introduce too many undesirable side effects, including reduced contrast (Yang et al., 2010).

In transform domain methods the medical images are converted to transform coefficients, the fusion is based on the transform coefficients, and the fused images are obtained back using inverse transform. All transform domain techniques are utilizing multi-scale Pyramid methods. But, all transform-based methods failed to provide directional details and poor signal to noise ratio (SNR). Hence, the method-based wavelet transform is proposed in this chapter to obtain clear details from the medical image. Many wavelet transform-based fusion techniques are discussed in the literature. The most famous and commonly used fusion transformation is a Discrete Wavelet Transform (DWT) (Li et al., 1995). Some advanced curvelet and contourlet based transform techniques are utilized in the fusion methods used for medical images like Non-Subsampled Contourlet Transform (NSCT), curvelet transform (CT) and contourlet transform to provide better medical image fusion performance over wavelet transform. But these advanced transform methods require high computation complexity and memory space (Valdimir & Costas, 2004).

Different sensor images have provided information about different features and the regions. Computer Tomography (CT) images provide better information about disease and details about denser tissues with lessor distortion (Borsdorf et al., 2008). To provide clearer details about anatomical and pathological information the Magnetic Resonance Imaging technique is utilized. Positron Emission Tomography images are utilized to obtain brain motor and speech region functional information. Single-Photon Emission Computed Tomography imaging technique provides clear details on the change in metabolic information. Therefore, every modality has its drawbacks in providing required details to doctors in assessing clinical conditions and each modality utilizes different acquisition techniques. Hence, a doctor needs to analyze the different modality images. The contrast of the individual CT and MRI scan image can be improved by contrast enhancement technique, but it is very difficult to solve the different modality imaging problems (Ganasala & Kumar, 2014).

The multimodal image fusion technique is used to combine different modality medical images such as SPECT-CT, SPECT-MRI, and PET-CT, etc. The Multimodal fused image provides clear information in comparison with individual images of different modality. Image fusion reduces redundancies produced by various sensors and increases the effectiveness in the assessment of medical problems. It further provides better visual and machine perception details. It is easy for further analysis and image processing purposes.

Some basic fundamental steps to be followed during the fusion process in medical imaging are: The important requirement is to retain most of the important features in the original input images. The multimodal image fusion technique image should provide better visibility and machine recognition details, and for subsequent analysis for image processing. It should contain a minimum of insignificant information and lessor noise levels. In the proposed technique image transform coefficients are derived from medical images using Stationary Wavelet Transform (SWT). The transform coefficients are utilized to derive appropriate parameters for fusion such as MAX, MIN, MEAN, and Principal Component Analysis (PCA). This chapter also suggests a better fusion rule by analyzing various analysis parameters evaluated for different DWT techniques.

FUSION RULES

Based on the image acquisition technique and processing levels the fusion methods are classified into two categories. Depending upon the purpose of fusion and input image acquisition techniques, four different kinds of medical image fusion methods are classified as Multi-sensor, Multi-temporal, Multi-focus, and Multi-view fusion. There are four different stages used in the fusion procedure stages, depending upon the purpose of fusion and the input image acquisition techniques and also based on the required area the fusion methods are grouped into four types as Pixel, Feature, Decision, and Block level.

Max Fusion Rule

Two-column vectors are formed using input images obtained from MRI technique i1(x, y) and i (x, y) and the corresponding empirical maximum value is calculated. The fusion process image is formed by

$$I_f(x, y) = \max i_1(x, y) + \max i_2(x, y) \tag{1}$$

Min Fusion Rule

Two-column vectors are formed using input images obtained from MRI technique i1(x, y) and i2(x, y) and the corresponding empirical minimum value is calculated. The fusion process image is formed by

$$I_f(x, y) = \min i_1(x, y) + \min i_2(x, y) \tag{2}$$

Mean Fusion Rule

Two-column vectors are formed using input images obtained from MRI technique i1(x, y) and i2(x, y) and the corresponding empirical mean value is calculated. The fusion process image is formed by

$$I_f(x, y) = \text{mean } i_1(x, y) + \text{mean} i_2(x, y) \tag{3}$$

PCA Fusion Rule

For analysis purposes, multidimensional data is converted into lower dimensions using PCA. It transforms correlated variables into uncorrelated variables. It provides improved structural details about the data for the fusion process. Two-column vectors are formed using input MRI images i_1 (x, y) and i_2 (x, y) and corresponding empirical means are subtracted. The eigenvalues and eigenvectors are identified from the obtained vector with a size of n × 2 (n is the length of each image vector), and the eigenvectors related to the maximum eigenvalue is achieved. The computation of normalized components p1 and p2 (i.e., p1 + p2 = 1) are achieved from the resultant eigenvector. The resultant image is given by

$$I_f(x, y) = p_1 i_1(x, y) + p_2 i_2(x, y) \tag{4}$$

Where p1and p2 is the normalized components

The generic process for a fusion of images of input images 1 and 2 and their coefficients p1 and p2 are calculated and a fused image is given by if.

Improved NLM Based Fusion Rule

Non-local means algorithm derived in Section 3.2, the weight is adjusted by the principal component as shown in Figure 1.

NLM filter smoothens the low-frequency component and highlights the edges. PCA matches the pattern, identify the similarities and reduce the information loss. For analysis purposes, multidimensional data is converted into lower dimensions using PCA. It transforms correlated variables into uncorrelated variables. It provides better structural information about the data for the fusion process. The optimal data set description is computed using PCA. The variance of the maximum data set is recorded using the first component of PCA. The consecutive PCA components record the variance of the maximum of the remaining data set. The first PCA component is appropriated with the maximum variance direction. The second PCA component is limited to subspace perpendicular to the first PCA component. The third PCA component records the maximum variance direction and normal to the initial PCA components. The PCA analysis is further known as the Karhunen-Loève transform (KL Transform) and the hotelling transform.

Figure 1. Improved NLM based image fusion rule

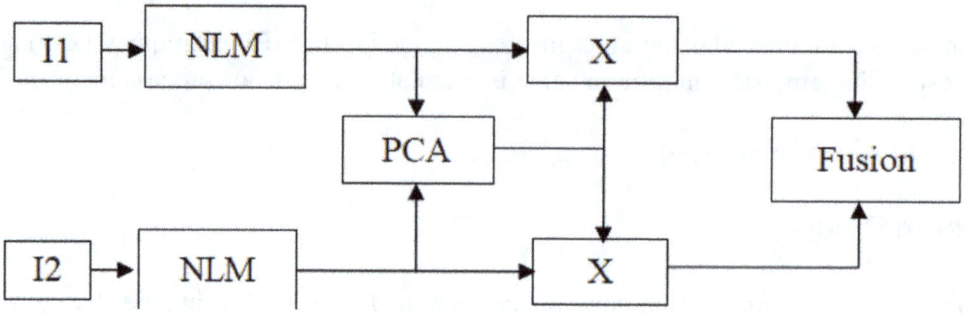

STATIONARY WAVELET TRANSFORM (SWT)

The undecimated wavelet transform method is familiarly known as SWT and it is mainly used to overcome the shift or translation-invariant drawback of the DWT by eliminating the downsampling process. The input MRI image is divided into two sub-bands using SWT. The low sub-band components are known as approximation coefficients and the high sub-band components are called as detailed coefficients. The SWT provides a good time and frequency localization for the fused image and is also useful for detecting curved shapes more precisely than the DWT. The filter bank digital implementation of DWT is given in Figure 2(a). For each of the coefficients, the downsampling is done by a factor in this transform. The SWT implementation is given in Figure 2(b).

The MRI Brain images reveal interspaces at the lines, curves, and edges. Edge enhancement and keeping intact are vital in the medical image analysis and hence stationary wavelet-based transformation is extended to image fusion. Besides, the NLM filter enhances better image feature extraction as exhibits in Figure 3. The improved curvelet transform is good for curve discontinuities and better edge preservation than wavelet transform.

HYBRID FUSION ALGORITHM

The amalgamation of SWT-PCA- Fast Discrete Curvelet Transform Non-Local Means Filter Shrinkage Rule (FDCTNLMSR) to the fusion of image is described below:

Figure 2. Filter bank coefficients of DWT & SWT

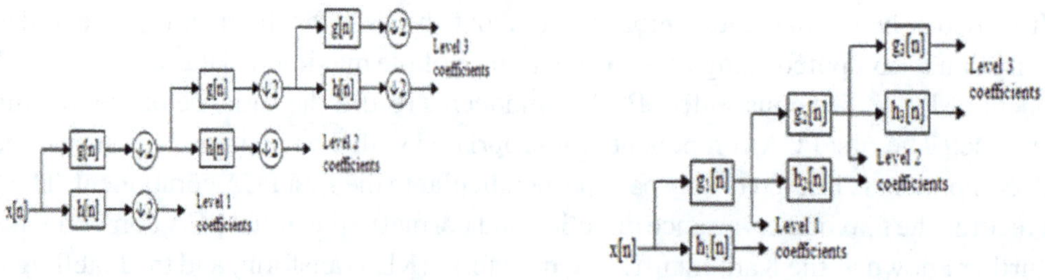

Figure 3. Block diagram of Improved NLM SWT Image Fusion

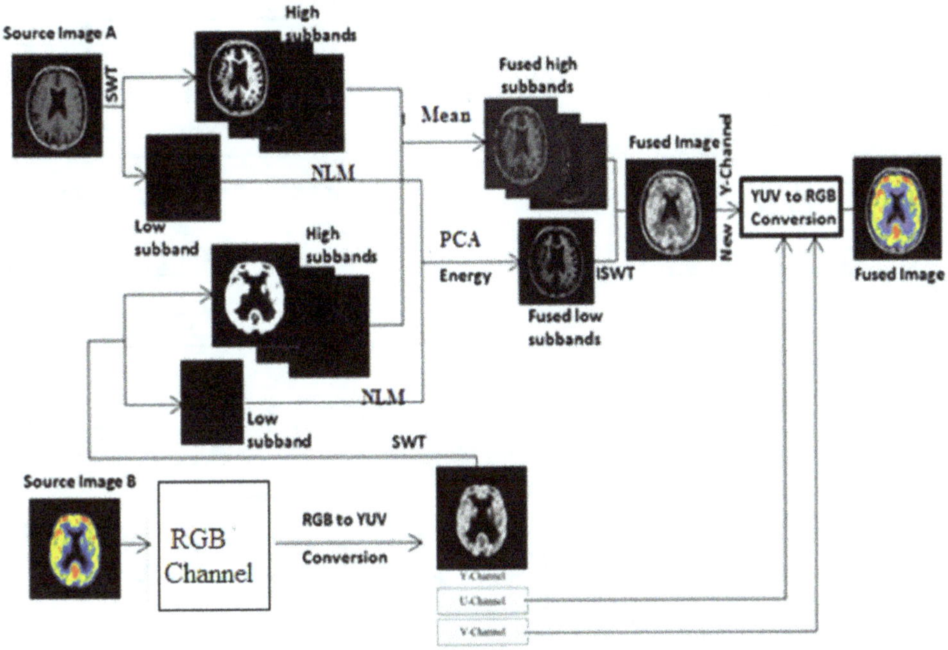

a. The registered MRI T1-T2 brain images consider I1 and I2. Brain images are mapped RGB to gray colors and resize 256×256 dimensions for the reduction of computational cost.
b. SWT algorithm applies to obtain a set of four sub-band coefficients for MRI images. Approximations are first frequency band coefficients.
c. In first sub-band coefficients, Fast Discrete CT (FDCT) wrapping transformation is applied to obtain curvelet descriptors of all scaled coefficients.
d. PCA fusion rule uses to combine the coefficients.
e. Sets of frequency bands are regenerated by inverse FDCT wrapping coefficients.
f. From step (b), to select horizontal and vertical coefficients as second and third frequency band coefficients. The mid frequencies fused by mean fusion rule which preserves the details.
g. From step (b), select diagonal coefficients as the fourth frequency band coefficient.
h. The MAX fusion rule combines the coefficients to get lead spatial-spectral information.

The final fused image F (Figure 4) is reconstructed using inverse SWT with four fused frequency components. The aspect of the fused image assessed using statistical parameters.

IMPROVED SIMILARITY BASED FUZZY C MEANS (FCM) ALGORITHM

The improved similarity-based FCM algorithm flow diagram is shown in Figure 5. In improved similarity-based FCM clustering method is as proceeds:

i) The fuzzy partition matrix (FPM) is initialized.

Figure 4. Improved curvelet self-similarity-based hybrid image fusion

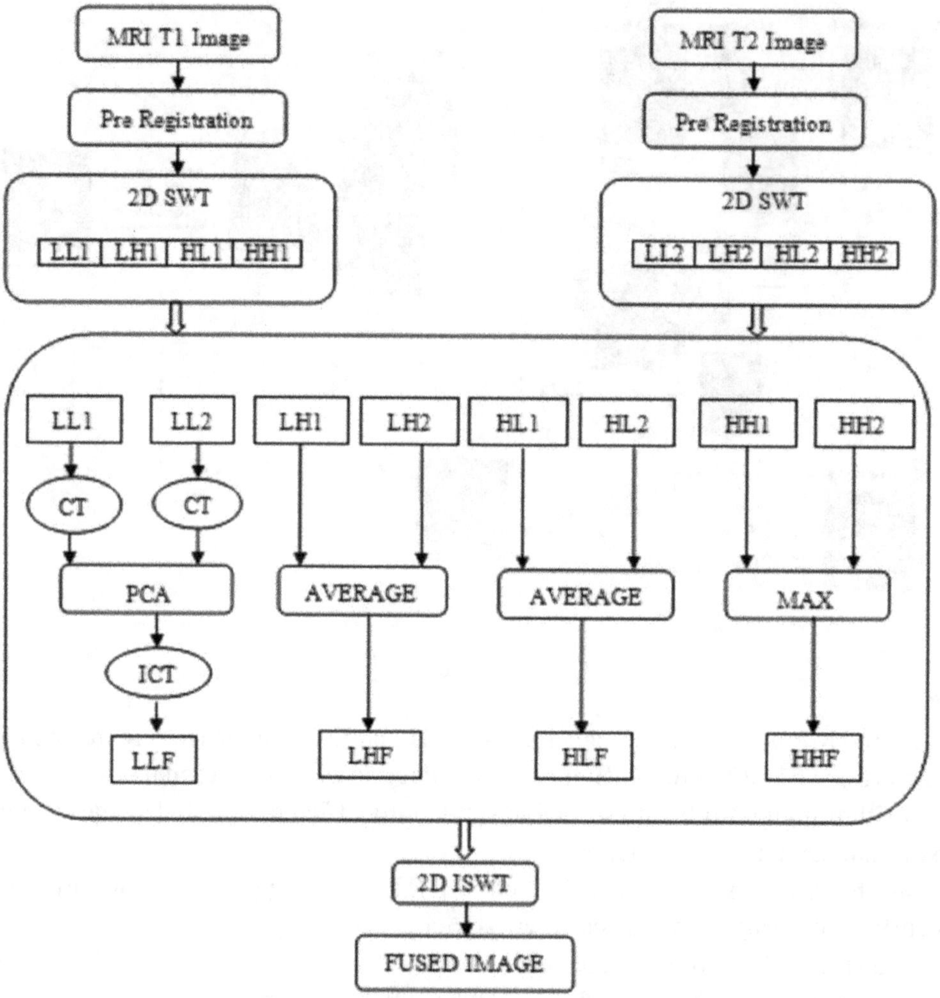

ii) Similarity-based weights are initialized using feature vectors.
iii) The membership function is computed as,

$$M(i,j) = \frac{FPM}{\sum FPM} \tag{5}$$

iv) The center is selected for each cluster which is expressed as,

$$C(i,j) = \frac{M(i,j) * I_f(i,j)}{\sum_{i=0}^{m} \sum_{j=0}^{n} M(i,j)} \tag{6}$$

Distant updates between the center and fused image

$$D_{ij} = \left| I_f(i,j) - C_{ij} \right| \tag{7}$$

v) To achieve the cost function minimum, the iteration process should be continued until the end.

STATISTICAL PERFORMANCE EVALUATION

The evaluations of fusion methods performance are done using the following statistical parameters.

Figure 5. Flow diagram of Improved Similarity measure in FCM based segmentation

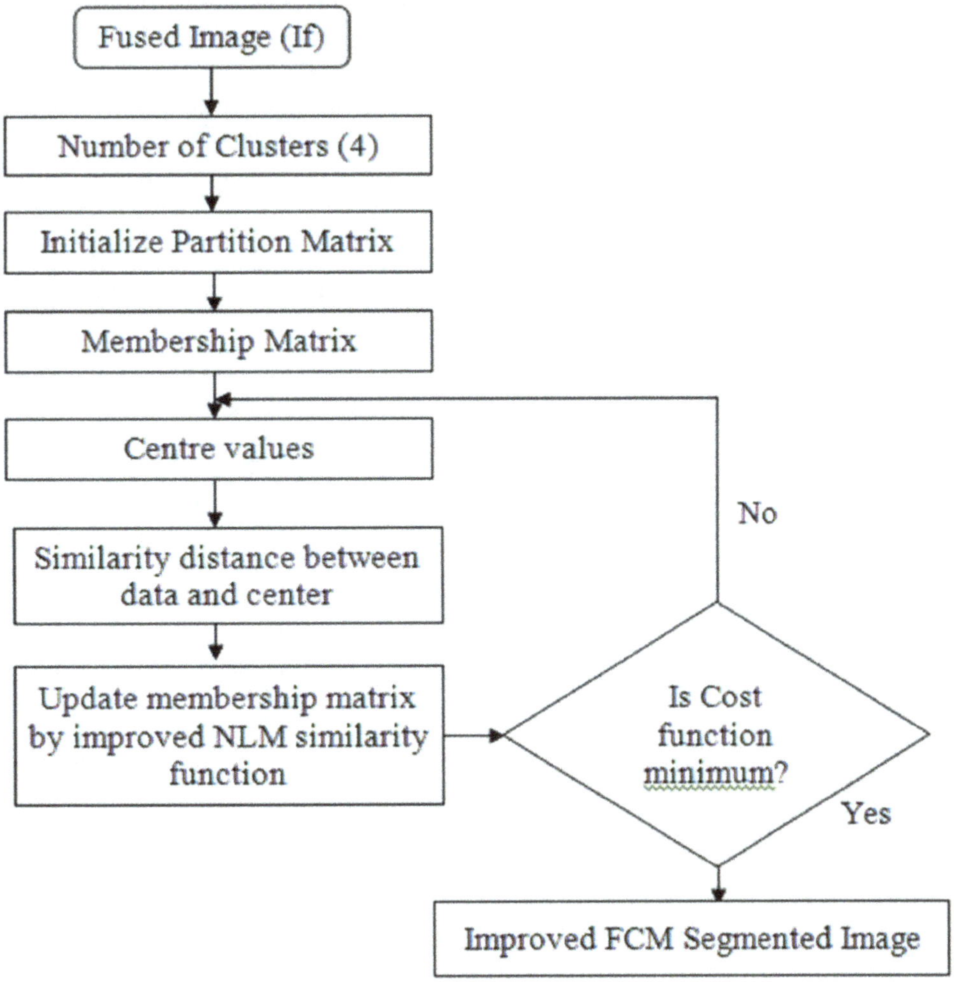

Entropy (EN)

The fused image information content is measured using entropy (Wang &Chang, 2011). If EN value is high, it shows that the fused image information content is more.

$$E_f = \sum_{i=0}^{L} P_{If}(i) \log P_{If}(i) \tag{8}$$

L- Number of gray levels and P_1 - a ratio of the number of pixels with gray value l to the total number of pixels.

The proposed method is applied to the axial brain image from brain slice+83 to -41. This method reduces irrelevant spatial and temporal information and highlighted the significant information shown in Figure 6.

Average Pixel Intensity (API)

The spatial resolution retention is computed using mean analysis (Cao et al., 2003). The fused image mean value is computed by

$$\mu = \frac{1}{MN} \sum_{x,y=0}^{m,n} I_f(x,y) \tag{9}$$

M, N is the image size

Since the obtained mean value is high as shown in Figure 7, the image obtains higher resolution.

Figure 6. Performance analysis of EN

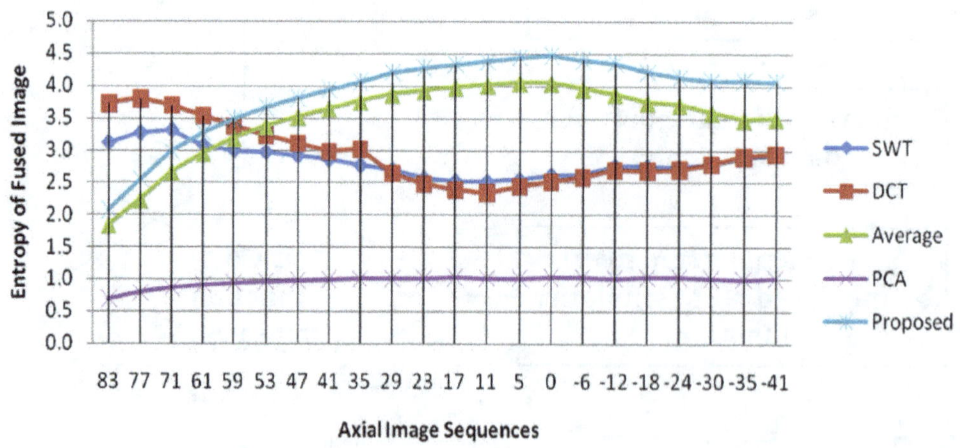

Figure 7. Performance analysis of Average Pixel Intensity

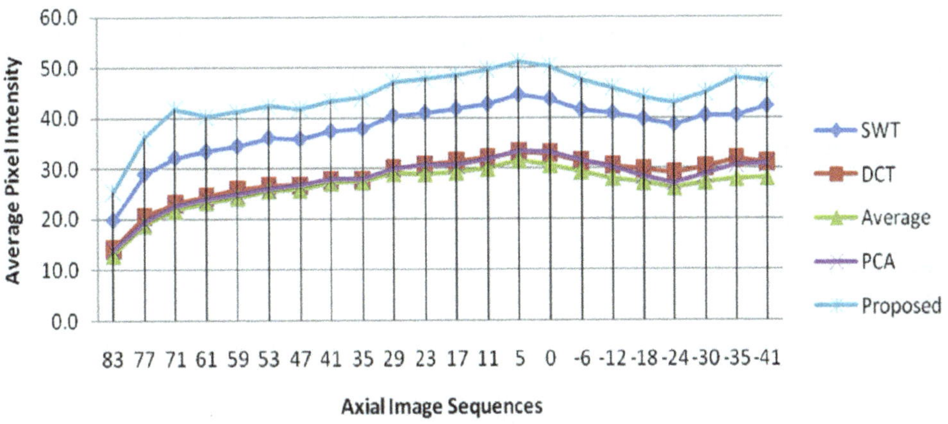

Standard Deviation (SD)

The fused image overall contrast is computed using SD.

$$\sigma = \sqrt{\frac{1}{MN}\sum_{x=1}^{m}\sum_{y=1}^{n}(I_f(x,y)-\mu)^2} \tag{10}$$

where μ is the mean

The fused image quality is correlated with the SD values and also more features extraction.

The improved curvelet based self-similarity method is applied to hybrid image fusion which identifies the high contrast of fused MRI T1-T2 by high standard deviation as shown in Figure 8.

Figure 8. Performance analysis of Standard Deviation

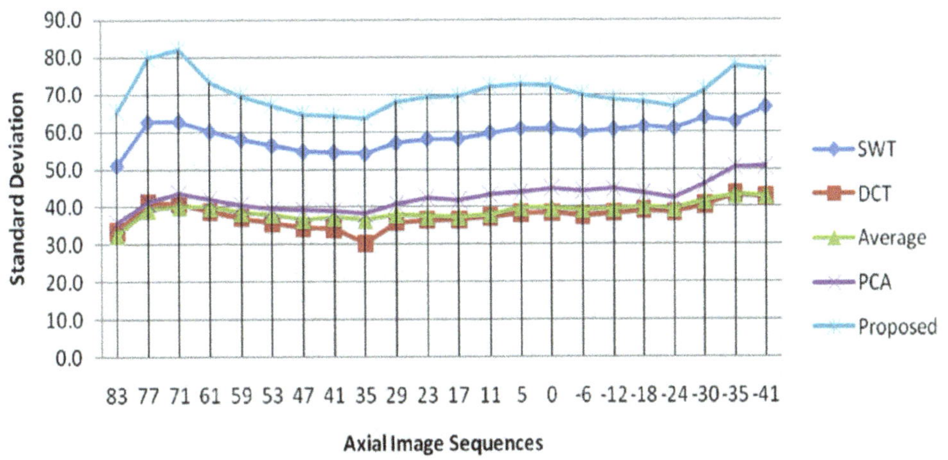

Correlation Coefficient (CC)

The proximity of the fused image with the actual image is computed using CC. CC varies between -1 and +1 while the highly similar images are indicated to the values close to +1 while the highly dissimilar images are indicated close to -1.

The CC is expressed as

$$CC = \frac{\sum_{x,y}(I_1(x,y)-\mu_1)(I_2(x,y)-\mu_2)}{\sqrt{\sum_{x,y}(I_1(x,y)-\mu_1)^2\sum_{x,y}(I_2(x,y)-\mu_2)^2}} \tag{11}$$

Where μ_1 μ_2 are mean of MRI T1and T2 Images

Edge Similarity Measure

It is mainly for a subjective score, Edge Similarity measure is expressed as

$$Q^{I_1I_2/F} = \frac{\sum_{x=1}^{M}\sum_{y=1}^{N}[Q^{I_1F}(x,y)w^1(x,y)+Q^{I_2F}(x,y)w^2(x,y)]}{\sum_{x=1}^{M}\sum_{y=1}^{N}[w^1(x,y)+w^2(x,y)]} \tag{12}$$

where $Q^{I_1F}(x,y)$ and $Q^{I_2F}(x,y)$ are edge preservations and weighted by $w^1(x,y)$ and $w^2(x,y)$.

RESULTS AND DISCUSSION

The fusion process for the multimodal image is implemented utilizing MRI T1-T2 2D axial images from a 3D volume and those images are shown in Figure 11. The MRI T1-T2 is preprocessed by NLM Filter

Figure 9. Performance analysis of CC

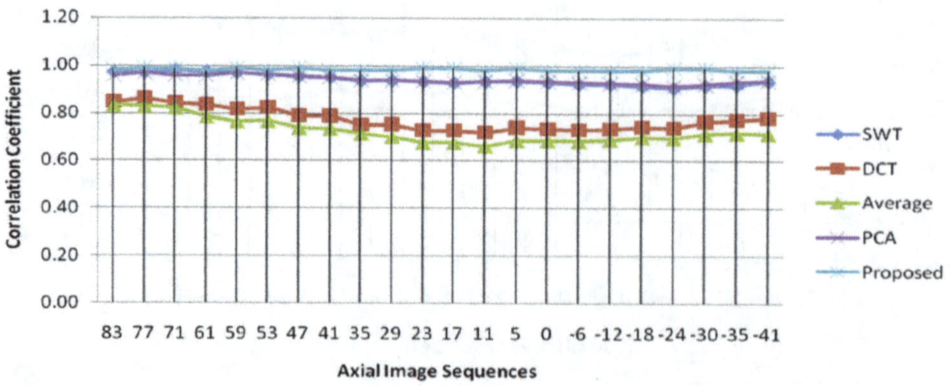

Figure 10. Performance analysis of Edge-based similarity

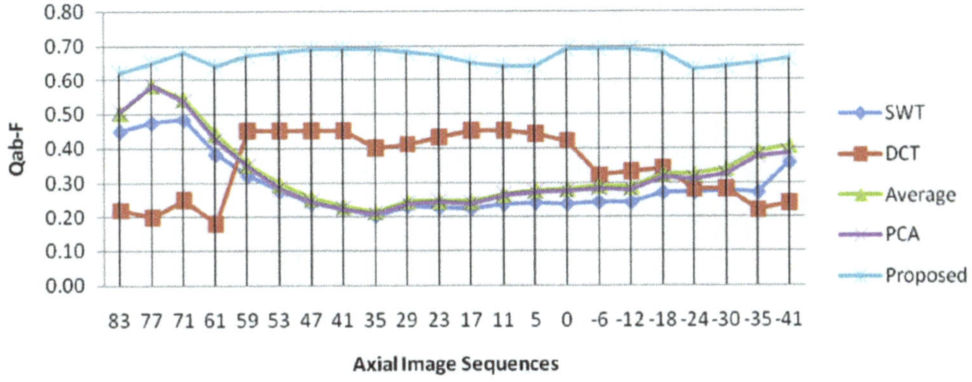

and resized by 256×256. The 2D SWT is applied to preprocessed MRI T1 & T2 images, the 2D SWT coefficients as approximation, and horizontal, vertical and diagonal details of brain sequences.

The approximation coefficient of MRI T1 and MRI T2 suffers from line discontinuities which are overcome by improved FDCT. The curvelet coefficients with different directions are fused by the Principal Component Analysis (PCA) for improving low-frequency information. It has highlighted the similarities and differences of the MRI T1-T2 easily, a powerful tool to analyze data.

The Horizontal and vertical components are fused by using the average fusion rule. The maximum fusion rule is used to fuse details for retaining the maximum intensity of high-frequency information. The input MRI T1&T2 and fused image outputs are shown in Figure 11.

This research work provides a better brain image feature extraction. Using the comparative analysis of different fusion techniques, the proposed improved curvelet based NLM is applied in the hybrid image fusion method which provides improved results both visually and statistically.

Figure 11. Results for MRI T1-T2 image fusion using SWT-FDCT-PCA

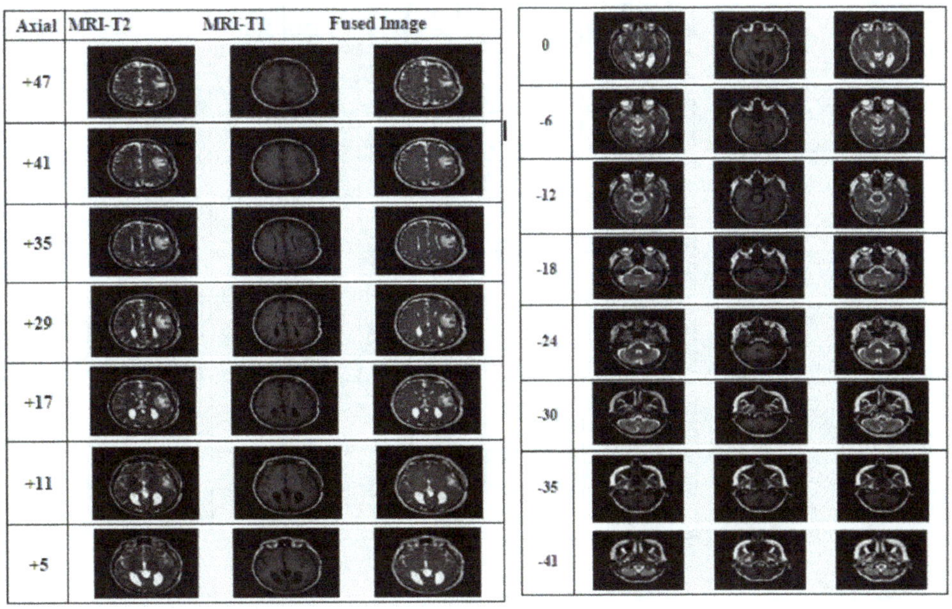

Table 1. Comparative Evaluation of Entropy, Standard Deviation and Average Pixel Intensity in Different Types of image Fusion Rules

Axial Sequences	Entropy of Fused Image					Standard Deviation					Average Pixel Intensity				
	SWT (Nowak R 1999)	DCT ((Jianwei Ma 2010)	AVERAGE (Hu *et al.* 2017)	PCA (Hu *et al.* 2017)	SWT+FDCT+PCA (Proposed)	SWT (Nowak R 1999)	DCT ((Jianwei Ma 2010)	AVERAGE (Hu *et al.* 2017)	PCA (Hu *et al.* 2017)	SWT+FDCT+PCA (Proposed)	SWT (Nowak R 1999)	DCT ((Jianwei Ma 2010)	AVERAGE (Hu *et al.* 2017)	PCA (Hu *et al.* 2017)	SWT+FDCT+PCA (Proposed)
47	2.9	3.1	3.5	1.0	3.8	54.5	34.2	36.4	39.0	64.5	35.8	26.6	25.8	26.8	41.8
41	2.8	3.0	3.6	1.0	3.9	54.2	34.0	36.9	38.7	64.1	37.3	27.6	27.2	27.9	43.4
35	2.8	3.0	3.8	1.0	4.1	53.9	30.1	36.3	38.1	63.6	37.8	27.7	27.4	28.0	44.1
29	2.7	2.6	3.9	1.0	4.2	56.8	35.6	37.7	40.6	67.9	40.3	30.1	29.0	30.0	47.0
23	2.6	2.5	3.9	1.0	4.3	57.8	36.3	37.2	42.1	69.1	40.9	30.7	28.9	30.7	47.6
17	2.5	2.4	4.0	1.0	4.3	57.9	36.4	37.0	41.5	69.4	41.7	31.3	29.3	30.6	48.4
11	2.5	2.3	4.0	1.0	4.4	59.5	37.1	37.7	43.0	72.0	42.6	31.9	29.9	31.8	49.5
5	2.5	2.4	4.0	1.0	4.4	60.5	38.1	39.5	43.7	72.7	44.5	33.2	31.6	33.5	51.1
0	2.6	2.5	4.0	1.0	4.5	60.7	38.3	39.4	44.8	72.1	43.7	32.9	30.7	33.2	50.2
-6	2.6	2.6	4.0	1.0	4.4	59.7	37.5	39.0	44.1	69.9	41.6	31.2	29.3	31.5	47.6
-12	2.7	2.7	3.9	1.0	4.4	60.4	38.2	39.2	44.5	68.6	40.8	30.5	28.0	30.2	45.8
-18	2.7	2.7	3.7	1.0	4.2	61.1	38.8	39.9	43.5	67.9	39.7	29.8	27.2	28.5	44.1
-24	2.7	2.7	3.7	1.0	4.1	60.6	38.2	39.2	42.2	66.7	38.6	29.1	26.1	27.1	42.8
-30	2.8	2.8	3.6	1.0	4.1	63.5	40.2	41.3	46.0	71.1	40.4	30.2	27.3	28.8	45.0
-35	2.9	2.9	3.5	1.0	4.1	62.4	43.2	42.9	50.5	77.5	40.4	31.8	27.9	30.7	48.0
-41	2.9	2.9	3.5	1.0	4.1	66.3	42.4	42.7	50.6	76.6	42.3	31.1	28.1	30.8	47.3

Table 2. Comparative Evaluation of Correlation coefficient and Edge Similarity measure in Different Types of image Fusion Rules

Axial Sequences	Correlation Coefficient					Edge Similarity Measure				
Chapter 1	SWT Chapter 1	DCT Chapter 2	AVERAGE Chapter 3	PCA Chapter 4	SWT+FDCT+PCA Chapter 5	SWT Chapter 6	DCT Chapter 7	AVERAGE Chapter 8	PCA Chapter 9	SWT+FDCT+PCA Chapter 10
47	0.95	0.79	0.74	0.95	0.99	0.24	0.45	0.25	0.24	0.69
41	0.95	0.79	0.74	0.95	0.98	0.22	0.45	0.23	0.22	0.69
35	0.94	0.75	0.71	0.94	0.98	0.20	0.40	0.21	0.21	0.69
29	0.94	0.75	0.70	0.94	0.98	0.23	0.41	0.25	0.24	0.68
23	0.93	0.73	0.67	0.94	0.99	0.23	0.43	0.25	0.24	0.67
17	0.93	0.73	0.68	0.93	0.99	0.22	0.45	0.24	0.24	0.65
11	0.93	0.72	0.66	0.94	0.98	0.24	0.45	0.26	0.26	0.64
5	0.94	0.74	0.68	0.94	0.99	0.24	0.44	0.28	0.27	0.64
0	0.93	0.73	0.69	0.94	0.98	0.24	0.42	0.28	0.27	0.69
-6	0.92	0.73	0.68	0.93	0.98	0.24	0.32	0.29	0.28	0.69
-12	0.92	0.74	0.69	0.93	0.98	0.24	0.33	0.29	0.28	0.69
-18	0.92	0.74	0.70	0.92	0.98	0.27	0.34	0.32	0.32	0.68
-24	0.91	0.74	0.69	0.92	0.99	0.27	0.28	0.32	0.31	0.63
-30	0.92	0.77	0.71	0.93	0.99	0.28	0.28	0.34	0.32	0.64
-35	0.92	0.77	0.72	0.94	0.98	0.27	0.22	0.39	0.38	0.65
-41	0.94	0.78	0.71	0.94	0.98	0.36	0.24	0.41	0.38	0.66

The entropy of the NLM method is higher while comparing with other methods (Table 1). The optimal entropy is obtained in axial slice 41and visually identified the abnormality. The standard deviation between anatomical MRI T1 and fused image extracts more brain spatial information. The mean value of all intensity leads to the average pixel intensity. The abnormality is caused by the mid-range of mean intensity values. From Table 2, the correlation coefficient of the proposed method reaches 0.99 that shows the positive way of diagnosing and identification of abnormality. The edge similarity value is evaluated as 0.69 which is depicted that more edges preserved from the proposed methodology.

The approximation detail coefficients are analyzed using the PCA fused rule; the horizontal and vertical detail coefficients are analyzed using the average fused and the diagonal detail coefficients are analyzed using the maximum fused rule. The coefficients are composed using the inverse SWT. The proposed method provides increased entropy, standard deviation, average pixel intensity, correlation coefficient and edge similarity measure for the fused image shown in Tables 5.1 and 5.2.

The experiments were carried out with 50 normal and 100 abnormal subjects with neurodegenerative symptoms (Age group of 20-70 years) due to alcoholic history. The MRI images were obtained from the radiology department, Stanley medical college. Reference MRI images of individuals used in this study received from Allen Brain Atlas shown in Table 3.

Brain specimens of case number 1015 showed histopathology as a moderate quantity of hemosiderin-laden macrophages identified in Virchow-robin spaces in cerebral lobes. Brain specimens of case numbers 1009 and 2001 had normal and abnormal micro neuropathology and were taken as controls for this study. The MRI image is 2D function denoted as s(i,j). Different biomarker gene-based localization of brain imaging should be assessed in the number of patients for image development. Image registration and analysis tools are applied to the reliability of the image. The maximum value to signal to noise ratio is reduced due to the medical image integrated noise effect and the value of root means square error increases. The proposed curvet and wavelet-based transform filtering exhibit better results over the wavelet-based method. The results have proved that the new method removes the noises efficiently, increases the enhancement factor of image and considerably reduces the noise level.

Table 3. MRI Image references used in this study

Case	Age (Years)	Clinical History	Neuro micro pathology
1009	57	Atherosclerosis	AD
2001	24	Asthma	Normal

Figure 12. Proposed DCTNLMSR Fuzzy C Means Clustering

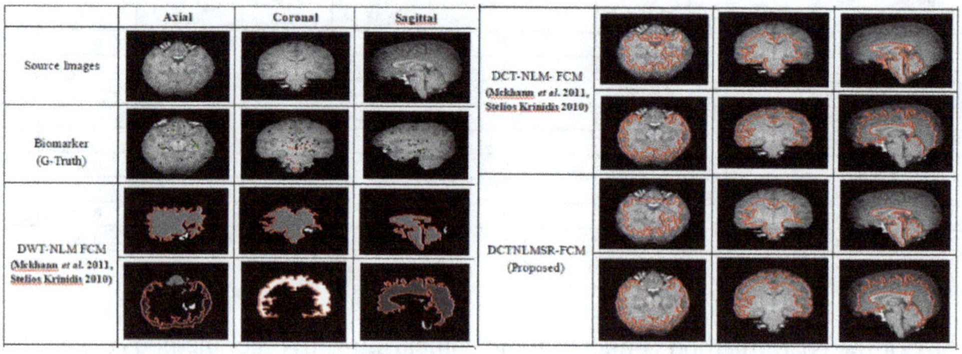

The multimodality fusion of different types of images such as MRI and CT are also possible by this analysis for better interpretation. Microarray gene expression specified sites were taken as MRI images in brain explorer from Allen brain atlas data. These images were analyzed using a discrete curve transform for AD localization. Imaging standardization using these large numbers of data based on gene expression sites will be helpful for the development of simple, reliable imaging techniques using DCT which in turn useful in early AD diagnosis and treatment shown in Figure 12.

SUMMARY

In this chapter, the proposed improved curvelet based NLM applies to hybrid image fusion and FCM clustering. The proposed hybrid image fusion reduces redundancies, enhances better visual perception and feature extraction. The proposed hybrid image fusion retains brain patterns; the brain image feature extraction is mainly useful for accurate disease diagnosis.

REFERENCES

Algorri, M. E., & Mangas, F. F. (2004). Classification of Anatomical Structures in MR Brain Images using Fuzzy parameters. *IEEE Transactions on Biomedical Engineering*, *51*(9), 1892–1894. doi:10.1109/TBME.2004.827532 PMID:15376508

Anbumozhi, S., & Manoharan, P. S. (2014). Performance Analysis of Medical Image Fusion Using Multimodal Graph Cut Algorithm. *International Journal of Advanced Research in Computer Engineering & Technology*, *3*(3), 802–807.

Arathi, T., & Parameswaran, L. (2013). An image fusion technique using Slantlet transform and phase congruency for MRI/CT. *International Journal of Biomedical Engineering and Technology*, *13*(1), 160–164. doi:10.1504/IJBET.2013.057715

Babu, G., & Sivakumar, R. (2017). Comparative Analysis of MRI-PET Brain Image Fusion Using Discrete Wavelet Transform. In *Proceedings of the 2017 Proceedings of the International Conference on Graphics and Signal Processing ICGSP '17* (pp. 48-54). Academic Press.

Barillot, C., & Lemine, D. (1993). Data fusion in medical imaging: Merging multimodal and multipatient images, identification of structures and 3D display aspects. *European Journal of Radiology*, *17*(1), 22–27. doi:10.1016/0720-048X(93)90024-H PMID:8348908

Bhateja, V., Krishn, A., Patel, H., & Sahu, A. (2015). Medical Image Fusion in Wavelet and Ridgelet Domains: A Comparative Evaluation. *International Journal of Rough Sets and Data Analysis*, *2*(2), 78–91. doi:10.4018/IJRSDA.2015070105

Borsdorf, A., Raupach, R., Flohr, T., & Hornegger, J. (2008). Wavelet-based Noise Reduction in CT- Images using Correlation Analysis. *IEEE Transactions on Medical Imaging*, *1*(1), 1–20. PMID:19033085

Buades, A., Coll, B., & Morel, J.-M. (2011). Non-Local Means Denoising. *Image Processing On Line*, *1*(1), 208–212.

Chang, S., & Yu, B. (2000). Adaptive wavelet thresholding for image denoising and compression. *IEEE Transactions on Image Processing*, *9*(9), 1532–1546. doi:10.1109/83.862633 PMID:18262991

Coatelen, J., & Qin, Y. (2011). *Image Registration on GPU*. University of Blaise Pascal-CSIRO.

Cootes, T. F., Taylor, C. J., Cooper, D. H., & Graham, J. (1992). Training models of shape from sets of examples. In *Proceedings of the British Machine Vision Conference* (pp. 9-18). Springer. 10.5244/C.6.2

Das, S., & Kundu, M. K. (2013). A Neuro-Fuzzy Approach for Medical Image Fusion. *IEEE Transactions on Biomedical Engineering*, *60*(12), 3347–3353. doi:10.1109/TBME.2013.2282461 PMID:24058012

Dwith, C. Y. N., Angoth, V., & Singh, A. (2013). Wavelet-Based Image Fusion for Detection of Brain Tumor. *I.J. Image. Graphics and Signal Processing*, *1*(1), 25–31. doi:10.5815/ijigsp.2013.01.04

El-Gamal, F. E.-Z. A., Elmogy, M., & Atwan, A. (2016). Current trends in medical image registration and fusion. *Egyptian Information Journal*, *17*(1), 99–124. doi:10.1016/j.eij.2015.09.002

Ferris, S., De Leon, M. J., Wolf, A. P., Farkas, T., Christman, D. R., Reisberg, B., ... Rampal, S. (1980). Positron emission tomography in the study of aging and senile dementia. *Neurobiology of Aging*, *1*(2), 127–131. doi:10.1016/0197-4580(80)90005-6 PMID:24279935

Friston, K. Ash bumer, J., Kiebel, S. J., Nichols, T. E., & Penny, W. D. (2007). Statistical Parameter Mapping: The Analysis of Functional Brain Images. Academic Press.

Ganasala, P., & Kumar, V. (2014). CT and MR image fusion scheme in nonsubsampled contourlet transform domain. *Journal of Digital Imaging*, *27*(1), 407–418. doi:10.100710278-013-9664-x PMID:24474580

Goshtasby, A. A. (2005). *2D and 3D image registration for medical, remote sensing and industrial applications*. Wiley.

Gudjartsson, H., & Patz, S. (1995). The rician distribution of noisy MRI data. *Magnetic Resonance in Medicine*, *34*(6), 910–914. doi:10.1002/mrm.1910340618 PMID:8598820

Hill, P., Achim, A., Al-Mualla, M. E., & Bull, D. (2016). Contrast Sensitivity of the Wavelet, Dual-Tree Complex Wavelet, Curvelet, and Steerable Pyramid Transforms. *IEEE Transactions on Image Processing*, *25*(6), 2739–2751. doi:10.1109/TIP.2016.2552725 PMID:27093623

Hou, Y., Dan, X., Babbar, M., Wei, Y., Hasselbalch, S. G., Croteau, D. L., & Bohr, V. A. (2019). Ageing as a risk factor for neurodegenerative disease. *Nature Reviews. Neurology*, *15*(10), 565–581. doi:10.103841582-019-0244-7 PMID:31501588

Katzman, R., Brown, T., Thal, L. J., Fuld, P. A., Aronson, M., Butters, N., ... Terry, R. D. (1988). Comparison of Rate of Annual Change of Mental Status Score in Four Independent Studies of Patients with Alzheimer's Disease. *Annals of Neurology*, *24*(3), 384–389. doi:10.1002/ana.410240306 PMID:3228273

Kirankumar, Y., & Shenbaga Devi, S. (2007). Transform-based medical image fusion'. *International Journal of Biomedical Engineering and Technology*, *1*(1), 101–110. doi:10.1504/IJBET.2007.014140

Krinidis, S., & Chatzis, V. (2010). A Robust Fuzzy Local Information C Means Clustering Algorithm. *IEEE Transactions on Image Processing*, *19*(5), 1057–1071. doi:10.1109/TIP.2010.2040763 PMID:20089475

Krishnamoorthy, S., & Soman, K. P. (2010). Implementations and Comparative study of image fusion algorithms. *International Journal of Computers and Applications*, *9*(2), 25–35. doi:10.5120/1357-1832

Li, H., Manjunath, B. S., & Mitra, S. K. (1995). Multisensor image fusion using the wavelet transform. *Graphical Models and Image Processing*, *57*(1), 235–245. doi:10.1006/gmip.1995.1022

Li, S., Yang, B., & Hu, J. (2011). Performance comparison of different multi-resolution transform for image fusion. *Journal Information Fusion*, *12*(2), 74–84. doi:10.1016/j.inffus.2010.03.002

Liu, Z., Yin, H., Chai, Y., & Yang, S. X. (2014). A novel approach for multimodal medical image fusion. *Expert Systems with Applications*, *41*(16), 7425–7435. doi:10.1016/j.eswa.2014.05.043

Bashiri, F. S., Baghaie, A., Rostami, R., Yu, Z., & D'Souza, R. M. (2019). Multi-Modal Medical Image Registration with Full or Partial Data: A Manifold Learning Approach. *Journal of Imaging*, *5*(5). doi:10.3390/jimaging5010005

Mzoughi, H., Njeh, I., Ben Slima, M., Ben Hamida, A., Mhiri, C., & Ben Mahfoudh, K. (2019). Denoising and contrast-enhancement approach of magnetic resonance imaging glioblastoma brain tumors. *Journal of Medical Imaging (Bellingham, Wash.)*, *6*(4), 044002. doi:10.1117/1.JMI.6.4.044002 PMID:31620548

Nygard, L. (2003). Instrumental Activities of Daily Living: A Stepping-Stone Towards Alzheimer's Disease Diagnosis in subjects with Mild Cognitive Impairment. *Acta Neurologica Scandinavica*, *179*(s179), 42–46. doi:10.1034/j.1600-0404.107.s179.8.x PMID:12603250

Padmavathi, K., Asha, C. S., & Maya, V. K. (2019). A novel medical image fusion by combining TV-L1 decomposed textures based on adaptive weighting scheme. *Engineering Science and Technology, an International Journal*. doi:10.1016/j.jestch.2019.03.008

Peter, A. (1998). MR Image Texture analysis applied to the diagnosis and tracking of Alzheimer's Disease. *IEEE Transactions on Medical Imaging*, *17*(3), 475–478. doi:10.1109/42.712137 PMID:9735911

Petersen, R. C. (2004). Mild cognitive impairment as a diagnostic entity. *Journal of Internal Medicine*, *256*(3), 183–194. doi:10.1111/j.1365-2796.2004.01388.x PMID:15324362

Piao, J., Chen, Y., & Shin, H. (2019). A New Deep Learning-Based Multi-Spectral Image Fusion Method. *Entropy (Basel, Switzerland)*, *21*(570). doi:10.3390/e21060570

Pritika, S. B., & Budhiraja, S. (2016). Multimodal medical image fusion based on guided filtered multiscale decomposition. *International Journal of Biomedical Engineering and Technology*, *20*(4), 285–301. doi:10.1504/IJBET.2016.076604

Sivakumar, R. (2007). Denoising of Computer Tomography Images using Curvelet Transform. *Journal of Engineering and Applied Sciences (Asian Research Publishing Network)*, *2*(1), 21–27.

Srivastava, R., Prakash, O., & Khare, A. (2016). Local energy-based multimodal medical image fusion in curvelet domain. *IET Computer Vision*, *10*(6), 513–527. doi:10.1049/iet-cvi.2015.0251

Valdimir, S. (2004). Gradient-based multiresolution Image Fusion. *IEEE Transactions on Image Processing*, *13*(2), 228–237. doi:10.1109/TIP.2004.823821 PMID:15376943

Wadhwa, A., Bhardwaj, A., & Verma, V. S. (2019). Review on brain tumor segmentation of MRI images. *Magnetic Resonance Imaging*, *61*, 247–259. doi:10.1016/j.mri.2019.05.043 PMID:31200024

Yang, B., Zing, Z. L., & Zhao, H. (2010). Review of Pixel Level Image Fusion. *Journal of Shanghai Jiao tong University*, *15*(1), 6-12.

Yang, Y., Tong, S., Huang, S., Lin, P., & Fang, Y. (2017). A Hybrid Method for Multi-focus Image Fusion Based on Fast Discrete Curvelet Transform. *IEEE Access*, *5*, 14898–14913. doi:10.1109/ACCESS.2017.2698217

Zhang, W., Huang, T., & Chen, J. (2019). A Robust Bias-Correction Fuzzy Weighted C-Ordered-Means Clustering Algorithm. *Mathematical Problems in Engineering*. doi:10.1155/2019/5984649

Compilation of References

Abadi, M., Chu, A., Goodfellow, I., McMahan, H. B., Mironov, I., Talwar, K., & Zhang, L. (2016). Deep Learning with Differential Privacy. In *Proceedings of the 2016 ACM SIGSAC Conference on Computer and Communications Security* (pp. 308–318). ACM. 10.1145/2976749.2978318

Abiyev, R. H. & Ma'aitah, M. K.S. (2018). Deep Convolutional Neural Networks for Chest Diseases Detection. *Journal of Healthcare Engineering.*

Acharya, U. R., Oh, S. L., Hagiwara, Y., Tan, J. H., & Adeli, H. (2017). Deep convolutional neural network for the automated detection and diagnosis of seizure using EEG signals. *Computers in Biology and Medicine*. doi:10.1016/j.comp-Biomed.2017.09.017 PMID:28974302

Agarwal, S. P., Goel, D. S., Ichhpujani, R. L., Salhan, R. N., & Shrivastava, S. (1946). *Mental Health An Indian Perspective Directorate General of Health Services Ministry of Health and Family Welfare New Delhi*. Retrieved from https://s3.amazonaws.com/academia.edu.documents/38096568/MENTAL_HEALTH_-INDIA.pdf?AWSAccessKeyId=AKIAIWOWYYGZ2Y53UL3A&Expires=1557355752&Signature=gmg4Gum%2Fh5cENamksdHfPZpuii8%3D&response-content-disposition=inline%3Bfilename%3DPostgraduate_psychiatric_

Agnes, G., Venet, O., Gernot, B., Jose, C., Stefan, O., Oscar, M., ... Paul, L. (2014). Using smart phone mobility traces for the diagnosis of depressive and manic episodes in bipolar patients. In *Proceedings of the 5th Augmented Human International Conference*. ACM. doi:10.1145/2582051.2582089

Aharony, N., Pan, W., Ip, C., Khayal, I., & Pentland, A. (2011). Social fMRI: Investigating and shaping social mechanisms in the real world. *Pervasive and Mobile Computing*, *7*(6), 643–659. doi:10.1016/j.pmcj.2011.09.004

Aitor, A., & Gorka, A. (2018). Predicting human behavior with recurrent neural networks. *Applied Sciences Journal*, *8*(2), 305. doi:10.3390/app8020305

Alba, M. (2017). How the Internet of Things is Changing Product Lifecycle Management"

Algorri, M. E., & Mangas, F. F. (2004). Classification of Anatomical Structures in MR Brain Images using Fuzzy parameters. *IEEE Transactions on Biomedical Engineering*, *51*(9), 1892–1894. doi:10.1109/TBME.2004.827532 PMID:15376508

Aljarah, I., Faris, H., & Mirjalili, S. (2018). Optimizing connection weights in neural networks using the whale optimization algorithm. *Soft Computing*, *22*(1), 1–15.

Allen, C., Tsou, M., Aslam, A., Nagel, A., & Gawron, J. (2016). Applying GIS and Machine Learning Methods to Twitter Data for Multiscale Surveillance of Influenza. *PLoS One*, *11*(7), e0157734. doi:10.1371/journal.pone.0157734 PMID:27455108

Alshammari, T., Alshammari, N., & Sedky, M. (2018). Evaluating machine learning techniques for activity classification in smart home environments. *International Journal of Information and Communication Engineering*, *12*, 2.

Al-Shayea, Q. K. (2011). Artificial neural networks in medical diagnosis. *International Journal of Computer Science Issues*, *8*(2), 150–154.

Amato, F., López, A., Peña-Méndez, E. M., Vaňhara, P., Hampl, A., & Havel, J. (2013). Artificial neural networks in medical diagnosis.

Amato, F., López, A., Pena-Méndez, E. M., Vanhara, P., Hampl, A., & Havel, J. (2013). Artificial neural networks in medical diagnosis. *Journal of Applied Biomedicine*, *11*(2), 47–58. doi:10.2478/v10136-012-0031-x

American Society for Testing and Materials (ASTM). (1991). Standard Guide for Description for Content and Structure of an automatic Primary Record of Care. Standard E, 1384-91.

Analytic Insight. (n.d.). Advancing healthcare industry robotic process automation. Retrieved from https://www.analyticsinsight.net/advancing-healthcare-industry-robotic-process-automation/

Anbumozhi, S., & Manoharan, P. S. (2014). Performance Analysis of Medical Image Fusion Using Multimodal Graph Cut Algorithm. *International Journal of Advanced Research in Computer Engineering & Technology*, *3*(3), 802–807.

Arathi, T., & Parameswaran, L. (2013). An image fusion technique using Slantlet transform and phase congruency for MRI/CT. *International Journal of Biomedical Engineering and Technology*, *13*(1), 160–164. doi:10.1504/IJBET.2013.057715

Auffray, C., Balling, R., Barroso, I., Bencze, L., Benson, M., Bergeron, J., ... Zanetti, G. (2016). Making sense of big data in health research: Towards an EU action plan. *Genome Medicine*, *8*(1), 71. doi:10.118613073-016-0323-y PMID:27338147

Augmented Mental Health. (n.d.). Retrieved from https://www.augmentedmentalhealth.com/

Awais, M., Chiari, L., Ihlen, E. A. F., Helbostad, J., & Palmerini, L. (2019). Physical activity classification for elderly people in free-living conditions. *IEEE Journal of Biomedical and Health Informatics*, *23*(1), 197–207. doi:10.1109/JBHI.2018.2820179 PMID:29994291

Babu, G., & Sivakumar, R. (2017). Comparative Analysis of MRI-PET Brain Image Fusion Using Discrete Wavelet Transform. In *Proceedings of the 2017 Proceedings of the International Conference on Graphics and Signal Processing ICGSP '17* (pp. 48-54). Academic Press.

Babu, G. S., Zhao, P., & Li, X. L. (2016, April). Deep convolutional neural network based regression approach for estimation of remaining useful life. In *Proceedings of the International conference on database systems for advanced applications* (pp. 214-228). Springer.

Bachani, D., & Srivastava, R. (2012). Burden of NCDs, Policies and Programme for Prevention and Control of NCDs in India. *Indian Journal of Community Medicine*, *36*(5), 7. doi:10.4103/0970-0218.94703 PMID:22628916

Badawi, O., Brennan, T., Celi, L. A., Feng, M., Ghassemi, M., Ippolito, A., & Moses, C. (2014). Making big data useful for health care: A summary of the inaugural mit critical data conference. *JMIR Medical Informatics*, *2*(2), e22. doi:10.2196/medinform.3447 PMID:25600172

Badjatiya, P., Gupta, S., Gupta, M., & Varma, V. (2017). Deep learning for hate speech detection in tweets. In *Proceedings of the 26th International Conference on World Wide Web Companion* (pp. 759–760). 10.1145/3041021.3054223

Bagheri, M., & Movahed, S. H. (2016). The Effect of the Internet of Things (IoT) on Education Business Model. In *Proceedings of the International Conference on Signal-Image Technology & Internet-Based Systems* (pp. 435-441). IEEE. 10.1109/SITIS.2016.74

Bajor, J. M., & Lasko, T. A. (2016). Predicting medications from diagnostic codes with recurrent neural networks. In *Proceedings of the International Conference on Learning Representations*. Academic Press.

Barillot, C., & Lemine, D. (1993). Data fusion in medical imaging: Merging multimodal and multi-patient images, identification of structures and 3D display aspects. *European Journal of Radiology*, *17*(1), 22–27. doi:10.1016/0720-048X(93)90024-H PMID:8348908

Barnett, G. O. (1984). The application of computer-based medical-record systems in mobile observe. *The New England Journal of Medicine*, *310*(25), 1643–1650. doi:10.1056/NEJM198406213102506 PMID:6427610

Bashiri, F. S., Baghaie, A., Rostami, R., Yu, Z., & D'Souza, R. M. (2019). Multi-Modal Medical Image Registration with Full or Partial Data: A Manifold Learning Approach. *Journal of Imaging*, *5*(5). doi:10.3390/jimaging5010005

Bauer, H., Patel, M., & Veira, J. (2016). The Internet of Things: sizing up the opportunity. McKinsey & Company. Retrieved from http://www.mckinsey.com/industries/hightech/our-insights/the-internet-of-things-sizing-up-theopportunity

Bayani, M., Leiton, K., & Loaiza, M. (2017). Internet of things (IoT) advantages on E-learning in the smart cities. *International Journal of Development Research*, *7*(12), 17747–17753.

Bazi, Y., & Melgani, F. (2006). Towards an optimal SVM classification system for hyperspectral remote sensing images. *IEEE Transactions on Geoscience and Remote Sensing*, *44*(11), 3374–3385. doi:10.1109/TGRS.2006.880628

Belle, A., Thiagarajan, R., Soroushmehr, S. M., Navidi, F., Beard, D. A., & Najarian, K. (2015). Big data analytics in healthcare. *BioMed Research International*. PMID:26229957

Belmaker, R. H. (2004). Bipolar disorder. *The New England Journal of Medicine*, *351*(5), 476–486. doi:10.1056/NEJMra035354 PMID:15282355

Ben-Ari, J., Zimlichman, E., Adi, N., & Sorkine, P. (2010). Contactless respiratory and heart rate monitoring: Validation of an innovative tool. *Journal of Medical Engineering & Technology*, *34*(7-8), 393–398. doi:10.3109/03091902.2010.503308 PMID:20698739

Benson, C. (2016). The internet of things, IoT systems, and higher education. *EDUCAUSE Review*, *51*(4), 6.

Berrouiguet, S., Perez-Rodriguez, M. M., Larsen, M., Baca-García, E., Courtet, P., & Oquendo, M. (2018). From eHealth to iHealth: Transition to participatory and personalized medicine in mental health. *Journal of Medical Internet Research*, *20*(1), 1–8. doi:10.2196/jmir.7412 PMID:29298748

Bhateja, V., Krishn, A., Patel, H., & Sahu, A. (2015). Medical Image Fusion in Wavelet and Ridgelet Domains: A Comparative Evaluation. *International Journal of Rough Sets and Data Analysis*, *2*(2), 78–91. doi:10.4018/IJRSDA.2015070105

Bhatia, D.M. & Mittal, D.M. (2017). Big Data & Deep Data: Minding the Challenges. *Deep Learning for Image Processing Applications*, *31*, 177.

Bhuvaneswari, P., & Therese, A. B. (2015). Detection of cancer in lung with k-nn classification using genetic algorithm. *Procedia Materials Science*, *10*, 433–440. doi:10.1016/j.mspro.2015.06.077

Birla, N. (2019). Mental health in India: 7.5% of country affected; less than 4,000 experts available. The Economic Times. Retrieved from https://economictimes.indiatimes.com/magazines/panache/mental-health-in-india-7-5-of-country-affected-less-than-4000-experts-available/articleshow/71500130.cms?from=mdr

Bloom, D. E., Cafiero, E. T., Jane-Llopis, E., Abrahams-Gessel, S., & Bloom, L.R. (2011). The Global Economic Burden of Non-Communicable Diseases. Geneva, Switzerland: World Economic Forum.

Bodenreider, O. (2004). The Unified Medical Language System (UMLS): Integrating biomedical terminology. *Nucleic Acids Research*, *32*(Database issue), D267–D270. doi:10.1093/nar/gkh061 PMID:14681409

Borsdorf, A., Raupach, R., Flohr, T., & Hornegger, J. (2008). Wavelet-based Noise Reduction in CT- Images using Correlation Analysis. *IEEE Transactions on Medical Imaging*, *1*(1), 1–20. PMID:19033085

Bowden, G. J. (2002). Optimal division of data for neural network models in water resources applications. *Water Recourses*, *38*, 1–11.

Bowonder, B., Bansal, M., & Sharnitha Giridhar, A. (2005). A telemedicine platform: A case study of Apollo hospitals telemedicine project. *International Journal of Services Technology and Management*, *6*(3-5), 449–466. doi:10.1504/IJSTM.2005.007420

Boyi, X., Li Da, X., Hongming, C., Cheng, X., Jingyuan, H., & Fenglin, B. (2014). Ubiquitous Data Accessing Method in IoT-Based Information System for Emergency Medical Services. Industrial Informatics. *IEEE Transactions on*, *10*(2), 1578–1586.

Braun, W., & Menth, M. (2014). Software-defined networking using OpenFlow: Protocols, applications and architectural design choices. *Future Internet*, *6*(2), 302–336. doi:10.3390/fi6020302

Brause, R. W. (2001, October). Medical analysis and diagnosis by neural networks. In *Proceedings of the International Symposium on Medical Data Analysis* (pp. 1-13). Springer. 10.1007/3-540-45497-7_1

Brown, J., Kurichi, J. E., Xie, D., Pan, Q., & Stineman, M. G. (2013). Instrumental activities of daily living staging as a possible clinical tool for falls risk assessment in physical medicine and rehabilitation. *PM & R*, *6*(4), 316–323. doi:10.1016/j.pmrj.2013.10.007 PMID:24140738

Brownlee, J. (2015). Practice Machine Learning with Datasets from the UCI Machine Learning Repository. Machine learning mastery. Retrieved from https://machinelearningmastery.com/practice-machine-learning-with-small-in-memory-datasets-from-the-uci-machine-learning-repository/

Buades, A., Coll, B., & Morel, J.-M. (2011). Non-Local Means Denoising. *Image Processing On Line*, *1*(1), 208–212.

Bychkov, D., Linder, N., Turkki, R., Nordling, S., Kovanen, P. E., Verrill, C., ... Lundin, J. (2018). Deep learning-based tissue analysis predicts outcome in colorectal cancer. *Scientific Reports*, *8*(1), 3395. doi:10.103841598-018-21758-3 PMID:29467373

Canary Health. (n.d.). Retrieved from http://www.canaryhealth.com/

Centers for Disease Control and Prevention. (n.d.). Lifestyle change program details. Retrieved from http://www.cdc.gov/diabetes/prevention/lifestyle-program/experience/index. html

Chandrashekar, P. (2018). Do mental health mobile apps work: Evidence and recommendations for designing high-efficacy mental health mobile apps. *mHealth*, *4*, 6–6. doi:10.21037/mhealth.2018.03.02 PMID:29682510

Chang, H. A., Chang, C. C., Tzeng, N. S., Kuo, T. B. J., Lu, R. B., & Huang, S. Y. (2014). Heart rate variability in unmedicated patients with bipolar disorder in the manic phase. *Psychiatry and Clinical Neurosciences*, *68*(9), 674–682. doi:10.1111/pcn.12178 PMID:24612182

Chang, S., & Yu, B. (2000). Adaptive wavelet thresholding for image denoising and compression. *IEEE Transactions on Image Processing*, *9*(9), 1532–1546. doi:10.1109/83.862633 PMID:18262991

Chan, M., Estève, D., Fourniols, J.-Y., Escriba, C., & Campo, E. (2012). Smart wearable systems: Current status and future challenges. *Artificial Intelligence in Medicine*, *56*(3), 137–156. doi:10.1016/j.artmed.2012.09.003 PMID:23122689

Chan, V., Ray, P., & Parameswaran, N. (2008). Mobile e-Health monitoring: An agent-based approach. *IET Communications*, *2*(2), 223–230. doi:10.1049/iet-com:20060646

Che, C., Xiao, C., Liang, J., Jin, B., Zho, J., & Wang, F. (2017). An RNN architecture with dynamic temporal matching for personalized predictions of Parkinson's disease. In *Proceedings of the 2017 SIAM International Conference on Data Mining* (pp. 198–206). Academic Press. 10.1137/1.9781611974973.23

Chen, M., Ma, Y., Song, J., Lai, C. F., & Hu, B. (2016). Smart clothing: Connecting human with clouds and big data for sustainable health monitoring. *Mobile Networks and Applications*, *21*(5), 825–845. doi:10.100711036-016-0745-1

Chen, X.-W., & Lin, X. (2014). Big data deep learning: Challenges and perspectives. *IEEE Access*, *2*, 514–525. doi:10.1109/ACCESS.2014.2325029

Che, Z., Kale, D., Li, W., Bahadori, M. T., & Yan, L. (2015). Computational Phenotyping. In *Proceedings of the 21st ACM SIGKDD Conference on Knowledge Discovery and Data Mining* (pp. 507-516). ACM Press. 10.1145/2783258.2783365

Choi, E., Bahadori, M. T., Schuetz, A., Stewart, W. F., & Sun, J. (2016). Doctor AI: predict-ing clinical events via recurrent neural networks. In *JMLR Workshop Conference proceedings* (pp. 301-318). Academic Press.

Choi, E., Schuetz, A., Stewart, W., F., & Sun, J., (2016). Medical Concept Representation Learning from Electronic Health Records and its Application on Heart Failure Prediction.

Christophe, A., D'Alché-Buc, F., & Grandvalet, Y. (2001). Semi-supervised margin boost. In Advances in neural information processing systems (pp. 553–560). Academic Press.

Cline, G. (2017). Integrated Product Lifecycle Management in the Era of IoT.

Coatelen, J., & Qin, Y. (2011). *Image Registration on GPU*. University of Blaise Pascal-CSIRO.

Cooper, D. L., Smith, G. E., Regan, M., Large, S., & Groenewegen, P. P. (2008). Tracking the spatial diffusion of influenza and norovirus using telehealth data: A spatiotemporal analysis of syndromic data. *BMC Medicine*, *6*(1), 16. doi:10.1186/1741-7015-6-16 PMID:18582364

Cootes, T. F., Taylor, C. J., Cooper, D. H., & Graham, J. (1992). Training models of shape from sets of examples. In *Proceedings of the British Machine Vision Conference* (pp. 9-18). Springer. 10.5244/C.6.2

Coudray, N., Ocampo, P. S., Sakellaropoulos, T., Narula, N., Snuderl, M., Fenyö, D., ... Tsirigos, A. (2018). Classification and mutation prediction from non–small cell lung cancer histopathology images using deep learning. *Nature Medicine*, *24*(10), 1559–1567. doi:10.103841591-018-0177-5 PMID:30224757

Covell, D. G., & Uman, G. C. (1985). Manning PR Information desires in workplace practice: Are they being met. *Annals of Internal Medicine*, *103*(4), 596–599. doi:10.7326/0003-4819-103-4-596 PMID:4037559

Cruz, J. A., & Wishart, D. S. (2006). Applications of machine learning in cancer prediction and prognosis. *Cancer Informatics*, *2*. doi:10.1177/117693510600200030 PMID:19458758

Cuba-Gyllensten, I., Gastelurrutia, P., Riistama, J., Aarts, R., Nunez, J., Lupon, J., & Bayes-Genis, A. (2014). A novel wearable vest for tracking pulmonary congestion in acutely decompensated heart failure. *International Journal of Cardiology*, *177*(1), 199–201. doi:10.1016/j.ijcard.2014.09.041 PMID:25499378

Cunningham, P., Carney, J., & Jacob, S. (2000). Stability problems with artificial neural networks and the ensemble solution. *Artificial Intelligence in Medicine*, *20*(3), 217–225. doi:10.1016/S0933-3657(00)00065-8 PMID:10998588

Dagon, D., Gu, G., Lee, C. P., & Lee, W. (2007, December). A taxonomy of botnet structures. In *Proceedings of the Twenty-Third Annual Computer Security Applications Conference (ACSAC 2007)* (pp. 325-339). IEEE. 10.1109/ACSAC.2007.44

Dakappa, P. H., Prasad, K., Rao, S. B., Bolumbu, G., Bhat, G. K., & Mahabala, C. (2018). Classification of infectious and noninfectious diseases using artificial neural networks from 24-hour continuous tympanic temperature data of patients with undifferentiated fever. *Critical Reviews in Biomedical Engineering*, *46*(2).

Dandıl, E. (2018). A Computer-Aided Pipeline for Automatic Lung Cancer Classification on Computed Tomography Scans. *Journal of Healthcare Engineering*. PMID:30515286

Daoud, M., & Mayo, M. (2019). A Survey of Neural Network-based Cancer Prediction Models from Microarray Data. *Artificial Intelligence in Medicine*, *97*, 204–214. doi:10.1016/j.artmed.2019.01.006 PMID:30797633

Dargazany, A. R., Stegagno, P., & Mankodiy, K. (2018, November). WearableDL: Wearable Internet-of-Things and Deep Learning for Big Data Analytics—Concept, Literature, and Future, Mobile. *Information Systems*, (2), 1–20. doi:10.1155/2018/8125126

Das, S., & Kundu, M. K. (2013). A Neuro-Fuzzy Approach for Medical Image Fusion. *IEEE Transactions on Biomedical Engineering*, *60*(12), 3347–3353. doi:10.1109/TBME.2013.2282461 PMID:24058012

Debes, C., Merentitis, A. S., Sukhanov, S., Niessen, M., Frangiadakis, N., & Bauer, A. (2016). Monitoring activities of daily living in smart homes: Understanding human behavior. *IEEE Signal Processing Magazine*, *33*(2), 81–94. doi:10.1109/MSP.2015.2503881

Deng, J., Dong, W., Socher, R. L., Li, J., Li, K., & Fei, F. (2009). Imagenet: A large-scale hierarchical image database. In *Proceedings of the 2009 IEEE Conference on Computer Vision and Pattern Recognition*. IEEE. 10.1109/CVPR.2009.5206848

Deng, L. (2016). Deep learning: From speech recognition to language and multimodal processing. *APSIPA Transactions on Signal and Information Processing*, *5*, E1. doi:10.1017/ATSIP.2015.22

Dhar, S. K., Bhunia, S., & Mukherjee, N. (2014). Interference Aware Scheduling of Sensors in IoT Enabled Health Care Monitoring Systems. In *Proceedings of the Fourth International Conference of Emerging Applications of Information Technology* (pp. 152-157). Academic Press. 10.1109/EAIT.2014.50

Dick, R. S., Steen, E. B., & Detmer, D. E. (Eds.). (1997). *The computer-based patient record: an essential technology for health care*. National Academies Press.

Dimitrov, D. V. (2016). Medical internet of things and big data in healthcare. *Healthcare Informatics Research*, *22*(3), 156–163. doi:10.4258/hir.2016.22.3.156 PMID:27525156

Dinesen, B., Nonnecke, B., Lindeman, D., Toft, E., Kidholm, K., Jethwani, K., ... Gutierrez, M. (2016). Personalized telehealth in the future: A global research agenda. *Journal of Medical Internet Research*, *18*(3), e53. doi:10.2196/jmir.5257 PMID:26932229

Divakaran, S., Manukonda, L., Sravya, N., Morais, M. M., & Janani, P. (2017, September). IOT clinic-Internet based patient monitoring and diagnosis system. In *Proceedings of the 2017 IEEE International Conference on Power, Control, Signals and Instrumentation Engineering (ICPCSI)* (pp. 2858-2862). IEEE. 10.1109/ICPCSI.2017.8392243

Dua, D., & Graff, C. (2019). *UCI Machine Learning Repository*. Irvine, CA: University of California, School of Information and Computer Science.

Dubey, H., Yang, J., Constant, N., Amiri, A. M., Yang, Q., & Makodiya, K. (2015, October). Fog data: Enhancing telehealth big data through fog computing. In *Proceedings of the ASE Big Data & Social Informatics 2015* (p. 14). ACM.

Dwith, C. Y. N., Angoth, V., & Singh, A. (2013). Wavelet-Based Image Fusion for Detection of Brain Tumor. *I.J. Image. Graphics and Signal Processing*, *1*(1), 25–31. doi:10.5815/ijigsp.2013.01.04

Dwolatzky, T., Dimant, L., Simon, E., & Doniger, G. (2010). Validity of a short computerized assessment battery for moderate cognitive impairment and dementia. *International Psychogeriatrics*, *22*(5), 795–803. doi:10.1017/S1041610210000621 PMID:20519066

Dzubur, E., Li, M., Kawabata, K., Sun, Y., McConnell, R., Intille, S., & Dunton, G. F. (2015). Design of a smartphone application to monitor stress, asthma symptoms, and asthma inhaler use. *Annals of Allergy, Asthma & Immunology*, *114*(4), 341–2.e2. doi:10.1016/j.anai.2014.12.017 PMID:25661657

El-Gamal, F. E.-Z. A., Elmogy, M., & Atwan, A. (2016). Current trends in medical image registration and fusion. *Egyptian Information Journal*, *17*(1), 99–124. doi:10.1016/j.eij.2015.09.002

Elprocus. (n.d.). Automatic wireless health monitoring system circuit. Retrieved from https://www.elprocus.com/automatic-wireless-health-monitoring-system-circuit/

Ercolano, G., Riccio, D., & Rossi, S. (2017). Two deep approaches for ADL recognition: A multi-scale LSTM and a CNN-LSTM with a 3D matrix skeleton representation. In *Proceedings of the IEEE International Symposium on Robot and Human Interactive Communication (RO-MAN)* (pp. 877-882). IEEE Press. 10.1109/ROMAN.2017.8172406

Esteva, A., Kuprel, B., Novoa, R. A., Ko, J., Swetter, S. M., Blau, H. M., & Thrun, S. (2017). Dermatologist-level classification of skin cancer with deep neural networks. *Nature*, *542*(7639), 115–118. doi:10.1038/nature21056 PMID:28117445

European Commission. (2014). Clinical trials - regulation EU No 536/2014. Brussels: European Commission. Retrieved from: http://ec.europa.eu/health/human-use/clinical-trials/regulation/index_en.htm

Fadlullah, Z. M., Tang, F., Mao, B., Kato, N., Akashi, O., Inoue, T., & Mizutani, K. (2017). State-of-the-Art Deep Learning: Evolving Machine Intelligence towards Tomorrow's Intelligent Network Traffic Control Systems. *IEEE Communications Surveys and Tutorials*, *19*(4), 2432–2455. doi:10.1109/COMST.2017.2707140

Famm, K., Litt, B., Tracey, K. J., Boyden, E. S., & Slaoui, M. (2013). Drug discovery: A jump-start for electroceuticals. *Nature*, *496*(7444), 159–161. doi:10.1038/496159a PMID:23579662

Faust, O., Hagiwara, Y., Hong, T. J., Lih, O. S., & Acharya, U. R. (2018). Deep learning for healthcare applications based on physiological signals: A review. *Computer Methods and Programs in Biomedicine*, *161*, 1–13. doi:10.1016/j.cmpb.2018.04.005 PMID:29852952

Ferris, S., De Leon, M. J., Wolf, A. P., Farkas, T., Christman, D. R., Reisberg, B., ... Rampal, S. (1980). Positron emission tomography in the study of aging and senile dementia. *Neurobiology of Aging*, *1*(2), 127–131. doi:10.1016/0197-4580(80)90005-6 PMID:24279935

Filkins, B. L., Kim, J. Y., Roberts, B., Armstrong, W., Miller, M. A., Hultner, M. L., ... Steinhubl, S. R. (2016). Privacy and security in the era of digital health: what should translational researchers know and do about it? *American journal of translational research*, *8*(3), 1560. 1580. PMID:27186282

Fioravante, D., & Byrne, J. H. (2011). Protein degradation and memory formation. *Brain Research Bulletin*, *85*(1–2), 14–20. doi:10.1016/j.brainresbull.2010.11.002 PMID:21078374

Flores, M., Glusman, G., Brogaard, K., Price, N. D., & Hood, L. (2013). P4 medicine: How systems medicine will transform the healthcare sector and society. *Personalized Medicine*, *10*(6), 565–576. doi:10.2217/pme.13.57 PMID:25342952

Foley, P., Steinberg, D., Levine, E., Askew, S., Batch, B. C., Puleo, E. M., ... Bennett, G. G. (2016). Track: A randomized controlled trial of a digital health obesity treatment intervention for medically vulnerable primary care patients. *Contemporary Clinical Trials*, *48*, 12–20. doi:10.1016/j.cct.2016.03.006 PMID:26995281

Foody, G. M., Mathur, A., Hernandez, C. H., & Boyd, D. S. (2006). Training set size requirements for the classification of a specific class. *Remote Sensing of Environment*, *104*(1), 1–14. doi:10.1016/j.rse.2006.03.004

Forbes, G., Massie, S., & Craw, S. (2019). Fall prediction using behavioral modeling from sensor data in smart homes. *Artificial Intelligence Review*, 1–21.

Forman, G., & Cohen, I. (2004). Learning from little: comparison of classifiers given little training. In *Proceedings of the European Conference on Principles of Data Mining and Knowledge Discovery* (pp. 161–172). Academic Press. 10.1007/978-3-540-30116-5_17

Friston, K. Ash bumer, J., Kiebel, S. J., Nichols, T. E., & Penny, W. D. (2007). Statistical Parameter Mapping: The Analysis of Functional Brain Images. Academic Press.

Gabriela, J.E.B. & Silvia, G. (2011). A framework for overcoming challenges in designing persuasive monitoring and feedback systems for mental illness. In *Proceedings of the 5th International Conference on Pervasive Computing Technologies for Healthcare (PervasiveHealth)*. IEEE. doi:10.4108/icst.pervasivehealth.2011.246097

Gaetano, S. V., Narayanaswami, C., & Menning, W. (2007). Guest Editors' Introduction Pervasive Computing in Healthcare. *IEEE Pervasive Computing*, *6*(1), 17–19. doi:10.1109/MPRV.2007.11

Gagnon, M. P., Lamothe, L., Fortin, J. P., Cloutier, A., Godin, G., Gagné, C., & Reinharz, D. (2005). Telehealth adoption in hospitals: An organisational perspective. *Journal of Health Organization and Management*, *19*(1), 32–56. doi:10.1108/14777260510592121 PMID:15938601

Gale, N. K., Heath, G., Cameron, E., Rashid, S., & Redwood, S. (2013). Using the framework method for the analysis of qualitative data in multi-disciplinary health research. *BMC Medical Research Methodology*, *13*(1), 117. doi:10.1186/1471-2288-13-117 PMID:24047204

Galiano, M. C., Valdivia, M. T. M., & Lopez, U. (2009). Query expansion with a medical ontology to improve a multimodal information retrieval system. *Computers in Biology and Medicine*, *39*(4), 396–403. doi:10.1016/j.compbiomed.2009.01.012 PMID:19268924

Ganapathy, N., Swaminathan, R., & Deserno, T. (2018). Deep Learning on 1-D Biosignals: A Taxonomy-based Survey. *IMIA Yearbook of Medical Informatics*, *27*(1), 98–109. doi:10.1055-0038-1667083 PMID:30157512

Ganasala, P., & Kumar, V. (2014). CT and MR image fusion scheme in nonsubsampled contourlet transform domain. *Journal of Digital Imaging*, *27*(1), 407–418. doi:10.100710278-013-9664-x PMID:24474580

Garcia-Ceja, E., Riegler, M., Nordgreen, T., Jakobsen, P., Oedegaard, K. J., & Tørresen, J. (2018). Mental health monitoring with multimodal sensing and machine learning: A survey. *Pervasive and Mobile Computing*, *51*, 1–26. doi:10.1016/j.pmcj.2018.09.003

Gartner. (2015). Says 6.4 Billion Connected Things Will Be in Use in 2016. Retrieved from http://www.gartner.com/newsroom/id/3165317

Gastaldi, L., & Corso, M. (2012). Smart healthcare digitalization: Using ICT to effectively balance exploration and exploitation within hospitals. *International Journal of Engineering Business Management*, *4*, 4–9.

Gianvecchio, S., Xie, M., Wu, Z., & Wang, H. (2008, July). Measurement and Classification of Humans and Bots in Internet Chat. In Proceedings of the USENIX security symposium (pp. 155-170). Academic Press.

Giraldo-Rodriguez, L., Torres-Castro, S., Martinez-Ramirez, D., Gutierrez-Robledo, L. M., & Perez-Cuevas, R. (2013). Tele-care and tele-alarms for the elderly: Preliminary experiences in Mexico. *Revista de Saude Publica*, *47*(4), 711–717. doi:10.1590/S0034-8910.2013047004574 PMID:24346662

Gokalp, H., & Clarke, M. (2013). Monitoring activities of daily living of the elderly and the potential for its use in telecare and telehealth. *Telemedicine Journal and e-Health*, *19*(12), 910–923. doi:10.1089/tmj.2013.0109 PMID:24102101

Goldberger, A., Amaral, L. A. N., Glass, L., Hausdorff, J. M., Ivanov, P. C., Mark, R. G., ... Stanley, H. E. (2000, June 13). PhysioBank, PhysioToolkit, and PhysioNet: Components of a new research resource for complex physiologic signals. *Circulation*, *101*(23), E215–E220. doi:10.1161/01.CIR.101.23.e215 PMID:10851218

Goodfellow, I., Bengio, Y. & Courville, A. (2016). Deep Learning (1st ed.). Cambridge, MA: The MIT Press.

Goshtasby, A. A. (2005). *2D and 3D image registration for medical, remote sensing and industrial applications*. Wiley.

Graf, C. (2008). The Lawton instrumental activities of daily living scale. *The American Journal of Nursing*, *108*(4), 52–62. doi:10.1097/01.NAJ.0000314810.46029.74 PMID:18367931

Granville, V. (n.d.). Difference Between Machine Learning, Data Science, AI, Deep Learning, and Statistics. Data science central. Retrieved from https://www.datasciencecentral.com/profiles/blogs/difference-between-machine-learning-data-science-ai-deep-learning.

Greco, F. A., & Oldham, R. K. (1979). Small-cell lung cancer. *The New England Journal of Medicine*, *301*(7), 355–358. doi:10.1056/NEJM197908163010704 PMID:223051

Greenhalgh, T., Procter, R., Wherton, J., Sugarhood, P., & Shaw, S. (2012). The organising vision for telehealth and telecare: Discourse analysis. *BMJ Open*, *2*(4), e001574. doi:10.1136/bmjopen-2012-001574 PMID:22815469

Griffiths, D. (1986). Pit construction by ant-lion larvae: A cost-benefit analysis. *Journal of Animal Ecology*, *55*(1), 39–57. doi:10.2307/4691

Grossi, E., & Suzuki, K. (2011). Artificial neural networks and predictive emedicine: a revolutionary paradigm shift. In Artificial Neural Networks-Methodological Advances and Biomedical Applications (pp. 139-150). Academic Press.

Gudjartsson, H., & Patz, S. (1995). The rician distribution of noisy MRI data. *Magnetic Resonance in Medicine*, *34*(6), 910–914. doi:10.1002/mrm.1910340618 PMID:8598820

Gulshan, V., Peng, L., Coram, M., Stumpe, M.C., Wu, D., Narayanaswamy, A., … Webster, D.R. (2016). Development and validation of a deep learning algorithm for detection of diabetic retinopathy in retinal fundus photographs. In Innovations In Health Care Delivery. American Medical Association.

Gupta, A., & Shrivastava, M. (2012). Performance of ANN using Back Propagation Algorithm for Medical Diagnosis System. *International Journal of Advanced Computer Research (IJACR)*, 2.

Gurjit, K., & Neena, G. (2006). E-health: A New Perspective on Global Health (india). *Journal of Evolution and Tenhnology*, *15*(1), 23–35.

Hackl, W. O. (2016). Intelligent re-use of nursing routine data: Opportunities and challenges. *Studies in Health Technology and Informatics*, *225*, 727–728. PMID:27332320

Han, J., & Kamber, M. (2005). Data mining: Concepts and techniques. San Francisco, CA: Kaufmann.

Hang, Y., Chen, R., Tang, J., Stewart, W. F., & Sun, J. (2017). LEAP: learning to prescribe effective and safe treatment combinations for multimorbidity. In *Proceedings of the 23rd ACM SIGKDD International Conference on Knowledge Discovery and Data Mining* (pp. 1315–1324). ACM.

Hartigan, I. (2007). A Comparative review of the Katz ADL and the Barthel Index in assessing the activities of daily living of older people. *International Journal of Older People Nursing*, *2*(3), 204–212. doi:10.1111/j.1748-3743.2007.00074.x PMID:20925877

Hasumi, T., Ahsan, F., Couper, C. M., Aguayo, J. L., & Jacobsen, K. H. (2012). Parental involvement and mental well-being of Indian adolescents. *Indian Pediatrics*, *49*(11), 915–918. doi:10.100713312-012-0218-y PMID:22728626

Hauptmann, A., Arridge, S., R., Lucka, F., R., Muthurangu, V., & Steeden. J., A. (2018), Real-time Cardiovascular MR with Spatio-temporal De-aliasing using Deep Learning, Proof of Concept in Congenital Heart Disease.

Haykin, S. S. (1999). *Neural networks: A comprehensive foundation*. Upper Saddle River, NJ: Prentice Hall.

Hebert, M. A., Korabek, B., & Scott, R. E. (2006). Moving research into practice: A decision framework for integrating home telehealth into chronic illness care. *International Journal of Medical Informatics*, *75*(12), 786–794. doi:10.1016/j.ijmedinf.2006.05.041 PMID:16872892

He, F., Hu, Z., Zhang, W., Cai, L., Cai, G., & Aoyagi, K. (2017). Construction and evaluation of two computational models for predicting the incidence of influenza in Nagasaki Prefecture, Japan. *Scientific Reports*, *7*(1), 7192. doi:10.103841598-017-07475-3 PMID:28775299

Hendy, J., Chrysanthaki, T., Barlow, J., Knapp, M., Rogers, A., Sanders, C., ... Newman, S. (2012). An organisational analysis of the implementation of telecare and telehealth: The whole systems demonstrator. *BMC Health Services Research*, *12*(1), 403. doi:10.1186/1472-6963-12-403 PMID:23153014

HereIsMyData. (n.d.). Radboud University Medical Center. Retrieved from http://www.hereismydata.com/

Hillestad, R., Bigelow, J., Bower, A., Girosi, F., Meili, R., Scoville, R., & Taylor, R. (2005). Can electronic medical record systems transform health care? Potential health benefits, savings, and costs. *Health Affairs*, *24*(5), 1103–1117. doi:10.1377/hlthaff.24.5.1103 PMID:16162551

Hill, P., Achim, A., Al-Mualla, M. E., & Bull, D. (2016). Contrast Sensitivity of the Wavelet, Dual-Tree Complex Wavelet, Curvelet, and Steerable Pyramid Transforms. *IEEE Transactions on Image Processing*, *25*(6), 2739–2751. doi:10.1109/TIP.2016.2552725 PMID:27093623

Hornik, K., Stinchcombe, M., & White, H. (1989). Multilayer feedforward networks are universal approximators. *Neural Networks*, *2*(5), 359–366. doi:10.1016/0893-6080(89)90020-8

Hosseini, M. P., Tuyen, X. T., Pompili, D., & Zadeh, H. (2017). Deep Learning with Edge Computing for Localization of Epileptogenicity using Multimodal rs-fMRI and EEG Big Data. In *Proceedings of the IEEE International Conference on Autonomic Computing* (pp. 83-92). 10.1109/ICAC.2017.41

Hou, Y., Dan, X., Babbar, M., Wei, Y., Hasselbalch, S. G., Croteau, D. L., & Bohr, V. A. (2019). Ageing as a risk factor for neurodegenerative disease. *Nature Reviews. Neurology*, *15*(10), 565–581. doi:10.103841582-019-0244-7 PMID:31501588

Hsu, C. W., & Lin, C. J. (2002). A comparison of methods for multiclass support vector machines. *IEEE Transactions on Neural Networks*, *13*(2), 415–425. doi:10.1109/72.991427 PMID:18244442

https://www.cancer.net/cancer-types/lung-cancer-non-small-cell/stages

Huang, M., & Chen, Y. (2018). Guest Editorial: Internet of things and intelligent devices and services. *CAAI Trans. Intell. Technol.*, *3*(2), 73–74.

Hudson, D. L., & Cohen, M. E. (2000). *Neural networks and artificial intelligence for biomedical engineering*. New York: IEEE.

Hu, Z., Tang, J., Wang, Z., Zhang, K., Zhang, L., & Sun, Q. (2018). Deep Learning for Image-based Cancer Detection and Diagnosis—A Survey. *Pattern Recognition*, *83*, 134–149. doi:10.1016/j.patcog.2018.05.014

IBEF. (n.d.). Healthcare India. Retrieved from https://www.ibef.org/industry/healthcare-india.aspx

ICS. (n.d.). Datasets. Retrieved from https://archive.ics.uci.edu/ml/datasets.html

Idtechex. (n.d.). Digital health 2019 trends opportunities and outlook. Retrieved from https://www.idtechex.com/en/research-report/digital-health-2019-trends-opportunities-and-outlook/660

IEEE. (2016). Standard for an Architectural Framework for the Internet of Things (IoT).

Ilahi, L., & Ghannouchi, S. A. (2013). Improving telemedicine processes via BPM. *Procedia Technology*, *9*, 1209–1216. doi:10.1016/j.protcy.2013.12.135

India is the most depressed country in the world. (2018). India Today. Retrieved from https://www.indiatoday.in/education-today/gk-current-affairs/story/india-is-the-most-depressed-country-in-the-world-mental-health-day-2018-1360096-2018-10-10

India Times. (n.d.). Indian healthcare in 2018 and forecast for 2019. Retrieved from https://health.economictimes.indiatimes.com/news/industry/indian-healthcare-industry-in-2018-and-forecast-for-2019/6726959

IndiaPKI. (n.d.). Patient Admission & Discharge. Retrieved from www.indiapki.org

INNT Foundation. (n.d.). Retrieved from https://www.innit.foundation

Islam, S. R., Kwak, D., Kabir, M. H., Hossain, M., & Kwak, K. S. (2015). The internet of things for health care: A comprehensive survey. *IEEE Access: Practical Innovations, Open Solutions*, *3*, 678–708. doi:10.1109/ACCESS.2015.2437951

Jagannatha, A.N. & Yu, H. (2016). Bidirectional Recurrent Neural Networks for Medical Event Detection in Electronic Health Records.

Jagannatha, A.N. & Yu, H. (2016). Structured prediction models for RNN based sequence labeling in clinical text.

James, N. (2019). Mental health is the elephant in the rooms of corporate India. The Hindu Business Line. Retrieved from https://www.thehindubusinessline.com/blink/cover/mental-health-the-elephant-in-the-rooms-of-corporate-india/article30211327.ece

Jia, F., Lei, Y., Lin, J., Zhou, X., & Lu, N. (2016, May). Deep neural networks: A promising tool for fault characteristic mining and intelligent diagnosis of rotating machinery with massive data. *Mechanical Systems and Signal Processing*, *72*, 303–315. doi:10.1016/j.ymssp.2015.10.025

Jiang, F., Jiang, Y., Zhi, H., Dong, Y., Li, H., Ma, S., ... Wang, Y. (2017). Artificial intelligence in healthcare: Past, present and future. *Stroke and Vascular Neurology.*, *2*(4). doi:10.1136vn-2017-000101 PMID:29507784

Jiang, N., & Xu, X. (2019). Exploring the survival prognosis of lung adenocarcinoma based on the cancer genome atlas database using artificial neural network. *Medicine*, *98*(20), e15642. doi:10.1097/MD.0000000000015642 PMID:31096483

Jin, J., Gubbi, J., Marusic, S., & Palaniswami, M. (2014). An information framework for creating a smart city through Internet of Things. *IEEE Internet of Things Journal*, *1*(2), 112–121. doi:10.1109/JIOT.2013.2296516

Johnson, J. L. (2011). *Probability and Statistics for Computer Science*. New York: Wiley.

Johnson, R., & Zhang, T. (2007). On the effectiveness of Laplacian normalization for graph semi-supervised learning. *Journal of Machine Learning Research*, *8*(July), 1489–1517.

Jossinet, J. (1998). The impedivity of freshly excised human breast tissue. *Physiological Measurement*, *19*(1), 61–75. doi:10.1088/0967-3334/19/1/006 PMID:9522388

Kamdar, M., & Wu, M. (2017). PRISM: A data-driven platform for monitoring mental health. *Physiology & Behavior*, *176*(1), 139–148. doi:10.1016/j.physbeh.2017.03.040 PMID:28363838

Kam, H. J., & Kim, H. Y. (2019). Learning representations for the early detection of sepsis with deep neural networks. *Computers in Biology and Medicine*, *89*, 248–255. doi:10.1016/j.compbiomed.2017.08.015 PMID:28843829

Kashf, D. W. A., Okasha, A. N., Sahyoun, N. A., El-Rabi, R. E., & Abu-Naser, S. S. (2018). Predicting DNA Lung Cancer using Artificial Neural Network. *International Journal of Academic Pedagogical Research*, *2*(10), 6–13.

Katzman, R., Brown, T., Thal, L. J., Fuld, P. A., Aronson, M., Butters, N., ... Terry, R. D. (1988). Comparison of Rate of Annual Change of Mental Status Score in Four Independent Studies of Patients with Alzheimer's Disease. *Annals of Neurology*, *24*(3), 384–389. doi:10.1002/ana.410240306 PMID:3228273

Katz, S. (1983). Assessing self-maintenance: Activities of daily living, mobility and instruments of daily living. *Journal of the American Geriatrics Society*, *31*(12), 721–726. doi:10.1111/j.1532-5415.1983.tb03391.x PMID:6418786

Kaur, B., & Singh, W. (2014). Review on Heart Disease Prediction System using Data Mining Techniques. *International Journal on Recent and Innovation Trends in Computing and Communication*, *2*(10), 3003–3008.

Khovanova, N. A., Mallick, K. K., & Shaikhina, T. (2015). Neural networks for analysis of trabecular bone in osteoarthritis. *Bioinspir Biomim Nanobiomater*, *4*(1), 90–100. doi:10.1680/bbn.14.00006

Kinthada, M. R., Bodda, S., & Mande, S. B. K. (2016). EMedicare: MHealth solution for Patient Medication Guidance and Assistance. In *Proceedings of the International conference on Signal Processing, Communication, Power and Embedded System* (pp. 657-661). Academic Press. 10.1109/SCOPES.2016.7955523

Kirankumar, Y., & Shenbaga Devi, S. (2007). Transform-based medical image fusion'. *International Journal of Biomedical Engineering and Technology*, *1*(1), 101–110. doi:10.1504/IJBET.2007.014140

Kirtana, R. N., & Lokeswari, Y. K. (2017). An IoT Based Remote HRV Monitoring System for Hypertensive Patients. In *Proceedings of the IEEE International Conference on Computer, Communication, and Signal Processing*. IEEE Press. 10.1109/ICCCSP.2017.7944086

Klaus, R. (1986). Vocal affect expression: A review and a model for future research. *Psychological Bulletin*, *99*(2), 143–165. doi:10.1037/0033-2909.99.2.143 PMID:3515381

Koch, S. (2006). Home telehealth—Current state and future trends. *International Journal of Medical Informatics*, *75*(8), 565–576. doi:10.1016/j.ijmedinf.2005.09.002 PMID:16298545

Kose, U. (2018). An Ant-Lion optimizer-trained artificial neural network system for chaotic electroencephalogram (EEG) Prediction. *Applied Sciences*, *8*(9), 1613. doi:10.3390/app8091613

Kreutz, D., Ramos, F. M., Verissimo, P. E., Rothenberg, C. E., Azodolmolky, S., & Uhlig, S. (1995). Software-defined networking: A comprehensive survey. *Proceedings of the IEEE*, *103*(1), 14–76.

Krinidis, S., & Chatzis, V. (2010). A Robust Fuzzy Local Information C Means Clustering Algorithm. *IEEE Transactions on Image Processing*, *19*(5), 1057–1071. doi:10.1109/TIP.2010.2040763 PMID:20089475

Krishnamoorthy, S., & Soman, K. P. (2010). Implementations and Comparative study of image fusion algorithms. *International Journal of Computers and Applications*, *9*(2), 25–35. doi:10.5120/1357-1832

Kruse, C. S., Kothman, K., Anerobi, K., & Abanaka, L. (2016). Adoption factors of the electronic health record: A systematic review. *JMIR Medical Informatics*, *4*(2), e19. doi:10.2196/medinform.5525 PMID:27251559

Kumar, A., & Hancke, G. P. (2015). A zigbee-based animal health monitoring system. *IEEE Sensors Journal*, *15*(1), 610–617. doi:10.1109/JSEN.2014.2349073

Kumar, P. D., Kumar, R. S., Sujatha, K., Ponmagal, R. S., & Rajavarman, V. N. (2016). Big data Analytics of IoT based Health Care Monitoring System. In *Proceedings of the International Conference on Electrical, Computer and Electronics Engineering* (pp. 55-60). Academic Press.

Kuruvilla, J., & Gunavathi, K. (2014). Lung cancer classification using neural networks for CT images. *Computer Methods and Programs in Biomedicine*, *113*(1), 202–209. doi:10.1016/j.cmpb.2013.10.011 PMID:24199657

Lanata, A., Valenza, G., Nardelli, M., Gentili, C., & Scilingo, E. P. (2015). Complexity index from a personalized wearable monitoring system for assessing remission in mental health. *IEEE Journal of Biomedical and Health Informatics*, *19*(1), 132–139. doi:10.1109/JBHI.2014.2360711 PMID:25291802

Larburu, N., Artetxe, A., Escolar, V., Lozano, A., & Kerexeta, J. (2018). Artificial Intelligence to Prevent Mobile Heart Failure Patients Decompensation in Real Time: Monitoring-Based Predictive Model. Mobile Information Systems.

Lawton, P. M., & Brody, E. M. (1969). Assessment of older people: Self-maintaining and instrumental activities of daily living. *The Gerontologist*, *9*(3), 179–18. doi:10.1093/geront/9.3_Part_1.179 PMID:5349366

LeBaron, B., & Weigend, A. S. (1998). A bootstrap evaluation of the effect of data splitting on financial time series. *IEEE Transactions on Neural Networks*, *9*(1), 213–220. doi:10.1109/72.655043 PMID:18252443

LeCun, Y., Bengio, Y., & Hinton, G. (2015). Deep learning. *Nature*, *521*(7553), 436–444. doi:10.1038/nature14539 PMID:26017442

Lee, H. A., Chao, L. R., Rau, H. H., & Hsu, C. Y. (2018, July). Constructing Prediction Model of Lung Cancer Treatment Survival. In *Proceedings of the International Conference on Frontier Computing* (pp. 1925-1933). Springer Singapore.

Lee, J. G., Jun, S., Cho, Y. W., Lee, H., Kim, G. B., Seo, J. B., & Kim, N. (2017). Deep Learning in Medical Imaging: General Overview. *Korean Journal of Radiology*, *18*(4), 570–584. doi:10.3348/kjr.2017.18.4.570 PMID:28670152

Li, D. C., Wu, C. S., Tsai, T. I., & Lina, Y. S. (2007). Using mega-trend-diffusion and artificial samples in small data set learning for early flexible manufacturing system scheduling knowledge. *Computers & Operations Research*, *34*(4), 966–982. doi:10.1016/j.cor.2005.05.019

Lightner, N. J. (2018). Advances in Human Factors and Ergonomics in Healthcare and Medical Devices. *Proceedings of the AHFE 2018 International Conference on Human Factors and Ergonomics in Healthcare and Medical Devices*. Springer.

Li, H., Manjunath, B. S., & Mitra, S. K. (1995). Multisensor image fusion using the wavelet transform. *Graphical Models and Image Processing*, *57*(1), 235–245. doi:10.1006/gmip.1995.1022

Li, L. J., Socher, R., & Fei-Fei, L. (2009, June). Towards total scene understanding: Classification, annotation and segmentation in an automatic framework. In *Proceedings of the 2009 IEEE Conference on Computer Vision and Pattern Recognition* (pp. 2036-2043). IEEE. doi:10.1109/CVPR.2009.5206718

Li, S., Yang, B., & Hu, J. (2011). Performance comparison of different multi-resolution transform for image fusion. *Journal Information Fusion*, *12*(2), 74–84. doi:10.1016/j.inffus.2010.03.002

Litjens, G., Kooi, T., Bejnordi, B. E., Setio, A. A. A., Ciompi, F., Ghafoorian, M., ... Sánchez, C. I. (2017). A Survey on Deep Learning in Medical Image Analysis. *Medical Image Analysis*, *42*, 60–88.

Litjens, G., Kooi, T., Bejnordi, B. E., Setio, A. A. A., Ciompi, F., Ghafoorian, M., ... Sánchez, C. I. (2017). A Survey on Deep Learning in Medical Image Analysis. *Medical Image Analysis*, *42*, 60–88. doi:10.1016/j.media.2017.07.005 PMID:28778026

Liu, S. (2017). Class-constrained Transfer LDA for Cross-view Action Recognition in Internet of Things. *IEEE Internet of things Journal, 5*(5), 3270-3277.

Liu, Z., Yin, H., Chai, Y., & Yang, S. X. (2014). A novel approach for multimodal medical image fusion. *Expert Systems with Applications, 41*(16), 7425–7435. doi:10.1016/j.eswa.2014.05.043

Lundervold, A. S., & Lundervold, A. (2019). An Overview of Deep Learning in Medical Imaging Focusing on MRI. *Zeitschrift fur Medizinische Physik, 29*(2), 102–127. doi:10.1016/j.zemedi.2018.11.002 PMID:30553609

Macukow, B. (2016). *Neural Networks – State of Art, Brief History, Basic Models and Architecture* (pp. 3–14). Switzerland: Springer International Publishing. doi:10.1007/978-3-319-45378-1_1

Madu, C. N., Kuei, C. H., & Lee, P. (2017). Urban sustainability management: A deep learning perspective. *Sustainable Cities Society, 30*, 1–17. doi:10.1016/j.scs.2016.12.012

Mamoshina, P., Vieira, A., Putin, E., & Zhavoronkov, A. (2016). Applications of Deep Learning in Biomedicine. *Molecular Pharmaceutics, 13*(5), 1445–1454. doi:10.1021/acs.molpharmaceut.5b00982 PMID:27007977

Manoranjitham, S. D., Rajkumar, A. P., Thangadurai, P., Prasad, J., Jayakaran, R., & Jacob, K. S. (2010). Risk factors for suicide in rural south India. *The British Journal of Psychiatry, 196*(1), 26–30. doi:10.1192/bjp.bp.108.063347 PMID:20044655

Mantzaris, D. H., Anastassopoulos, G. C., & Lymberopoulos, D. K. (2008). Medical disease prediction using Artificial Neural Networks. In *Proceedings of the IEEE International Conference on BioInformatics and BioEngineering*. IEEE Press. . 8-10.10.1109/BIBE.2008.4696782

Maria, F. J., Brage, S., Vinberg, M., Christensen, E. M., Knorr, U., Jensen, H. M., & Kessing, L. V. (2012). Differences in psychomotor activity in patients suffering from a unipolar and bipolar affective disorder in the remitted or mild/moderate depressive state. *Journal of Affective Disorders, 141*(2), 457–463. doi:10.1016/j.jad.2012.02.020 PMID:22391514

Mark, A. H., Eibe, F., Holmes, G., Bernhard, P., & Reutemann, P., & Ian, H.W. (2009). The WEKA data mining software: an update. ACM SIGKDD explorations newsletter, 11(1), 10–18. doi:10.1145/1656274.1656278

Marsh, J. (2017). The Internet of Everything Manufacturing and Product Lifecycle Management.

Masood, S., Luthra, T., Sundriyal, H., & Ahmed, M. (2017). Identification of Diabetic Retinopathy in Eye Images Using Transfer Learning. In *Proceedings of the International Conference on Computing, Communication and Automation (ICCCA)*. Academic Press. 10.1109/CCAA.2017.8229977

Matheson, R. (2014). Mental-health monitoring goes mobile. MIT News. Retrieved from http://news.mit.edu/2014/mental-health-monitoring-goes-mobile-0716

Maurer, U., Smailagic, A., Siewiorek, D. P., & Deisher, M. (2006, April). Activity recognition and monitoring using multiple sensors on different body positions. In *Proceedings of the International Workshop on Wearable and Implantable Body Sensor Networks (BSN'06)* (pp. 4-pp). IEEE. doi:10.1109/BSN.2006.6

Max, K., & Kjell, J. (2013). Applied predictive modeling. Springer.

Mayo Magazine, . (1989). Old records never die: Medical records at the salad dressing clinic. *Mayo Magazine*.

McLean, S., Protti, D., & Sheikh, A. (2011). Telehealthcare for long term conditions. *BMJ (Clinical Research Ed.), 342*(5), 449–457. PMID:21292710

Michelle, E. M., & Michelle, C. F. (2016). Assessment of activities of daily living, self-care, and independence. *Archives of Clinical Neuropsychology, 31*(6), 506–516. doi:10.1093/arclin/acw049 PMID:27475282

Miotto, R., Wang, F., Wang, S., Jiang, X., & Dudley, J. T. (2017). Deep learning for healthcare: Review, opportunities and challenges. *Briefings in Bioinformatics*, *19*(6), 1236–1246. doi:10.1093/bib/bbx044 PMID:28481991

Mirjalili, S. (2015). The ant lion optimizer. *Advances in Engineering Software*, *83*, 80–98. doi:10.1016/j.advengsoft.2015.01.010

Moffatt, J. J., & Eley, D. S. (2010). The reported benefits of telehealth for rural Australians. *Australian Health Review*, *34*(3), 276–281. doi:10.1071/AH09794 PMID:20797357

Mohr, D. C., Burns, M. N., Schueller, S. M., Clarke, G., & Klinkman, M. (2013). Behavioral intervention technologies: Evidence review and recommendations for future research in mental health. *General Hospital Psychiatry*, *35*(4), 332–338. doi:10.1016/j.genhosppsych.2013.03.008 PMID:23664503

Mora, N., Grossi, F., Russo, D., Barsocchi, P., Hu, R., Brunschwiler, T., & Ciampolini, P. (2019). IoT-based home monitoring: supporting practitioner's assessment by behavioral analysis. *Sensors, 19*(14), 3238.

Mora, N., Matrella, G., & Ciampolini, P. (2018). Cloud-based behavioral monitoring in smart homes. *Sensors*, *18*(6), 1951.

Munten, G. (2013). An organisational analysis of the implementation of telecare and telehealth: The whole systems demonstrator1. *Nederlands Tijdschrift voor Evidence Based Practice*, *4*(11), 9–10. doi:10.100712468-013-0032-0

Murman, D. L. (2015). The impact of age on cognition. *Seminars in Hearing*, *36*(3), 111–121. doi:10.1055-0035-1555115 PMID:27516712

MyDario.com. (n.d.). Retrieved from http:// mydario.com/

Mythili, T. Mukherji, D. Padalia, N. & Naidu, A. (2013). A Heart Disease Prediction Model using SVM-Decision Trees-Logistic Regression (SDL). *International Journal of Computer Applications,* 68(16).

MyTomorrows. (n.d.). Retrieved from https://mytomorrows.com

Mzoughi, H., Njeh, I., Ben Slima, M., Ben Hamida, A., Mhiri, C., & Ben Mahfoudh, K. (2019). Denoising and contrast-enhancement approach of magnetic resonance imaging glioblastoma brain tumors. *Journal of Medical Imaging (Bellingham, Wash.)*, *6*(4), 044002. doi:10.1117/1.JMI.6.4.044002 PMID:31620548

Nall, R. (2018). What to know about lung cancer. Medical News Today. Retrieved from https://www.medicalnewstoday.com/articles/323701.php

Naresh, P., & Shettar, D. R. (2014). Early Detection of Lung Cancer Using Neural Network Techniques. *Prashant Naresh Int. Journal of Engineering Research and Applications*, 4.

National Health Portal, India. (n.d.). Retrieved from https://www.nhp.gov.in/

NEC. (2016). NEC Helps Toshiba Machine Enhance Trouble Free Operations by Detecting Malfunctions of Machines before They Occur. Retrieved from http://www.nec.com/en/case/toshibamachine/index.html

Nevon Projects. (n.d.). Iot based ICU patient monitoring system. Retrieved from https://nevonprojects.com/iot-based-icu-patient-monitoring-system/

Nicola, V., Guidi, A., Gentili, C., Werner, S., Bertschy, G., Valenza, G., . . . Scilingo, E. P. (2012). Speech analysis for mood state characterization in bipolar patients. In *Proceedings of the 2012 Annual International Conference of the IEEE Engineering in Medicine and Biology Society (EMBC)* (pp. 2104–2107). IEEE. doi:10.1109/EMBC.2012.6346375

NIDEC. (2016). Nidec and IBM Japan to Jointly Develop IoT Technology. Retrieved from http://www.nidec.com/enNA/product/news/2015/news0622-01/

Nie, L., Wang, M., Zhang, L., Yan, S., Zhang, B., & Chua, T. S. (2017). Disease inference from health-related questions via sparsely connected deep learning, knowledge and data engineering. *IEEE Transactions*, *27*(87), 2107–2119.

Nuffield Bioethics. (n.d.). Artificial intelligence in healthcare and research. Retrieved from https://nuffieldbioethics.org/wp-content/uploads/Artificial-Intelligence-AI-in-healthcare-and-research.pdf

Nygard, L. (2003). Instrumental Activities of Daily Living: A Stepping-Stone Towards Alzheimer's Disease Diagnosis in subjects with Mild Cognitive Impairment. *Acta Neurologica Scandinavica*, *179*(s179), 42–46. doi:10.1034/j.1600-0404.107.s179.8.x PMID:12603250

Olutayo, O. & Singhal, G. (2009). Piecewise Multi-Classification Support Vector Machines, In *Proceedings of International Joint Conference on Neural Networks*. Academic Press.

Ong, M. E. H., Ng, C. H. L., Goh, K., Liu, N., Koh, Z. X., Shahidah, N., ... Lin, Z. (2012). Prediction of cardiac arrest in critically ill patients presenting to the emergency department using a machine learning score incorporating heart rate variability compared with the modified early warning score. *Critical Care (London, England)*, *16*(3), R108. doi:10.1186/cc11396 PMID:22715923

Padmavathi, K., Asha, C. S., & Maya, V. K. (2019). A novel medical image fusion by combining TV-L1 decomposed textures based on adaptive weighting scheme. *Engineering Science and Technology, an International Journal*. doi:10.1016/j.jestch.2019.03.008

Pantelopoulos, A., & Bourbakis, N. (2008, August). A survey on wearable biosensor systems for health monitoring. In *Proceedings of the 2008 30th Annual International Conference of the IEEE Engineering in Medicine and Biology Society* (pp. 4887-4890). IEEE. doi:10.1109/iembs.2008.4650309

Park, J., & Lee, Y. J. (2017). Patterns of instrumental activities of daily living and association with predictors among community-dwelling older women: A latent class analysis. *BMC Geriatrics*, *17*(1), 158. doi:10.118612877-017-0557-6 PMID:28732473

Patel, R., Belousov, M., Jani, M., Dasgupta, N., Winokur, C., Nenadic, G., & Dixon, W. G. (2018). Frequent discussion of insomnia and weight gain with glucocorticoid therapy: An analysis of Twitter posts. *NPJ digital medicine, 1*, 20177. doi:10.103841746-017-0007-z

Paul, Y., Hickok, E., Sinha, A., Tiwari, U., Mohandas, S., Ray, S. … Bidare, P.M. (2018). *Artificial Intelligence in the Healthcare Industry in India*. Retrieved from https://cis-india.org/internet-governance/files/ai-and-healtchare-report

Peter, A. (1998). MR Image Texture analysis applied to the diagnosis and tracking of Alzheimer's Disease. *IEEE Transactions on Medical Imaging*, *17*(3), 475–478. doi:10.1109/42.712137 PMID:9735911

Petersen, R. C. (2004). Mild cognitive impairment as a diagnostic entity. *Journal of Internal Medicine*, *256*(3), 183–194. doi:10.1111/j.1365-2796.2004.01388.x PMID:15324362

Piao, J., Chen, Y., & Shin, H. (2019). A New Deep Learning-Based Multi-Spectral Image Fusion Method. *Entropy (Basel, Switzerland)*, *21*(570). doi:10.3390/e21060570

Pinto, S., Cabral, J., & Gomes, T. (2017, March). We-care: An IoT-based health care system for elderly people. In *Proceedings of the 2017 IEEE International Conference on Industrial Technology (ICIT)* (pp. 1378-1383). IEEE. 10.1109/ICIT.2017.7915565

Prajapati, S. A., Nagaraj, R., & Mitra, S. (2017). Classification of dental diseases using CNN and transfer learning. In *Proceedings of the IEEE 5th International Symposium on Computational and Business Intelligence (ISCBI)*. IEEE Press. doi:10.1109/ISCBI.2017.8053547

Price, M., Yuen, E. K., Goetter, E. M., Herbert, J. D., Forman, E. M., Acierno, R., & Ruggiero, K. J. (2014). mHealth: A mechanism to deliver more accessible, more effective mental health care. *Clinical Psychology & Psychotherapy*, *21*(5), 427–436. doi:10.1002/cpp.1855 PMID:23918764

Pritika, S. B., & Budhiraja, S. (2016). Multimodal medical image fusion based on guided filtered multi-scale decomposition. *International Journal of Biomedical Engineering and Technology*, *20*(4), 285–301. doi:10.1504/IJBET.2016.076604

Priyanka, K., & Kulennavar, N. (2014). A survey on big data analytics in health care. *International Journal of Computer Science and Information Technologies*, *5*(4), 5865–5868.

Qiang, L., Daqing, Z., Liming, C., Hongbo, N., & Xingshe, Z. (2014). Managing elders wandering behavior using sensors-based solutions: A survey. *International Journal of Gerontology*, *8*(2), 49–55. doi:10.1016/j.ijge.2013.08.007

Qin, N., Ana, B., Garcia, H., & Ivan, P. (2015). The elderly's independent living in smart homes: A characterization of activities and sensing infrastructure survey to facilitate services development. *Sensors (Basel)*, *15*(5), 11312–11362. doi:10.3390150511312 PMID:26007717

Raento, M., Oulasvirta, A., Petit, R., & Toivonen, H. (2005). ContextPhone: A prototyping platform for context-aware mobile applications. *IEEE Pervasive Computing*, *4*(2), 51–59. doi:10.1109/MPRV.2005.29

Ranked Health. (n.d.). Retrieved from http:// www.rankedhealth.com/about/

Ran, L., Jiang, X., Li, B., Kong, H., Du, M., Wang, X., ... Liuf, Q. (2017). Association among activities of daily living, instrumental activities of daily living and health-related quality of life in elderly ethnic minority. *BMC Geriatrics*, *17*(1), 74. doi:10.118612877-017-0455-y PMID:28330442

Rao, P. B., & Uma, S. K. (2015). Raspberry Pi home automation with wireless sensors using smart phone. *International Journal of Computer Science and Mobile Computing*, *4*(5), 797–803.

Ravì, D., Wong, C., Deligianni, F., Berthelot, M., Andreu-Perez, J., Lo, B., & Yang, G. Z. (2017). Deep learning for health informatics. *IEEE Journal of Biomedical and Health Informatics*, *21*(1), 4–21. doi:10.1109/JBHI.2016.2636665 PMID:28055930

Rayid, G., & Nigam, K. P. (2000). Analyzing the effectiveness and applicability of training. In *Proceedings of the ninth international conference on Information and knowledge management* (pp. 86–93). ACM. doi:10.1145/354756.354805

Richard , O.D., Peter, E.H., & Stork, D.G. (1997). Pattern Classification. John Wiley & Sons.

Richard, M. (2004). The early warning symptom intervention for patients with the bipolar affective disorder. *Advances in Psychiatric Treatment*, *10*(1), 18–26. doi:10.1192/apt.10.1.18

Roine, R., Ohinmaa, A., & Hailey, D. (2001). Assessing telemedicine: A systematic review of the literature. *Canadian Medical Association Journal*, *165*(6), 765–771. PMID:11584564

Rong, H. J., Huang, G. B., Sundararajan, N., & Saratchandran, P. (2009). Online Sequential Fuzzy Extreme Learning Machine for Function Approximation and Classification Problems, IEEE Transactions on Systems, Man, and Cybernetics. *Part B*, *39*, 1067–1072. PMID:19336333

Sanders, C., Rogers, A., Bowen, R., Bower, P., Hirani, S., Cartwright, M., ... Chrysanthaki, T. (2012). Exploring barriers to participation and adoption of telehealth and telecare within the Whole System Demonstrator trial: A qualitative study. *BMC Health Services Research*, *12*(1), 220. doi:10.1186/1472-6963-12-220 PMID:22834978

Sannino, G., Bouguila, N., De Pietro, G., & Celesti, A. (2019). *Artificial intelligence for mobile health data analysis and processing*. Mobile Information Systems; doi:10.1155/2019/2673463

Sanyal, V. (2018). Why India needs to focus on mental health and wellbeing. Yourstory. Retrieved from https://yourstory.com/2018/10/india-needs-focus-mental-health-wellbeing

Sarchiapone, M., Gramaglia, C., Iosue, M., Carli, V., Mandelli, L., Serretti, A., ... Zeppegno, P. (2018). The association between electrodermal activity (EDA), depression and suicidal behaviour: A systematic review and narrative synthesis. *BMC Psychiatry*, *18*(1), 22. doi:10.118612888-017-1551-4 PMID:29370787

Scheen, A. J. (2016). Precision medicine: The future in diabetes care? *Diabetes Research and Clinical Practice*, *117*, 12–21. doi:10.1016/j.diabres.2016.04.033 PMID:27329017

Scheinkman, J. A., & LeBaron, B. (1989). Nonlinear dynamics and stock returns. *The Journal of Business*, *62*(3), 311–337. doi:10.1086/296465

Schmidhuber, J. (2015). Deep learning in neural networks: An overview. *Neural Networks*, *61*, 85–117. doi:10.1016/j.neunet.2014.09.003 PMID:25462637

Schneier, B., Kelsey, J., Whiting, D., Wagner, D., Hall, C., & Ferguson, N. (1998). Twofish: A 128-bit block cipher. *NIST AES Proposal*, *15*(1), 23–91.

Schneier, B., Kelsey, J., Whiting, D., Wagner, D., Hall, C., & Ferguson, N. (1999). *The Twofish encryption algorithm: a 128-bit block cipher*. John Wiley & Sons, Inc.

Schreiber, T., & Schmitz, A. (1996). Improved surrogate data for nonlinearity tests. *Physical Review Letters*, *77*(4), 635–638. doi:10.1103/PhysRevLett.77.635 PMID:10062864

Selvanambi, R., Natarajan, J., Karuppiah, M., Islam, S. H., Hassan, M. M., & Fortino, G. (2018). Lung cancer prediction using higher-order recurrent neural network based on glowworm swarm optimization. *Neural Computing & Applications*, 1–14.

Selvi, S. T., Arumugam, S., & Ganesan, L. (2000). BIONET: An Artificial Neural Network model for diagnosis of diseases. *Pattern Recognition Letters*, *21*(8), 721–740. doi:10.1016/S0167-8655(00)00027-1

Senior, M. (2014). Novartis signs up for Google smart lens. *Nature Biotechnology*, *32*(9), 856. doi:10.1038/nbt0914-856 PMID:25203024

Sepah, S. C., Jiang, L., & Peters, A. L. (2015). Long-term outcomes of a Web-based diabetes prevention program: 2-year results of a single-arm longitudinal study. *Journal of Medical Internet Research*, *17*(4), e92. doi:10.2196/jmir.4052 PMID:25863515

Sethi, P., & Sarangi, S. R. (2017). Internet of things: Architectures, protocols, and applications. *Journal of Electrical and Computer Engineering*, 25. doi:10.1155/2017/9324035

Shaikhina, T., Khovanova, N., & Mallick, K. (2014). Artificial neural networks in hard tissue engineering: another look at age-dependence of trabecular bone properties in osteoarthritis. In *Proceedings of the IEEE EMBS Int. Conf. Biomed. Heal. Informatics* (pp. 622-625). IEEE Press. 10.1109/BHI.2014.6864441

Sharif, M., Khan, M. A., Rashid, M., Yasmin, M., Afza, F., & Tanik, U. J. (2018). Deep CNN and geometric features-based gastrointestinal tract diseases detection and classification from wireless capsule endoscopy images. *Journal of Experimental & Theoretical Artificial Intelligence*. doi:10.1080/0952813X.2019.1572657

Shen, D., Wu, G., & Suk, H. I. (2017). Deep learning in medical image analysis. *Annual Review of Biomedical Engineering*, *19*(1), 221–248. doi:10.1146/annurev-bioeng-071516-044442 PMID:28301734

Shin, H. C., Roth, H. R., Gao, M., Lu, L., Xu, Z., Nogues, I., & Summers, R. M. (2016, May). Deep Convolutional Neural Networks for Computer-Aided Detection: CNN Architectures, Dataset Characteristics and Transfer Learning. *IEEE Transactions on Medical Imaging*, *35*(5), 1285–1298. doi:10.1109/TMI.2016.2528162 PMID:26886976

Sikorska, J., Hodkiewicz, M. R., De Cruz, A., Astfalck, L., & Keating, A. (2016). A collaborative data library for testing prognostic models. *Presented at the 3rd European Conference of Prognostics Health Management Society*. Academic Press.

Simon, T., Goldberg, A., Daniel, A. L., Leykin, D., & Adini, B. (2014). Twitter in the CrossFire—The Use of Social Media in the Westgate Mall Terror Attack in Kenya. *PLoS One*, *9*(8), e104136. doi:10.1371/journal.pone.0104136

Sims, J., Smith, F., Duffy, A., & Hilton, S. (1999). The vagaries of self-reports of physical activity: a problem revisited and addressed in a study of exercise promotion in the over 65s in general practice. Family Practice, 16(2), 152–157. doi:10.1093/fampra/16.2.152

Singh, S. P., Kumar, A., Darbari, H., Singh, L., Rastogi, A., & Jain, S. (2017). Machine translation using deep learning: An overview. In *Proceedings of the 2017 International Conference on Computer, Communications and Electronics* (pp. 162–167). Academic Press. 10.1109/COMPTELIX.2017.8003957

Sivakumar, R. (2007). Denoising of Computer Tomography Images using Curvelet Transform. *Journal of Engineering and Applied Sciences (Asian Research Publishing Network)*, *2*(1), 21–27.

SleepBot. (n.d.). Retrieved from https://mysleepbot. com/

Small, M., Yu, D., & Harrison, R. G. (2001). Surrogate test for pseudo periodic time series. *Physical Review Letters*, *87*(18), 188101. doi:10.1103/PhysRevLett.87.188101

Smaradottir, B. F., Håland, J. A., & Martinez, S. G. (2018). *User Evaluation of the Smartphone Screen Reader VoiceOver with Visually Disabled Participants*. Mobile Information Systems; doi:10.1155/2018/6941631

Sodhroa, A. H., Pirbhulalc, S., & Sangaiahe, A. K. (2017). Convergence of IoT and Product Lifecycle Management in Medical Health Care. VIT University.

Song, J., Qin, S., & Zhang, P. (2016). Chinese text categorization based on deep belief networks. In *Proceedings of the 2016 IEEE/ACIS 15th International Conference on Computer and Information Science Computer and Information Science*. IEEE.

Srivastava, R., Prakash, O., & Khare, A. (2016). Local energy-based multimodal medical image fusion in curvelet domain. *IET Computer Vision*, *10*(6), 513–527. doi:10.1049/iet-cvi.2015.0251

Suryadevara, N. K., Mukhopadhya, S. C., Wang, R., & Rayudu, R. K. (2013). Forecasting the behavior of an elderly using wireless sensors data in a Smart Home. *Engineering Applications of Artificial Intelligence*, *26*(10), 2641–2652. doi:10.1016/j.engappai.2013.08.004

Suzuki, K. (2017, September). Overview of deep learning in medical imaging. *Radiological Physics and Technology*, *10*(3), 257–273. doi:10.100712194-017-0406-5 PMID:28689314

Szegedy, C., Liu, W., Jia, Y., Sermanet, P., Reed, S., Anguelov, D., Erhan, D., Vanhoucke, V., & Rabinovich, A. (2014). Going deeper with convolutions.

Szegedy, C., Wei, L., Yang, J., Sermanet, P., Reed, S., Anguelov, D., . . . Rabinovich, A. (2015). Going deeper with convolutions. In *Proceedings of the IEEE Conference on Computer Vision and Pattern Recognition*. IEEE Press.

Tafti, A., Zotti, R., & Jank, W. (2016). Real-Time Diffusion of Information on Twitter and the Financial Markets. *PLoS One*, *11*(8), e0159226. doi:10.1371/journal.pone.0159226 PMID:27504639

Teramoto, A., Tsukamoto, T., Kiriyama, Y., & Fujita, H. (2017). Automated classification of lung cancer types from cytological images using deep convolutional neural networks. *BioMed Research International*. PMID:28884120

Tharwat, A., & Hassanien, A. E. (2018). Chaotic antlion algorithm for parameter optimization of support vector machine. *Applied Intelligence*, *48*(3), 670–686. doi:10.100710489-017-0994-0

Theiler, J., Eubank, S., Longtin, A., Galdrikian, B., & Doyne, F. J. (1992). (. Testing for nonlinearity in time series: The method of surrogate data. *Physica*, *58*(1–4), 77–94.

Thorsten, J. (1999). Transductive inference for text classification using support vector machines. In *Proceedings of the Sixteenth International Conference on Machine Learning (ICML)* (pp. 200–209). Academic Press.

Tian, T., Liu, C., Guo, Q., Yuan, Y., Li, W., & Yan, Q. (2018). An improved ant lion optimization algorithm and its application in hydraulic turbine governing system parameter identification. *Energies*, *11*(1), 95. doi:10.3390/en11010095

Timmer, J. (1998). Power of surrogate data testing with respect to nonstationary. *Phys. Rev. E.*, *58*(4), 5153-5156.

Tkacz, E. J., & Kostka, P. (2000). An application of a wavelet neural network for classification of patients with coronary artery disease based on HRV analysis. In *Proceedings of the 22nd Annual International Conference of the IEEE Engineering in Medicine and Biology Society* (Vol. 2, pp. 1391-1393). IEEE. 10.1109/IEMBS.2000.897999

Todder, D., Caliskan, S., & Baune, B. T. (2007). Longitudinal changes of day-time and night-time gross motor activity in clinical responders and non-responders of major depression. *The World Journal of Biological Psychiatry*, 1–9. doi:10.1080/15622970701403081 PMID:19921969

Travel trends Today. (n.d.). Medical tourism emerging as a next growth driver. Retrieved from https://www.traveltrendstoday.in/news/india-tourism/item/5792-medical-tourism-emerging-as-a-next-growth-driver

Tung, C. E., Su, D., Turakhia, M. P., & Lansberg, M. G. (2015). Diagnostic yield of extended cardiac patch monitoring in patients with stroke or TIA. *Frontiers in Neurology*, *5*, 266. doi:10.3389/fneur.2014.00266 PMID:25628595

Ullah, K., Shah, M. A., & Zhang, S. (2016). Effective Ways to Use Internet of Things in the Field of Medical and Smart Health Care. In *Proceedings of the 2016 International Conference on Intelligent Systems Engineering (ICISE)*. IEEE. doi:10.1109/INTELSE.2016.7475151

Uramoto, H., & Tanaka, F. (2014). Recurrence after surgery in patients with NSCLC. *Translational Lung Cancer Research*, *3*(4), 242. PMID:25806307

Valdimir, S. (2004). Gradient-based multiresolution Image Fusion. *IEEE Transactions on Image Processing*, *13*(2), 228–237. doi:10.1109/TIP.2004.823821 PMID:15376943

van Leeuwen, N., Swen, J. J., Guchelaar, H. J., & Hart, L. M. (2013). The role of pharmacogenetics in drug disposition and response of oral glucose-lowering drugs. *Clinical Pharmacokinetics*, *52*(10), 833–854. doi:10.100740262-013-0076-3 PMID:23719679

van Uem, J. M., Maier, K. S., Hucker, S., Scheck, O., Hobert, M. A., Santos, A. T., ... Maetzler, W. (2016, May 31). Twelve-week sensor assessment in Parkinson's disease: Impact on quality of life. *Movement Disorders*, *31*(9), 1337–1338. doi:10.1002/mds.26676 PMID:27241524

Vanus, J., Belesova, J., Martinek, R., Nedoma, J., Fajkus, M., Bilik, P., & Zidek, J. (2017). Monitoring of the daily living activities in smart home care. *Human Centric Computing and Information Sciences*, *7*(1), 30. doi:10.118613673-017-0113-6

Vashist, S., Schneider, E., & Luong, J. (2014). Commercial Smartphone-Based Devices and Smart Applications for Personalized Healthcare Monitoring and Management. *Diagnostics (Basel)*, *4*(3), 104–128. doi:10.3390/diagnostics4030104 PMID:26852680

Vepakomma, P., De, D., Das, S. K., & Bhansali, S. (2015). A-Wristocracy: Deep learning on wrist-worn sensing for recognition of user complex activities. In *Proceedings of the IEEE/SICE International Conference on Wearable and Implantable Body Sensor Networks (BSN)*. IEEE Press. 10.1109/BSN.2015.7299406

Vippalapalli, V., & Ananthula, S. (2016). Internet of things (IoT) based smart health care System. In *Proceedings of the International Conference on Signal Processing, Communication, Power and Embedded System* (pp. 1229-1233). Academic Press. 10.1109/SCOPES.2016.7955637

Volkers, A. C., Tulen, J. H. M., Van Den Broek, W. W., Bruijn, J. A., Passchier, J., & Pepplinkhuizen, L. (2003). Motor activity and autonomic cardiac functioning in major depressive disorder. *Journal of Affective Disorders*, *76*(1–3), 23–30. doi:10.1016/S0165-0327(02)00066-6 PMID:12943930

Volkova, S., Ayton, E., Porterfield, K., & Corley, C. D. (2017). Forecasting influenza-like illness dynamics for military populations using neural networks and social media. *PLoS One*, 12. PMID:29244814

Wadhwa, A., Bhardwaj, A., & Verma, V. S. (2019). Review on brain tumor segmentation of MRI images. *Magnetic Resonance Imaging*, *61*, 247–259. doi:10.1016/j.mri.2019.05.043 PMID:31200024

Wahyunggoro, O., Permanasari, A. E., & Chamsudin, A. (2013). Utilization of Neural Network for Disease Forecasting. In *Proceedings 59th ISI World Statistics Congress* (pp. 549- 554). Academic Press.

Wang, T., Qiu, R. G., & Yu, M. (2018). Predictive modeling of the progression of Alzheimer's disease with recurrent neural networks. *Scientific Reports*, *8*(1), 9161. doi:10.103841598-018-27337-w PMID:29907747

Wasserman, P. D. (1998). *Neural computing: theory and practice*. New York: Van Nostrand-Reinhold.

Wei, J. (2014). How wearables intersect with the cloud and the internet of things: Considerations for the developers of wearables. *IEEE Consumer Electronics Magazine*, *3*(3), 53–56. doi:10.1109/MCE.2014.2317895

Wei, J., He, J., Chen, K., Zhou, Y., & Tang, Z. (2017). Collaborative filtering and deep learning-based recommendation system for cold start items. *Expert Systems with Applications*, *69*, 29–39. doi:10.1016/j.eswa.2016.09.040

Welhenge, A., & Taparugssanagorn, A. (2018). Human activity classification using long short-term memory network. *Signal, Image and Video Processing*, *13*, 11.

Weng, C., Huang, T. C.-K., & Han, R.-P. (2016). Disease prediction with different types of neural network classifiers. *Telematics and Informatics*, *33*(2), 277–292. doi:10.1016/j.tele.2015.08.006

Wetzels, M., Ayoola, I., Bogers, S., Peters, P., Chen, W., & Feijs, L. (2018). Consume: A privacy-preserving authorisation and authentication service for connecting with health and wellbeing APIs. *Pervasive and Mobile Computing*, *43*, 20–26. doi:10.1016/j.pmcj.2017.11.002

Winnig, L. (2016). GE's big bet on data and analytics. *MIT Sloan Management Review*, *57*(3).

Winograd-Gurvich, C., Fitzgerald, P. B., Georgiou-Karistianis, N., Bradshaw, J. L., & White, O. B. (2006). Negative symptoms: A review of schizophrenia, melancholic depression and Parkinson's disease. *Brain Research Bulletin*, *70*(4–6), 312–321. doi:10.1016/j.brainresbull.2006.06.007 PMID:17027767

Win, S. L., Htike, Z. Z., Yusof, F., & Noorbatcha, I. A. (2014). Cancer recurrence prediction using machine learning. *International Journal of Computational Science and Information Technology*, *6*(1).

Wootton, R. (2001). Telemedicine. *BMJ (Clinical Research Ed.), 323*(7312), 557–560. doi:10.1136/bmj.323.7312.557 PMID:11546704

World Health Organization. (2007). *Monitoring and evaluation of mental health policies and plans.* Retrieved from http://www.who.int/mental_health/policy/services/14-monitoringevaluation_HKprinter.pdf

World Health Organization. (2017). Mental health in India. Retrieved from http://www.searo.who.int/india/topics/mental_health/about_mentalhealth/en/

Wu, Y. C., Wei, N. C., Hung, J. J., Yeh, Y. C., Su, L. J., Hsu, W. H., & Chou, T. Y. (2017). Generating a robust prediction model for stage I lung adenocarcinoma recurrence after surgical resection. *Oncotarget, 8*(45), 79712. doi:10.18632/oncotarget.19161 PMID:29108351

Xia, F., Su, X., Wang, W., Zhang, C., Ning, Z., & Lee, I. (2016). Bibliographic Analysis of Nature-Based on Twitter and Facebook Altmetrics Data. *PLoS One, 11*(12), e0165997. doi:10.1371/journal.pone.0165997 PMID:27906981

Xiaojin, Z. (2006). *Semi-Supervised Learning Literature Survey.* University of Wisconsin-Madison.

Xia, W., Wen, Y., Foh, C. H., Niyato, D., & Xie, H. (2015). A survey on software-defined networking. *IEEE Communications Surveys and Tutorials, 17*(1), 27–51. doi:10.1109/COMST.2014.2330903

Xie, Y., & Minna, J. D. (2008). Predicting the future for people with lung cancer. *Nature Medicine, 14*(8), 812–813. doi:10.1038/nm0808-812 PMID:18685594

Xu, B., Da Xu, L., Cai, H., Xie, C., Hu, J., & Bu, F. (2014). Ubiquitous data accessing method in IoT-based information system for emergency medical services. *IEEE Transactions on Industrial Informatics, 10*(2), 1578–1586. doi:10.1109/TII.2014.2306382

Xu, Q., Gel, Y. R., Ramirez, L. L., Nezafati, K., Zhang, Q., & Tsui, K. L. (2017). Forecasting influenza in Hong Kong with Google search Queries and statistical model fusion. *PLoS One*, 12. PMID:28464015

Yalçin, N., Alver, S., & Uluhatun, N. (2018). Classification of retinal images with deep learning for early detection of diabetic retinopathy disease. In *Proceedings of the 26th Signal Processing and Communications Applications Conference (SIU)*. Academic Press. 10.1109/SIU.2018.8404369

Yamany, W., Tharwat, A., Hassanin, M. F., Gaber, T., Hassanien, A. E., & Kim, T. H. (2015, September). A new multilayer perceptrons trainer based on an ant lion optimization algorithm. In *Proceedings of the 2015 Fourth international conference on information science and industrial applications (ISI)* (pp. 40-45). IEEE. 10.1109/ISI.2015.9

Yang, B., Zing, Z. L., & Zhao, H. (2010). Review of Pixel Level Image Fusion. *Journal of Shanghai Jiao tong University, 15*(1), 6-12.

Yang, C., & Hsu, Y. (2012). Remote monitoring and assessment of daily activities in the home environment. *Journal of Clinical Gerontology and Geriatrics, 3*(3), 97–104. doi:10.1016/j.jcgg.2012.06.002

Yang, G., Jiang, M., Ouyang, W., Ji, G., Xie, H., Rahmani, A. M., ... Tenhunen, H. (2018). IoT-Based Remote Pain Monitoring System: From Device to Cloud Platform. *IEEE Journal of Biomedical and Health Informatics, 22*(6), 1711–1719. doi:10.1109/JBHI.2017.2776351 PMID:29990259

Yang, Y., Tong, S., Huang, S., Lin, P., & Fang, Y. (2017). A Hybrid Method for Multi-focus Image Fusion Based on Fast Discrete Curvelet Transform. *IEEE Access, 5*, 14898–14913. doi:10.1109/ACCESS.2017.2698217

Yao, J., Wang, S., Zhu, X., & Huang, J. (2016, October). Imaging biomarker discovery for lung cancer survival prediction. In *Proceedings of the International Conference on Medical Image Computing and Computer-Assisted Intervention* (pp. 649-657). Springer. 10.1007/978-3-319-46723-8_75

Yoon, H. J., Ramanathan, A., & Tourassi, G. (2016). Multi-task deep neural networks for automated extraction of primary site and laterality information from cancer pathology reports. In P. Angelov, Y. Manolopoulos, L. Iliadis, A. Roy, & M. Vellasco (Eds.), *Advances in Big Data* (pp. 195–204). Cham: Springer.

Yousefi, A. M., & Hamey, L. (2017). Text summarization using unsupervised deep learning. *Expert Systems with Applications*, *68*, 93–105. doi:10.1016/j.eswa.2016.10.017

Yuan Jie, F., Yue Hong, Y., Li Da, X., Yan, Z., & Fan, W. (2014). IoT-Based Smart Rehabilitation System. *IEEE Transactions on Industrial Informatics*, *10*(2), 1568–1577. doi:10.1109/TII.2014.2302583

Yu, Z., Rennong, Y., Guillaume, C., Ximeng, X., & Zhenxing, Z. (2018). Deep residual bidir-LSTM for human activity recognition using wearable sensors. *Mathematical Problems in Engineering*.

Zanella, A., Bui, N., Castellani, A., Vangelista, L., & Zorzi, M. (2014). Internet of things for smart cities. *IEEE Internet Things J*, *1*(1), 22–32. doi:10.1109/JIOT.2014.2306328

Zhang, S., Zheng, D., Hu, X., & Yang, M. (2015). Bidirectional long short-term memory networks for relation classification. In *Proceedings of the 29th Pacific Asia Conference on Language, Information and Computation (PACLIC)* (pp. 73-78). Academic Press.

Zhang, W., & Li, Y. (2014). A Study on Consumer Behavior of Commercial Health and Fitness Club--A Case of Consumers in Liverpool. *American journal of industrial and business management, 4*(1), 58.

Zhang, W., Huang, T., & Chen, J. (2019). A Robust Bias-Correction Fuzzy Weighted C-Ordered-Means Clustering Algorithm. *Mathematical Problems in Engineering*. doi:10.1155/2019/5984649

Zheng, Y. L., Ding, X. R., Poon, C. C. Y., Lo, B. P. L., Zhang, H., Zhou, X. L., ... Zhang, Y. T. (2014). Unobtrusive sensing and wearable devices for health informatics. *IEEE Transactions on Biomedical Engineering*, *61*(5), 1538–1554.

Zhou, X., Gong, W., Fu, W., & Du, F. (2017). Application of deep learning in object detection. In *Proceedings of the 2017 IEEE/ACIS 16th International Conference on Computer and Information Science* (pp. 631-634). IEEE. 10.1109/ICIS.2017.7960069

Zhu, H., Chen, H., & Brown, R. (2018). A sequence-to-sequence model-based deep learning approach for recognizing activity of daily living for senior care. *Journal of Biomedical Informatics*, *84*, 148–158. doi:10.1016/j.jbi.2018.07.006 PMID:30004019

About the Contributors

Dinesh Goyal is a Professor of Cloud Computing and Security and Academic Dean of Suresh Gyan Vihar University, holding Ph.D. degree from Suresh Gyan Vihar University in 2014, also has 16 years of rich experience in teaching with 7 years in pure R&D sector of image processing, cloud computing/ information security and over 90 research papers in international publications followed by 21 papers presented in conferences, out of above 8 papers are SCI/Scopus/Web of Sciences/ Thomson Reuter Indexed Journals. Also, in order to have inquisitiveness for the current trends in technology, He has conducted and organized 4 conferences and 5 workshops followed by 5 national paper publications. In addition to this, he strove hard to guide mentor over 35 research scholars during his career followed by 8 doctoral guidance with 5 as supervisor and 3 as co-supervisor.

Vishal Jain is currently working as an Associate Professor with Bharati Vidyapeeth's Institute of Computer Applications and Management (BVICAM), New Delhi Affiliated to GGSIPU and Accredited by AICTE, since July 2017. He has joined BVICAM, New Delhi in year 2010 and worked as Assistant Professor from August 2010 to July 2017. Before joined BVICAM, New Delhi, he has worked four years in Guru Presmsukh Memorial College of Engineering, Affiliated to GGSIPU and Accredited by AICTE, from July 2004 to July 2008. He has more than 300 research citation indices with Google scholar h-index score 9 and i-10 index 9. His research area includes information retrieval, semantic web, ontology engineering, data mining, adhoc networks, and sensor networks. He has received Young Active Member award for the year 2012 – 13 from Computer Society of India.

S. Balamurugan is the Director - R&D, Intelligent Research Consultancy Services (iRCS), India. Formerly he was the Head of R&D at QUANTS IS & CS, India. He has published 45 books, 200 international journals/conferences and 35 patents. He is the Editor-in-Chief of the Book Series "Artificial Intelligence and Soft Computing for Industrial Transformation," Scrivener, John Wiley. He is the Editor-in-Chief of Information Science Letters, Natural Sciences Publishing, NSP and International Journal of Robotics and Artificial Intelligence, PRIRS, USA. He is Associate Editor of IEICE Transactions on Information and Systems-Oxford University Press, Cluster Computing- Springer, Simulation- Sage Publishing, Technology and Healthcare- IOS Press, Intelligent IoT Computing, Inderscience, World Journal of Engineering, Emerald. He is also in editorial of International Journal of Intelligent Unmanned Systems, Emerald, International Journal of Automation and Control, Inderscience Publishers, International Journal of Society, Systems and Science, Inderscience Publishers, IJSDA, IJSSMET, IJKSS which are journals of IGI Global.

* * *

Dileep Kumar Agarwal is currently working as an Assistance Professor, in BIET, Sikar. He is pursuing Ph.D in area of artificial intelligence from BTU, Bikaner. He has obtained his M.tech (Computer Science) degree from Rajasthan University, Kota. His areas of interest are artificial intelligence, machine learning, and Big Data.

Parul Agarwal is currently working as an Associate Professor in Jamia Hamdard. Has been associated in teaching for more than 17 years. have published more than 30 papers in indexed/ reputed journals and conferences which are indexed in SCIE, Scopus, Google scholar and a few are published by Springer Nature.

Alankrita Aggarwal is pursuing a PhD in Software Risk Control Strategies from IKGPTU, Jallandhar, India. She is an M.Tech and a BE in Computer science and engineering from Maharishi Dayanand University, India, with approximately 15 years of teaching, as well as research experience. Her areas of interest are soft computing, software engineering, and neural networks. She has published 22 research papers in reputed international journals and guided more than 12 M.tech dissertations. She also worked as the organizing secretary and coordinator of various Workshops. She is a member of the International Associations of Engineers (IAENG) also lifetime member of ISTE.

Jawed Ahmed is working as an Assistant Professor, Department of Computer Science & Engineering, School of Engineering Sciences and Technology Jamia Hamdard, New Delhi, India. His areas of research are algorithms, bioinformatics, and mathematical modeling. He has a total of 15 years of teaching experience.

Amit Kumar Arora is serving as an Assistant Professor in KIET School of Management, KIET Group of Institutions, Ghaziabad. He is pursuing his PhD from IGNOU, New Delhi. He is an Associate Member of Cost and Management Accountants (ACMA), UGC-NET, MBA (Finance), M.Com, M.A. (Eco.), P.hD(P). He has more than 15 years of academic and corporate experience. His areas of interest are cost, accounting, finance, and economics. He is the author of two textbooks titled Management of Working Capital and Financial Management. His various papers have been published in reputed research journals including journal of ICAI-CMA and SCOPUS.

Ayshwarya Balakumar is currently pursuing a Ph.D. from REVA University, Bangalore, and also her research works are related to lung cancer predictions in the field of data mining. She has more than a decade of teaching experience from Kristu Jayanti College, Bangalore, with subjects such as C, C++, JavaScript and other web development technologies. she has authored around 12 papers in national and international level journals and authored 2 books.

Madhulika Bhadauria is working as an Associate Professor in the Department of Computer Science and Engineering at Amity School of Engineering and Technology, Amity University, Noida, Faridabad, Haryana. She holds a diploma in Computer Science & Engineering, B.E. in Computer Science and Engineering, MBA in Information Technology, M.Tech in Computer Science and a Ph.D. from Amity University, Noida. She has total 13 years of Teaching experience. She published almost 29 research papers in national, international conferences and journals. She is also author of two books. She has filed two provisional patents. She attended and organized many workshops, guest lectures, and seminars. She is also member of many Technical societies like IET, ACM, UACEE. She reviewed for Elsevier-Heliyon, IGI Global, the Indian Journal of Science and Technology and completed an editorial for Springer Nature, Switzerland, and a book chapter in Data Visualization and Knowledge Engineering.

Nirbhay Kumar Chaubey is currently working as a Dean of Computer Science, Ganpat University, Gujarat, India. Prior to joining Ganpat University, he worked as an Associate Dean and Associate Professor of Computer Science at SSAICS College Code 554, Gujarat Technological University, Ahmedabad, Gujarat, India. Before joining as the Associate Professor, he was working as an Assistant Professor of Computer Science, at the Institute of Science & Technology for Advanced Studies & Research (ISTAR), Vallabh Vidyanagar, affiliated to the Sardar Patel University, Vallabh Vidyanagar and then to the Gujarat Technological University, Ahmedabad, Gujarat, India. Before that, he has worked as a Lecturer, Computer Science Department, C.U. Shah College of Engineering and Technology, Surendranagar, Saurastra University, Gujarat, India. Professor Chaubey also worked as an Officer on Special Duty (OSD) to the Gujarat Technological University (GTU) for year 2011-2012. Professor Nirbhay Chaubey received his Ph.D. in Computer Science, Faculty of Engineering, from Gujarat University, Ahmedabad, India. He has worked in the area of network communication and security for the past two decades. His research interests lie in the areas of computer and network security, cyber security, algorithms, wireless networks, sensor networks and Cloud computing. He has published several research papers in peered reviewed international journals and conferences, his published research works well cited by the research community worldwide which shows his exception research performance. Prof. Chaubey is a Senior Member of the IEEE, Senior Member of the ACM and a Life Member of Computer Society of India. He has been actively associated with the IEEE India Council and IEEE Gujarat Section and served IEEE in various volunteer positions. He has received numerous awards including IEEE Outstanding Volunteer Award- Year 2015 (IEEE Region 10 Asia Pacific), Gujarat Technological University (GTU) Pedagogical Innovation Awards (PIA) -2015, IEEE Outstanding Branch Counselor Award - Year 2010 (IEEE Region 10 Asia Pacific).

Kanwalvir Singh Dhindsa is a Professor in computer science and engineering department at Baba Banda Singh Bahadur Engineering College, Fatehgarh Sahib, Punjab, India, affiliated to IKGPTU Kapurthala Jallandhar Punjab (India). He has more than 20 years of industrial experience, and teaching as well as research experience. He has published research papers in reputed international journals and guided PhD as well as M.Tech students. His areas of interest are cloud computing, Big data, IoT, mobile computing, database and security, and web engineering. He is also a member of the Computer Society of India (CSI), the Indian Society of Technical education (ISTE), and the Institution of Engineers (IEI). He is also convener of various national and international conferences and workshops.

Nitesh Kumar Dixit is currently working as an Assistant Professor, at BIET, Sikar. He has submitted Ph.D. in the area of energy harvesting from VGU, Jaipur. He obtained his M.tech (Embedded Systems) degree from SRM university, Chennai and B.E. (ECE) from SEC, Dundlod (jhujhunu. Raj). His area of interest is VLSI, artificial intelligence, and renewal energy.

Vikas Garg is currently working as an Assistant Director, Executive Programs Management Domain at Amity University, Uttar Pradesh, India. He is UGC NET qualified with academic experience of 15 years. He also has an expertise in accounting and finance. His areas of interests are financial markets, financial reporting and analysis. He is associated with several universities as an external guide for research scholars. He is lifetime member of the Indian Commerce Association, the Indian Accounting Association, and the Indian Management Association. He is certified in Customer Relationship Management from IIM, Bangalore. As a Professor of Amity University, has been an efficient researcher who has published many research papers in various international and national journals. He is highly efficient in different spheres of work and producing quality work. He has in depth knowledge in the area of finance and accounting and has been consistent performer in delivering accuracy in his tasks. He has organized many seminars and workshops at different. He is very good team leader and always performs the task with creativity.

Richa Goel is an Assistant Professor-Economics and International Business at Amity International Business School, Amity University Noida. She is a Ph.D. in Management and has a journey of almost 18 years in academic and consistently striving to create a challenging and engaging learning environment where students become life-long scholars and learners. Imparting lectures using different teaching strategies, she is an avid teacher, researcher, and mentor. She has to her credit a number of publications in reputed national and international journals accompanied with participation in conferences. She is serving as a member of review committee for conferences journals and acting as Lead Editor of Annual International Referred Journal and Research Coordinator with Amity International Business School. Her area of interest includes economics, business law, human resource management, and diversity management.

Vijay Prakash Gupta is serving as an Assistant Professor at ITS, Ghaziabad, U.P. He is M.A (Eco.), MBA, UGC-NET, and Ph.D. He has about 11 years of experience including both corporate and academics. He has edited 3 books and contributed many chapters in books as well as contributed a variety of research papers in national and international journals. He is the member of Editorial Board of various journals like the Emperor International Journal of Finance and Management Research and the Journal of Accounting Finance and Marketing Technology.

Syed Imtiyaz Hassan works as an Associate Professor in the Department of CS & IT, Maulana Azad National Urdu University, Telangana, India. His professional experience spans over more than 18 years of teaching, research, and project supervision. He has supervised more than 90 students for interdisciplinary research and industrial projects. Over the years, he has published many research papers with national and international journals of repute. In addition to these, he is also in the editorial boards and reviewers' panels of various journals. His primary area of research is computational intelligence and sustainability. To meet the above objective, he explores the role of data science, machine learning, fog computing, and Internet of Things for developing sustainable systems in healthcare and smart city domains.

Mahendra Kumar is currently working as an Assistance Professor, in BIET, Sikar. He has obtained his M.tech (COMMUNICATION System) degree from MPUAT, university, Udaipur (RAJ.) and B.TECH. (ECE) from Sobhasaria Institute of Engineering and technology, Sikar. His areas of interest are communication and artificial intelligence.

Syed Khalid Mustafa completed a Ph.D. in Organic Chemistry in 2004 from the Department of Chemistry, Patna University, India. Presently, he is working in the Department of Chemistry, Faculty of Science, University of Tabuk, Saudi Arabia for the past several years. Published more than 25 research articles in various National and International Journals.

Shanthi Palaniappan completed her doctorate in the field of information retrieval. She has published international journal papers in the field of her specialisation. She has also published one book and two more book chapters in reputed publications.

Sivakumar Rajagopal is a Professor of the School of Electronics Engineering at VIT-Vellore Institute of Technology, Tamilnadu, India. He has been teaching in the Electronics and Communication field since 1997. He obtained his master's degree and PhD from College of Engineering Guindy, Anna University, Chennai. His research interests include Bio Signal Processing, Medical Image Processing, wireless body sensor networks and VLSI. He has published over 34 journal and 42 conference papers over the last several years. He has taught a wide variety of Electronics courses including Digital Image Processing, Multimedia Compression Techniques, VLSI Design, Medical Electronics and Electronic Circuits. Dr. Siva is a life member of the Indian Society of Technical Education, a member of IEEE. Dr. Siva has been invited to deliver Keynote Speech and Chair at various International conferences.

S. Senthil is a Professor and Director, School of Computer Science and Applications, REVA University, India. Previously, he worked as an Associate Professor and Head, Department of Computer Science, Vidyasagar College of Arts and Science, India. He obtained his B.Sc. (Applied Science – Computer Technology) from PSG College of Technology, India, in 1995, Master of Computer Applications from Bharathidasan University, India, in 1999, M.Phil. in Computer Science from Manonmaniam Sundaranar University, India, in 2002, and Ph.D. in Computer Science from Bharathiar University, India, in 2014. Another achievement is clearing SET in 2012. He has published 40 research papers in various reputed National and International Journals. He has presented a paper entitled "Lossless Preprocessing Algorithms for better Compression" in an IEEE International Conference at Zhangjiajie, China. His interest is in Database Systems, Data Mining, Data Compression, Machine Learning and Big Data Analytics.

Gurinder Singh, Group Vice Chancellor, Amity Universities, Director General, Amity Group of Institutions and Vice Chairman, Global Foundation for Learning Excellence. He has an extensive experience of more than 21 years in institutional building, teaching, consultancy, research, and industry. A renowned scholar and academician in the area of international business, he holds a prestigious Doctorate in the area along with a post graduate degree from Indian Institute of Foreign Trade where he illustriously topped with 7 merits. He holds the distinction of being the youngest Founder Pro Vice Chancellor of Amity University for two terms, the Founder Director General of Amity International Business School and the Founder CEO of Association of International Business School, London. He has been instrumental in establishing various Amity campuses abroad including at London, USA, Singapore, Mauritius and other parts of the world. He is internationally recognized as a known Professor in the area of management and is known in the field of academics as an institution builder, a writer, professor, distinguished academician, a top class trainer, international business expert, and the Champion of the Hearts of Students.

Meenakshi Srivastava is working as Assistant Professor at Amity Institute of Information Technology, Amity University, Uttar Pradesh, Lucknow Campus since 2005. She has done her Ph.D. in Engineering. Her area of teaching and research includes Web Mining, Data Structures, Business Intelligence, and Bioinformatics. She is having more than 18 years of teaching experience and 5 years of industry experience. She is having more than 40 national and international publications. She is an integral member of Amity Proctorial Board and member secretary Prevention of Sexual Harassment Cell, etc.

P. K. Suri is a former Professor, Dean Academic and Chairman of department of computer science and applications, Kurukshetra University, Kurukshetra, Haryana, India, and HCTM Technical Campus, Kaithal (Haryana), India. He has forty years of teaching and research experience with various designations in both institutes. He received his MSc Degree from IIT Roorkee (formerly known as University of Roorkee) in 1972. He completed his PhD Degree with the Faculty of Engineering, Kurukshetra University, Kurukshetra, in 1981. His research interests include simulation, cloud computing, Adhoc networks, wireless networks, distributed systems, software engineering. He has attended number of national and international conferences and published a number of research papers in national and international journals. He has guided more than 20 PhD research scholars.

Pooja Tiwari has 12 years of experience in teaching and research and 2.5 years of industrial experience in production. She has many national and international publications and takes active part in seminars, conferences and organizing workshops. Her area of interests is human resource management, Cross Cutler management, etc. She is an active member of various professional bodies and also a member of editorial board of many international journals. She is a sincere and committed academician and has authored various research papers in Scopus indexed journals and copyrights in her name. Her core strength lies in research, training and developing business and academic leaders. She is a good team leader and always performs various tasks with creativity.

Index

A

Active Daily Living (ADL) 115-122, 124-125, 129
Algorithms 48, 51, 58, 62, 76, 78, 80-82, 90, 94, 99-100, 106, 113, 115, 117, 119-121, 133-135, 147, 149, 152, 156, 168, 216
Alzheimer's Disease 116, 130, 197-199, 201, 216-217
Analytics 20, 25, 28-30, 33-36, 39, 41, 43, 47-49, 51, 68-69, 75, 85, 94, 115, 119, 122, 127
Ant Lion and Prediction 176
Artificial Intelligence (AI) 2, 7, 9, 18, 43, 46, 50-51, 55-56, 58-60, 67, 69, 71, 90, 96-97, 100, 113-114, 119, 129-130, 132, 145, 195
Augmented Mental Health 90, 94, 96
Automation 1-2, 4-13, 16-19, 38, 45, 51, 55-57, 61-67, 114, 117-118, 144
Automation Healthcare 55

B

Behavioural Healthcare 89
Big Data 12-13, 17-18, 29, 34-36, 39-43, 45-46, 48-50, 53, 55, 59, 68, 71, 73, 83, 85, 88, 96, 134

C

Cancer Re-Occurrence, Prediction of 176
Classification 7, 40, 65, 73, 80, 84, 91, 100, 105-107, 113-114, 121, 124-133, 135, 137, 145-146, 149-150, 152, 161, 164-166, 168, 173-179, 185, 188, 194-196, 199, 201, 214
Clustering 71, 178, 198, 200, 205, 214, 216-217
Convolution Neural Network (CNN) 38, 59, 70, 72, 80, 87, 99-100, 106-107, 109-114, 124, 178
Curvelet 197-201, 204-206, 209, 211, 214, 216-217

D

Deep Data 20, 28-30, 33-35, 39
Deep Learning 35-36, 38-39, 48, 59, 68, 70-76, 78-88, 99, 106-107, 113-115, 117-121, 123-125, 127-128, 130-135, 138, 140, 144, 178, 194
Detection 9, 42, 45, 70, 72-73, 80-81, 83, 85, 87-88, 90-91, 99-100, 106, 109, 113-114, 118, 120-123, 128, 137, 177, 181, 185, 194-195, 197, 199-200, 215
Digitalization 1-2, 6-7, 11, 16-18, 46

F

Fuzzy C Means (FCM) Algorithm 197-198, 205, 207, 214
Fuzzy-AHP 42

H

Health Informatics 14, 19, 55, 69, 71, 86, 89, 97, 129, 134, 144
Healthcare 1-18, 20, 23, 25-28, 30-31, 33-34, 39, 43, 45-46, 48, 50-51, 53, 55-61, 65, 69-72, 81-82, 84, 86, 89-90, 97-98, 100, 112-113, 116, 118, 120, 127, 132-133, 144, 148, 173-174, 195
Hybrid 31, 59, 197, 204, 206, 209, 211, 214, 217

I

Image Registration 73, 198-199, 213, 215-216
Information 2, 4, 6-8, 10-15, 21, 23-26, 28, 30-31, 34, 39, 41, 43-45, 47, 50-52, 55-56, 58-60, 63-65, 68-72, 74, 76, 81, 84, 87-88, 91, 94, 103, 119-124, 128, 130-131, 133-134, 145, 147-153, 156, 160, 162-166, 168, 170-171, 173-175, 178, 189, 196-198, 200-203, 205, 208, 211, 213, 215-216
Internet of Everything (IOE) 70, 72, 74-75
Internet of Things (IoT) 12-13, 17-18, 34, 42-46, 48, 50-52, 55-56, 58, 68-69, 73, 83-85, 87, 92, 118, 121, 132

K

k-means 99

L

Logistic Reasoning 132
Logistic Regression 99-100, 103, 125, 128, 178
Lung Cancer Classification 176, 195

M

Machine Algorithm 147
Machine Learning 20, 34, 41, 48, 51, 58-59, 70-73, 75, 80-83, 89-90, 94, 96, 100, 107, 113, 115, 117-120, 122, 124, 127-128, 132-134, 145, 147, 149, 173-176, 178-179, 194, 196
Magnetic Resonance Imaging 197-198, 201, 216-217
Medical Diagnosis and Treatment 70
Mental Health 30, 40, 90-98, 118, 147-148, 173-174

N

Neural Network 38, 59, 68, 71, 83, 99, 105-107, 110, 112, 114-115, 133-136, 138-140, 144-145, 176, 178-180, 190, 195-196, 200
Neural Network Optimization 176
NLM Filter 197, 203-204, 210

P

Pervasive Healthcare 89
Prediction 9, 29, 35, 41, 49, 56-57, 59, 70-74, 79, 81-82, 84-85, 90, 99-100, 105-106, 112-115, 120-124, 127-129, 132, 134-135, 143-144, 151-152, 168, 171, 176-179, 183, 189-191, 193-197
Principal Component Analysis 180, 202, 211

R

Recurrent Neural Network (RNN) 70, 73, 80-81, 83, 85, 115, 123

S

Segmentation 73, 81, 100, 106, 121, 148-149, 174, 198, 200-201, 207, 217
Semi-Supervised Learning 147, 149, 152, 168, 172-175
Sensors 12-15, 19, 28, 44, 47, 49, 55-56, 60, 70, 73-74, 76, 78-79, 84, 91, 97, 117-121, 125, 128, 130-131, 148, 162, 173-175, 202
Services 1-8, 10-17, 21-26, 29-31, 33, 39-43, 45-46, 48-50, 52, 56-57, 60, 62-64, 68-69, 82, 92, 94, 96, 98, 100, 115-119, 124, 130
Smart Home 115, 118, 120-121, 125, 128, 130
Smartphone 53, 56, 59, 69, 94-95, 147-148, 151, 153, 155, 164, 168, 171, 173-174
Stationary Wavelet Transform 197, 202, 204
Support Vector Machine 100, 115, 127, 145, 152-153

T

Technological Innovation 1
Telemedicine 2, 5-7, 14, 16-18, 20-22, 26, 28, 31-33, 35-36, 39, 41, 57-58, 61-62, 129
Transfer Learning Method 147

V

Validation 18, 106-107, 113, 132, 135, 140-144

W

Wearable Technology 55-56, 60, 91

www.ingramcontent.com/pod-product-compliance
Lightning Source LLC
LaVergne TN
LVHW080536300926
849162LV00007B/1625
* 9 7 8 1 7 9 9 8 2 1 0 1 4 *